Dear Jamie and family

Thank you so much for your unwavering support over the years which has allowed me to develop and extend the elements of humanism in medicine

As an editor of this volume, I was very cognizant of each author's idea of the approach to the patient and their hematologic problems

Hope to get together soon.

Fred

Consultative Hematology

Guest Editors

FRED SCHIFFMAN, MD
ANTHONY MEGA, MD

HEMATOLOGY/ONCOLOGY CLINICS OF NORTH AMERICA

www.hemonc.theclinics.com

Consulting Editors
GEORGE P. CANELLOS, MD
NANCY BERLINER, MD

April 2012 • Volume 26 • Number 2

SAUNDERS an imprint of ELSEVIER, Inc.

W.B. SAUNDERS COMPANY
A Division of Elsevier Inc.

1600 John F. Kennedy Blvd. • Suite 1800 • Philadelphia, PA 19103-2899

http://www.theclinics.com

HEMATOLOGY/ONCOLOGY CLINICS OF NORTH AMERICA Volume 26, Number 2
April 2012 ISSN 0889-8588, ISBN 13: 978-1-4557-3875-5

Editor: Patrick Manley
Developmental Editor: Donald Mumford

Hematology/Oncology Clinics (ISSN 0889-8588) is published bimonthly by Elsevier Inc., 360 Park Avenue South, New York, NY 10010-1710. Months of issue are February, April, June, August, October, and December. Business and Editorial Offices: 1600 John F. Kennedy Blvd., Ste. 1800, Philadelphia, PA 19103–2899. Customer Service Office: 3251 Riverport Lane, Maryland Heights, MO 63043. Periodicals postage paid at New York, NY and at additional mailing offices. Subscription prices are $353.00 per year (domestic individuals), $576.00 per year (domestic institutions), $173.00 per year (domestic students/residents), $401.00 per year (Canadian individuals), $705.00 per year (Canadian institutions) $477.00 per year (international individuals), $705.00 per year (international institutions), and $233.00 per year (international and Canadian students/residents). International air speed delivery is included in all *Clinics* subscription prices. All prices are subject to change without notice. **POSTMASTER:** Send address changes to *Hematology/Oncology Clinics of North America*, Elsevier Health Sciences Division, Subscription Customer Service, 3251 Riverport Lane, Maryland Heights, MO 63043. Customer Service (orders, claims, online, change of address): Elsevier Health Sciences Division, Subscription Customer Service, 3251 Riverport Lane, Maryland Heights, MO 63043. Tel: 1-800-654-2452 (U.S. and Canada); 314-447-8871 (outside U.S. and Canada). Fax: 314-447-8029. E-mail: journalscustomerservice-usa@elsevier.com (for print support); journalsonlinesupport-usa@elsevier.com (for online support).

Reprints. For copies of 100 or more, of articles in this publication, please contact the Commercial Reprints Department, Elsevier Inc., 360 Park Avenue South, New York, New York 10010-1710; Tel.: 212-633-3813, Fax: 212-462-1935, E-mail: reprints@elsevier.com.

Hematology/Oncology Clinics of North America is covered in *MEDLINE/PubMed (Index Medicus), EMBASE/ Excerpta Medica, and BIOSIS.*

Printed in the United States of America.

Contributors

CONSULTING EDITORS

GEORGE P. CANELLOS, MD
William Rosenberg Professor of Medicine, Department of Medical Oncology, Dana-Farber Cancer Institute, Boston, Massachusetts

NANCY BERLINER, MD
Chief, Division of Hematology, Brigham and Women's Hospital; Professor of Medicine, Harvard Medical School, Boston, Massachusetts

GUEST EDITORS

FRED SCHIFFMAN, MD
Sigal Family Professor of Humanistic Medicine, Division of Hematology/Oncology, Warren Alpert Medical School of Brown University, The Miriam Hospital, Providence, Rhode Island

ANTHONY MEGA, MD
Associate Professor of Medicine (Clinical), Division of Hematology/Oncology, Warren Alpert Medical School of Brown University, The Miriam Hospital, Providence, Rhode Island

AUTHORS

ELISABETH M. BATTINELLI, MD, PhD
Instructor of Medicine, Hematology Division, Brigham and Women's Hospital/Dana-Farber Cancer Institute, Harvard Medical School, Boston, Massachusetts

GIADA BIANCHI, MD
Department of Internal Medicine, Mayo Clinic, Rochester, Minnesota

LOCKE J. BRYAN, MD
Clinical Instructor of Medicine, University of Vermont College of Medicine, Burlington, Vermont

JORGE J. CASTILLO, MD
Division of Hematology/Oncology, Warren Alpert Medical School of Brown University, The Miriam Hospital, Providence, Rhode Island

JAN CERNY, MD, PhD
Assistant Professor of Medicine, University of Massachusetts Medical School and University of Massachusetts Memorial Medical Center, Worcester, Massachusetts

NATHAN T. CONNELL, MD
Teaching Fellow in Hematology and Medical Oncology, Department of Medicine, Rhode Island and The Miriam Hospital, Warren Alpert Medical School of Brown University, Providence, Rhode Island

JEAN M. CONNORS, MD
Assistant Professor of Medicine, Hematology Division, Brigham and Women's Hospital/Dana-Farber Cancer Institute, Harvard Medical School, Boston, Massachusetts

IRENE M. GHOBRIAL, MD
Associate Professor of Medicine, Department of Medical Oncology, Dana-Farber Cancer Institute, Harvard Medical School, Boston, Massachusetts

RONALD HOFFMAN, MD
Albert A. and Vera G. List Professor of Medicine, Director, Myeloproliferative Disorders Research Program, Tisch Cancer Institute, Mount Sinai School of Medicine, New York, New York

PAULA D. JAMES, MD
Associate Professor and Hematologist, Department of Medicine, Queen's University, Kingston, Ontario, Canada

MARINA KREMYANSKAYA, MD, PhD
Department of Hematology/Oncology, Tisch Cancer Institute, Mount Sinai School of Medicine, New York, New York

JOHN MASCARENHAS, MD
Department of Hematology/Oncology, Tisch Cancer Institute, Mount Sinai School of Medicine, New York, New York

GABRIELA MOTYCKOVA, MD, PhD
Dana-Farber Cancer Institute and Harvard Medical School, Boston, Massachusetts

DEVON L. MURPHY, BS
Hematology Division, Brigham and Women's Hospital/Dana-Farber Cancer Institute, Harvard Medical School, Boston, Massachusetts

JOHN L. REAGAN, MD
Division of Hematology/Oncology, Warren Alpert Medical School of Brown University, The Miriam Hospital, Providence, Rhode Island

TINA RIZACK, MD, MPH
Assistant Professor of Medicine (Clinical), Women and Infants Hospital, Warren Alpert Medical School of Brown University, Providence, Rhode Island

MICHAL G. ROSE, MD
Associate Professor, Yale University School of Medicine and Cancer Center, Veterans Affairs Connecticut Healthcare System, West Haven, Connecticut

KAREN ROSENE-MONTELLA, MD
Professor of Medicine, The Miriam Hospital, Alpert Medical School of Brown University, Providence, Rhode Island

ALAN G. ROSMARIN, MD
Gladys Smith Martin Professor of Oncology, Director, Division of Hematology-Oncology, University of Massachusetts; Co-Director, UMass Memorial Cancer Center of Excellence, University of Massachusetts Medical School and University of Massachusetts Memorial Medical Center, Worcester, Massachusetts

NATALIA RYDZ, MD
Clinical Hemostasis Fellow, Department of Pathology and Molecular Medicine, Kingston, Ontario, Canada

DAVID P. STEENSMA, MD
Dana-Farber Cancer Institute and Harvard Medical School, Boston, Massachusetts

NANNA H. SULAI, MD
Department of Internal Medicine, Mayo Clinic, Rochester, Minnesota

JOSEPH D. SWEENEY, MD
Professor of Pathology and Laboratory Medicine, Department of Pathology and Laboratory Medicine, Rhode Island and The Miriam Hospital, Warren Alpert Medical School of Brown University, Providence, Rhode Island

AYALEW TEFFERI, MD
Division of Hematology, Department of Internal Medicine, Mayo Clinic, Rochester, Minnesota

ELLICE Y. WONG, MD
Assistant Professor, Yale University School of Medicine and Cancer Center, Veterans Affairs Connecticut Healthcare System, West Haven, Connecticut

NEIL A. ZAKAI, MD, MSc
Assistant Professor of Medicine and Pathology, University of Vermont College of Medicine, Burlington, Vermont

Contents

Preface   xiii

Fred Schiffman and Anthony Mega

Why is My Patient Anemic?   205

Locke J. Bryan and Neil A. Zakai

Anemia is a decreased number of circulating red blood cells and is a common medical condition faced in clinical practice. Anemia is caused by loss of red blood cells, destruction of red blood cells, decreased production of red blood cells, or a combination of these processes. Through a clinical history, physical examination, and laboratory evaluation the provider must identify the process by which the patient is anemic. Often the cause of anemia is straightforward; however, the cause can be challenging, requiring a thorough knowledge of both hematology and general medicine.

Why Does My Patient Have Thrombocytopenia?   231

Ellice Y. Wong and Michal G. Rose

Thrombocytopenia, usually defined as a platelet count of less than 150,000/μL, is a common reason for a hematology consult in both the inpatient and outpatient setting. In most patients, the cause of the thrombocytopenia can be identified and treated. This article reviews the clinical approach to the patient with thrombocytopenia, the mechanisms that underlie it, and the laboratory tests available to investigate it. A practical approach to the investigation and management of thrombocytopenia in the clinical settings commonly encountered by the hematology consultant is then described.

Why is My Patient Neutropenic?   253

John L. Reagan and Jorge J. Castillo

Neutropenia is a common reason for hematology consultations in the inpatient and outpatient settings and is defined as an absolute neutrophil count less than 1500 cells/μL. Neutropenia varies in severity, with more profound neutropenia being associated with higher rates of infections and infection-related deaths. The causes for neutropenia are diverse and include congenital and acquired conditions (ie, autoimmune, drugs, infection, and malignancy). This article outlines the most common causes of neutropenia and discusses differential diagnoses, treatment modalities, and the mechanisms by which neutropenia occurs.

Why Does My Patient Have Erythrocytosis?   267

Marina Kremyanskaya, John Mascarenhas, and Ronald Hoffman

Primary polycythemias are the result of intrinsic abnormalities of the hematopoietic progenitors that lead to constitutive overproduction of red cells accompanied by low erythropoietin (EPO) levels. Secondary polycythemias are caused by conditions resulting in increased EPO production. Polycythemia vera (PV) is a primary polycythemia, and is a chronic clonal progressive myeloproliferative neoplasm. A single recurrent point mutation in the pseudokinase domain of JAK2 molecule (JAK2^{V617F}) is present in >95% of patients with PV. The goal of therapy in PV is to normalize blood counts to minimize the risk of thrombotic events.

Why Does My Patient Have Thrombocytosis?

285

Nanna H. Sulai and Ayalew Tefferi

Thrombocytosis is a common clinical problem frequently encountered during routine evaluation. The diagnostic workup entails a step-by-step approach, which allows for an accurate assessment of the underlying cause. A thorough clinical history and physical examination may help differentiate thrombocytosis secondary to a reactive process versus an underlying clonal proliferation process. Once essential thrombocytosis is evident, relevant laboratory evaluation for an ongoing myeloproliferative disorder is paramount. Various treatment modalities have been proven to be beneficial. With further scientific investigation underway, molecular therapies may soon be cornerstones of therapy in essential thrombocytosis.

Why Does My Patient Have Leukocytosis?

303

Jan Cerny and Alan G. Rosmarin

Leukocytosis is one of the most common laboratory abnormalities in medicine, and one of the most frequent reasons for hematologic consultation. Effective evaluation of leukocytosis requires an attentive history, careful physical examination, meticulous review of the complete blood count and peripheral blood smear, judicious application of laboratory and radiologic testing, and thoughtful analysis. Definitive diagnosis may require bone marrow aspiration and biopsy, imaging studies, and specialized molecular tests. The differential diagnosis of leukocytosis includes physiologic responses to a broad range of infectious and inflammatory processes, as well as numerous primary hematologic disorders such as leukemias, lymphomas, and myeloproliferative neoplasms.

Why Is My Patient Bleeding Or Bruising?

321

Natalia Rydz and Paula D. James

The evaluation of a patient presenting with bleeding symptoms is challenging. Bleeding symptoms are frequently reported by a normal population, and overlap significantly with bleeding disorders, such as type 1 Von Willebrand disease. The history is subjective; bleeding assessment tools significantly facilitate an accurate quantification of bleeding severity. The differential diagnosis is broad, ranging from defects in primary hemostasis, coagulation deficiencies, to connective tissue disorders. Finally, despite significant clinical evidence of abnormal bleeding, many patients will have not an identifiable disorder. Clinical management of bleeding disorders is highly individualized and focuses on the particular symptoms experienced by the patient.

Venous Thromboembolism Overview   **345**

Elisabeth M. Battinelli, Devon L. Murphy, and Jean M. Connors

> This article gives a general overview of venous thromboembolism (VTE). Pathophysiology, presentation, diagnosis, and initial management of VTE are briefly reviewed. More difficult management problems are reviewed in greater depth, including duration of anticoagulation, treatment of superficial venous thrombosis, and controversies surrounding bridging therapy, with a brief review of currently available new oral anticoagulants.

Does My Patient Have a Life- or Limb-Threatening Thrombocytopenia?   **369**

Nathan T. Connell and Joseph D. Sweeney

> The diagnosis and management of severe thrombocytopenias can be difficult, but is necessary to avoid significant morbidity and mortality. The causes of severe thrombocytopenias, often with a platelet count of less than $10 \times 10^9/L$, include heparin-induced thrombocytopenia, the thrombotic microangiopathies, the catastrophic antiphospholipid syndrome, preeclampsia/HELLP, and posttransfusion purpura. This review provides a brief overview of the key clinical features of each of these major clinical entities, and strategies for their diagnostic workup and therapeutic management.

Does My Patient with a Serum Monoclonal Spike have Multiple Myeloma?   **383**

Giada Bianchi and Irene M. Ghobrial

> A monoclonal spike on serum protein electrophoresis is a frequent finding in the general population and pathognomonic of a plasma cell dyscrasia. In otherwise healthy individuals, it is diagnostic of two asymptomatic, premalignant conditions called monoclonal gammopathy of undetermined significance (MGUS) and smoldering multiple myeloma (SMM) which carry a lifelong risk of progression to multiple myeloma (MM) or related malignancy. This article discusses the criteria for diagnosis of MGUS, SMM, and MM; current recommendations for follow-up and risk factors for progression to MM of patients with MGUS and SMM; and diagnostic evaluation of suspected MM transformation.

Why Does My Patient Have Lymphadenopathy or Splenomegaly?   **395**

Gabriela Motyckova and David P. Steensma

> Lymph node or spleen enlargement may be innocent or the first sign of a serious disorder. Lymphadenopathy and splenomegaly can be found in symptomatic or asymptomatic patients. Lymph node enlargement in a single region or multiple sites can be seen in various diseases, including infections, noninfectious inflammatory conditions, or malignancies; a similar differential diagnosis applies to splenomegaly, but splenomegaly can also be caused by vascular abnormalities and hemolysis. Frequently, lymphadenopathy is detected incidentally during screening examinations or imaging procedures. This review focuses on causes of lymphadenopathy and splenomegaly and an appropriate diagnostic approach to patients with lymphadenopathy or splenomegaly.

Special Hematologic Issues in the Pregnant Patient   409

Tina Rizack and Karen Rosene-Montella

> Evaluation and treatment of hematologic disorders in pregnancy requires an understanding of normal physiologic changes during pregnancy. Hematologic disorders may be caused by preexisting conditions, normal physiologic changes, or can be acquired. A multidisciplinary approach is often necessary for monitoring and treatment of both the mother and the fetus. In general, outcomes are good for both the mother and the fetus.

Index   433

FORTHCOMING ISSUES

June 2012
New Drugs for Malignancy
Franco Muggia, MD,
Guest Editor

August 2012
Central Nervous System Malignancies
Jill Lacy, MD, and
Joachim M. Baehring, MD,
Guest Editors

October 2012
Non-CML Myeloproliferative Diseases
Ross Levine, MD,
Guest Editor

RECENT ISSUES

February 2012
Gynecologic Cancer
Ross S. Berkowitz, MD,
Guest Editor

December 2011
Acute Leukemia
Martin S. Tallman, MD,
Guest Editor

October 2011
Chronic Myelogenous Leukemia
Daniel J. DeAngelo, MD, PhD,
Guest Editor

THE CLINICS ARE NOW AVAILABLE ONLINE!

Access your subscription at:
www.theclinics.com

Preface

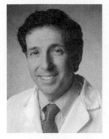 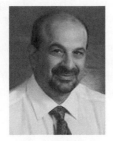

Fred Schiffman, MD   Anthony Mega, MD
Guest Editors

We are pleased to present a variety of topics in "Consultative Hematology" in this issue of *Hematology/Oncology Clinics of North America*. We chose our subject matter by compiling the nature of requests for hematologic advice by colleagues who have reached out to us over many decades of serving them as consultants, and also by polling hematologists throughout the country about their experience as consultants.

In this issue, we include articles that reflect common questions asked of hematologists—particularly about too many or too few red blood cells, white blood cells, platelets, and disorders of coagulation and immunoglobulins. We also have added information in response to questions we are often asked, about the special domains of hematologists (and oncologists): the lymph nodes and the spleen. For clarity and reinforcement, we have separated out life- or limb-threatening thrombocytopenias and also the pregnant patient with hematologic problems.

The methods and skills that should be demonstrated by all consultants are beautifully outlined in an article by Goldman, Lee, and Rudd entitled "Ten Commandments for Effective Consultations"[1] and include the following:

   I. Determine the question
  II. Establish urgency
 III. Look for [and at data] yourself
 IV. Be as brief as appropriate
  V. Be specific
 VI. Provide contingency plans
VII. Honor thy turf
VIII. Teach with tact
 IX. Talk is cheap … and effective
  X. Follow-up.

These precepts should be learned and demonstrated by all who consult and are especially pertinent for the hematology consultant.

We believe that this issue may be useful in several ways: first as a cueing device for any physician or caregiver whose patient demonstrates a hematologic problem; we

Hematol Oncol Clin N Am 26 (2012) xiii–xiv
doi:10.1016/j.hoc.2012.03.001
0889-8588/12/$ – see front matter © 2012 Elsevier Inc. All rights reserved.

hope that it will help to focus the nature of the consultative request and sharpen the questions to be posed to the hematologist. For example, "My patient who was started on heparin has a platelet count of 10,000/uL within 2 hours of beginning that medication, with no prior history of heparin use. Should we look for other causes of thrombocytopenia?" Yes!

Second, by reviewing the relevant chapter prior to the consultant's arrival, the requesting physician may be able to anticipate basic information the consultant may wish to obtain (eg, a *heparin induced thrombocytopenia* [HIT] IgG ELISA test or *a disintegrin and metalloproteinase with a thrombospondin type 1 motif, member 13* [ADAMTS 13] level). This will allow for more coherent discourse between caregivers, which can then move more quickly to a higher level of dialogue so that the patient's needs may be met more efficiently.

Furthermore, by anticipating some of the recommendations by the consulting hematologist, the requesting physician may avoid corruption of important laboratory studies. For example, in a patient with anemia, the knowledge that blood transfusion will affect serum and red blood cell test results might suggest to the requesting physician that transfusion be delayed, or that blood samples be drawn and saved before transfusion is given. In this way, important clinical clues would be preserved.

For certain conditions, it may be critical for the requesting physician to realize that transfusion may not only confound the data but be downright dangerous (eg, the transfusion of platelets in HIT and thrombotic thrombocytopenic purpura [TTP]).

For the consulting hematologist, we hope that this issue will serve as a resource about 1) the approach to the patient, 2) the appropriate differential diagnosis for hematologic problems, 3) critical testing to establish the diagnosis, and 4) general and specific therapeutic guidelines.

Finally, we hope that the references at the end of each article will allow both the requesting caregiver and the consulting hematologist the opportunity to obtain further detail about the information presented in these articles.

Fred Schiffman, MD
Anthony Mega, MD

Division of Hematology/Oncology
Warren Alpert Medical School of Brown University
The Miriam Hospital
164 Summit Avenue
Providence, RI 02906, USA

E-mail addresses:
fschiffman@lifespan.org (F. Schiffman)
amega@lifespan.org (A. Mega)

REFERENCE

1. Goldman L, Lee T, Rudd P. Ten commandments for effective consultations. Arch Int Med 1983;143:1753–5.

Why is My Patient Anemic?

Locke J. Bryan, MD[a], Neil A. Zakai, MD, MSc[b],*

KEYWORDS

- Anemia • Review • Clinical medicine • Blood cell count

Key Points

- Anemia is a common clinical question in consultative hematology.
- The causes and consequences of anemia have important implications for the care of patients.
- Anemia results from 1. red cell loss of sequestration, 2. red cell destruction, or 3. decreased red cell production.
- A systematic approach to the evaluation of anemia is needed to diagnose the cause of anemia.

Anemia is one of the most common clinical questions in consultative hematology.[1] The variety of causes and consequences of anemia reflects the key role of blood as a transport and messaging system for the entire body. Traditionally, anemia has been viewed as an innocent bystander, a marker of disease rather than a cause of disease, but emerging evidence suggests that anemia may affect quality of life, cardiovascular health, and mortality.[2]

Despite the association of anemia with a variety of diseases and with adverse clinical outcomes, the hemoglobin concentration that defines anemia is not established and variations within the normal range are associated with disease.[2,3] The World Health Organization (WHO) in 1958 defined sex-specific hemoglobin targets of 12 g/dL in women and 13 g/dL in men, but acknowledged that "[t]hese figures were chosen arbitrarily and it is still not possible to define normal precisely."[4] Most clinical laboratories define anemia as the bottom 2.5% of the distribution of hemoglobin values from a healthy population.[5]

The lack of a standard definition complicates the role of the clinician, because small changes in the definition of abnormal can change dramatically the number of people who are anemic. In certain situations, the patient serves as their own reference range

---

[a] University of Vermont College of Medicine, 111 Colchester Avenue, Smith Room 244, Burlington, VT 05401, USA
[b] Colchester Research Facility, University of Vermont College of Medicine, 208 South Park Drive, Colchester, VT 05446, USA
* Corresponding author.
E-mail address: Neil.Zakai@uvm.edu

Hematol Oncol Clin N Am 26 (2012) 205–230
doi:10.1016/j.hoc.2012.02.008
0889-8588/12/$ – see front matter © 2012 Elsevier Inc. All rights reserved.

and changes in hemoglobin over time may provide an indicator of health or illness. In this review, the epidemiology and risk factors for anemia are discussed and a clinical guide to the evaluation of anemia is presented.

WHAT IS ANEMIA?

The Merriam-Webster dictionary defines anemia as "a condition in which the blood is deficient in red blood cells (RBC), in hemoglobin, or in total volume."[2] In clinical practice, anemia has multiple clinical definitions, usually based on RBC volume or hemoglobin concentration. **Table 1** presents multiple standards that are reported for healthy populations; however, many more are available. Most clinical laboratories define abnormal as the bottom 2.5% of the gender-specific population distribution, occasionally including age-specific ranges for adults, and thus reference ranges differ based on the local population.[5]

WHAT ARE THE DETERMINANTS OF HEMOGLOBIN CONCENTRATION?

Hemoglobin concentration is a complex phenotype, controlled by both genetic and environmental factors. Although the environmental risk factors for anemia have been studied for years, we are only just beginning to understand the genetics of hemoglobin concentration.

Genetics

Previous analyses of the genetics of hemoglobin concentration have focused on disease states involving hemoglobin variants (ie, thalassemias, hemoglobin C, S, or E disease), red cell structural and metabolism protein defects (ie, hereditary spherocytosis), and iron metabolism (ie, hemochromatosis). In a recent genome-wide association study of healthy individuals, variations in multiple genes, some known to affect hematopoiesis and others novel, were found that affect hemoglobin concentration (**Table 2**).[6] These variants explain only some of the observed variation in hemoglobin concentration in individuals with European ancestry, and further work is under way in non-European ancestry populations.

Age

Age is a known risk factor for anemia, although the physiology is often not completely understood.[7] As we age, a greater proportion of our bone marrow is replaced with fat, leaving fewer hematopoietic elements.[8] In an apparently healthy elderly cohort

Table 1			
Hemoglobin reference ranges to define anemia in various populations			
	Men (g/dL)		Women (g/dL)
WHO[4]	13		12
Williams hematology[1]	14.0		12.3
Beutler & Waalen[5]	Age 20–59 y	Age 60 y+	All ages
White	13.7	13.2	12.2
Black	12.9	12.7	11.5
Boston, MA[62]	13.5		12.0
Togo[63]	11.9		10.2
Tanzania[64]	13.7		11.1
Ethiopia[65]	13.9		12.2

Table 2
Genetic determinants of hemoglobin concentration from the CHARGE consortium

Protein Name	Chromosome	Function
Protein C kinase ε	2p21	Phosphorylates a wide variety of protein targets in cellular signaling
Transmembrane protein 163	2q21	Unknown
Aminomethyltransferase	3p21	Glycene cleavage system
v-kit Hardy-Zuckerman 4 feline sarcoma viral oncogene homolog	4q11	Transmembrane protein, target for stem cell factor; mutations are associated with various tumors
Hereditary hemochromatosis protein	6p21	Controls iron absorption by regulating interaction between transferrin and the transferrin receptor
HBS1L-like v-myb myeloblastosis viral oncogene homolog	6q23	Guanosine triphosphate elongation factor; regulates hematopoiesis; intragenic region associated with modification of severity of sickle cell anemia and thalassemia/hemoglobin E disease
Erythropoietin	7q22	Regulates red cell production by promoting erythroid differentiation and initiating hemoglobin synthesis
Protein kinase, adenosine monophosphate-activated, γ2 noncatalytic subunit	7q36	Monitors cellular energy status and inactivates key enzymes involved in regulating synthesis of fatty acids and cholesterol
Hexokinase 1	10q22	Phosphorylates glucose to glucose-6-phosphate–energy metabolism
SH2B adaptor protein 3	12q24	Signaling protein believed to play a role in hematopoiesis
TSHZ3 teashirt zinc finger homeobox 3	19q12	Unknown
Transmembrane protease, serine 6	22q12	Hepatic protein, may be involved in regulating iron metabolism

Data from Ganesh SK, Zakai NA, van Rooij FJ, et al. Multiple loci influence erythrocyte phenotypes in the CHARGE Consortium. Nat Genet 2009;41(11):1191–8.

(age >64 years), the Cardiovascular Health Study, the prevalence of anemia (WHO criteria) at baseline was 8.5%.[3] In another study, for every 10-year increase in age, participants had a 30% increased odds of anemia using the WHO criteria.[9] Whether lower hemoglobin concentrations and increased anemia prevalence represents physiologic aging versus a condition of disease is poorly studied. Several studies in elderly individuals suggest hemoglobin decline is associated with increased mortality.[3,10,11]

Race

African Americans have lower hemoglobin levels and a nearly 3-fold increased odds of anemia than whites.[9,12] Some of the difference is associated with an increased prevalence of hemoglobin variants such as α-thalassemia.[12] When examining the distribution of hemoglobin between African Americans and whites (**Fig. 1**), the curves are almost identical except for a shift to lower hemoglobin values in African Americans. Whether African Americans tolerate lower hemoglobin concentrations better is not known. In one analysis of elderly individuals, anemia by the WHO criteria was just as poorly tolerated in blacks as in whites.[3]

Gender

Women have lower hemoglobin concentrations than men. Most anemia criteria use sex-specific ranges and thereby the prevalence of anemia differs only slightly between men and women. In younger women, this difference may be partially explained by menstrual blood losses; however, this differences persists into older ages. Again, apart from a shift to lower hemoglobin values, there is no evidence of a skewed distribution in women versus men (see **Fig. 1**). Although there are no outcomes data to support using different hemoglobin criteria for men and women

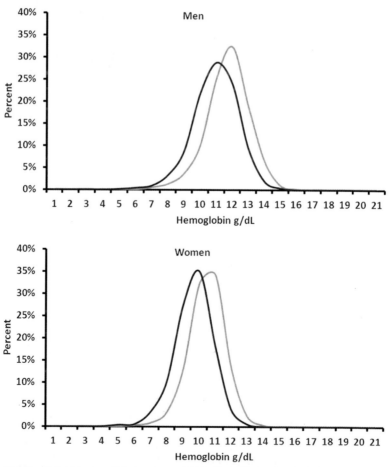

Fig. 1. Distribution of hemoglobin concentration for African American (*blue line*) and white (*green line*) men and women in the United States. (*Data from* Zakai NA, McClure LA, Prineas R, et al. Correlates of anemia in American blacks and whites: the REGARDS Renal Ancillary Study. Am J Epidemiol 2009;169(3):355–64.)

to define anemia, different ranges have been used for many years in clinical practice.

Geography

Environmental factors such as altitude have a profound effect on hemoglobin concentrations. At higher altitudes, decreased oxygen concentrations in the blood provoke a reactive polycythemia, potentially increasing hemoglobin concentrations by more than 2 g/dL in individuals acclimatized to sea level.[13] Polycythemia is seen in some populations native to high altitudes such as the Aymara in South America but not in others such as Tibetans in Asia, suggesting different genetic adaptations to altitude in different populations.[14] Recent studies indicate that there may be geographic differences in hemoglobin concentration independent of altitude, but the impact on health and anemia definitions have not been studied.[9] Apart from incorporating population-specific reference ranges in clinical laboratories serving discrete populations, no effort has been made to account for altitude and geography when establishing normal hemoglobin ranges.

Diseases and Medications

A variety of acute disease conditions affect hemoglobin concentration, but the role of chronic disease conditions is less recognized. Common medical conditions are independently associated with anemia, such as a history of stroke or myocardial infarction, diabetes mellitus, hypertension, and chronic kidney disease.[9] Some common medications such as angiotensin-converting enzyme inhibitors and antiandrogen medications are also associated with anemia.[15–18]

WHAT ARE THE CONSEQUENCES OF ANEMIA?

The effect of severe anemia on cardiovascular function is well recognized in clinical practice.[1] In contrast, less severe anemia has been considered a consequence of disease rather than a cause of disease.[2] A growing body of evidence suggests that anemia and even hemoglobin concentrations within the lower normal range are associated with increased morbidity and mortality in a variety of populations.[3,10] An alternate approach to defining anemia is to use the individual as their own reference range; a decreasing hemoglobin concentration, even within the normal range, has been shown to relate to future mortality in an elderly population.[11]

SUMMARY

A variety of factors both genetic and environmental can affect hemoglobin concentration and the prevalence of arbitrarily defined anemia. In most cases, a hemoglobin concentration less than 11 g/dL is abnormal. Hemoglobin concentrations between 11 g/dL and 14 g/dL may or may not be normal, depending on the clinical context. The role of the consulting hematologist is to help identify the cause of anemia and when appropriate recommend treatment options. Patients should be given transfusion support when experiencing severe anemia-related symptoms. However, there are no data to show that providing transfusion support for asymptomatic patients with the purpose of bringing hemoglobin concentrations into a specific normal range improves outcomes.

WHY IS MY PATIENT ANEMIC?

The reasons for anemia can be complex and multifactorial. To diagnose and manage anemia, the workup needs a systematic approach. Although there are innumerable immediate causes of anemia, there are only a few overarching reasons why someone is anemic:

1. Blood loss or sequestration
2. Increased destruction of RBC
3. Decreased production of RBC.

Determining which of these processes is occurring in the patient helps determine the cause of the anemia. An initial clinical and laboratory assessment must focus on determining which of these processes are active. An initial workup consisting of a complete blood count, reticulocyte count, a clinical history, and a physical examination can help guide the anemia workup.

Clinical History

A careful history to establish whether or not the patient has an unstable volume is warranted in all anemias. A history of gastrointestinal (GI), urinary, or respiratory blood loss is essential, with confirmatory testing for the presence of blood. A dietary and medication/drug history determines whether the patient is at risk for nutritional deficiencies. The physical examination may help direct the workup for anemia:

- Head and neck: the presence of scleral icterus and mucosal jaundice can indicate increased RBC destruction and increase of indirect bilirubin in the serum. Thyromegaly can suggest anemia caused by thyroid disease.
- Lymph nodes: lymphadenopathy can denote an underlying infection or malignancy leading to anemia.
- Cardiac: the detection of murmurs associated with valvular heart disease can lead to suspicion for increased RBC destruction. In the appropriate clinical scenario, assess for signs of endocarditis, which can lead to both diminished RBC production and increased RBC destruction.
- Respiratory: blood loss can present as a hemothorax yielding diminished breath sounds and dullness to percussion. Basilar crackles can suggest congestive heart failure, which is commonly associated with anemia.
- Abdominal: detection of an enlarged spleen or liver can signify a malignancy, increased RBC destruction, or RBC sequestration. The presence of a palpable mass is suggestive of malignancy. A fluid wave or shifting dullness in the abdomen also can suggest a malignancy associated with ascites or portal hypertension and cirrhosis. Abdominal distention with tenderness and abdominal wall ecchymosis can denote a retroperitoneal hematoma associated with RBC loss.
- Extremities: thigh swelling or ecchymosis can point to a site of bleeding. Joint swelling or deformity can hint at an infectious or rheumatologic process leading to anemia.
- Skin: jaundice can be a sign of increased RBC destruction. Rashes can be associated with diseases such as systemic lupus erythematosus or vasculitis, which can lead to anemia.

Laboratory Studies

Several initial laboratory studies guide the workup, as can review of the peripheral smear:

- Peripheral smear blood
  - RBC size: the RBC is a biconcave disc that appears as round to slightly ovoid on review of the peripheral smear. Approximately one-third of the center appears

paler than the surrounding periphery. A normal RBC is typically the size of the nucleus of a nonreactive lymphocyte, approximately 7 mm (**Fig. 2**A). A change in the cell size or amount of central pallor constitutes an abnormal RBC. RBC greater than 8.5 μm are called macrocytes (see **Fig. 2**E). Macrocytic RBC occur with nutritional deficiencies (eg, vitamin B_{12} or folic acid), primary bone marrow disorders (eg, myelodysplastic syndromes, multiple myeloma), hypothyroidism, medications (eg, hydroxyurea), excess alcohol consumption and reticulocytosis in response to bleeding or hemolysis. Small RBC, microcytes, are seen with iron deficiency, lead poisoning, thalassemias, abnormal hemoglobins (eg, sickle disease), and sideroblastic anemia (see **Fig. 2**C). Spherocytes are small RBC less than 6.5 μm with absent central pallor (see **Fig. 2**D) seen in hereditary spherocytosis and autoimmune hemolytic anemias.

○ RBC shape: when viewing the peripheral blood smear it is important to consider the shape of the RBC. Several distinct shapes can suggest a diagnosis. Schistocytes are small fragmented pieces of RBC caused by hemolysis (see **Fig. 2**B).

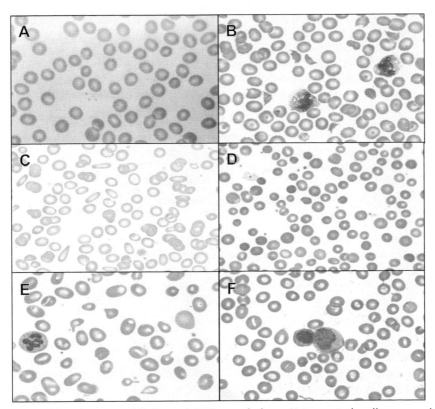

Fig. 2. Peripheral smears. (*A*) Normal RBC morphology. Note central pallor occupying approximately one-third of cell. (*B*) Schistocytes and burr cells consistent with microangiopathic hemolytic anemia. (*C*) Hypochromic microcytic RBC consistent with IDA. (*D*) Spherocytes as seen in hereditary spherocytosis or autoimmune hemolytic anemia. (*E*) Megaloblastic RBC with a hypersegmented neutrophil as seen in vitamin B_{12} deficiency. (*F*) Nucleated RBC and tear-drop cells consistent with leukoerythroblastic syndrome as seen in bone marrow infiltration. (*Courtesy of* John H. Lunde, Medical Director of the Hematology Lab.)

Target cells, codocytes, are small RBC with a central area of pigmentation. Target cells are present in the hemoglobinopathies and may also appear in iron-deficiency anemia (IDA). Dacrocytes, tear-drop cells, appear in the presence of myelophthisis or leukoerythroblastosis when the bone marrow is infiltrated by another process (see **Fig. 2**F). Sickle cells are present in the sickle hemoglobinopathies. Rouleaux formation or the appearance of RBC as a coin stack can be present in Waldenstrom macroglobulinemia, multiple myeloma, and inflammatory states. Clumping of RBC suggest cold antibodies.

- ○ Abnormal circulating cells: the peripheral smear can reveal crucial information beyond direct visualization of the RBC. Review of the circulating white blood cells (WBC) and platelets is essential. Hypersegmented neutrophils, neutrophils with greater than 6 nuclear lobes, may be present in vitamin B_{12} deficiency (see **Fig. 2**C). Immature lymphocytes or numerous lymphocytes can reveal the diagnosis of acute or chronic leukemias, respectively. Abnormal platelets can raise suspicion for the myelodysplastic or myeloproliferative disorders.

- Red cell distribution width (RDW): the RDW is a measure in the variation of the size of RBC, with an abnormally high RDW indicating increased RBC variation. An increased RDW is the first sign of an iron-depleted state and when noted in the setting of microcytosis is consistent with IDA. An increased RDW with macrocytosis can indicate a mixed nutritional deficiency (eg, combined iron and vitamin B_{12} or folic acid deficiency), or reticulocytosis in response to either RBC loss, RBC destruction, or correction of a nutritional deficiency.

- Reticulocyte count: a reticulocyte count helps differentiate anemias of increased RBC loss/destruction from anemias of decreased RBC production. Reticulocytes are young RBC forced into the circulation in response to increased RBC loss or destruction. A low reticulocyte count with anemia suggests decreased RBC production or inadequate time for RBC production to increase. Reticulocytes can be reported as either a percentage of RBC or as an absolute count. If the reticulocytes are presented as a percentage of RBC, a correction factor $\left(\text{corrected reticuocyte count} = \% \text{ reticulocytes} \times \left(\dfrac{\text{Patient Hct}}{\text{Normal Hct}} \right) \right)$ should be applied to adjust for the severity of anemia.[19]

- Other initial laboratory tests: increases in lactate dehydrogenase (LDH) and indirect bilirubin levels with a decrease in haptoglobin level are signs of increased RBC destruction. A positive direct antibody test (DAT) is suggestive of immune-mediated RBC destruction.

RED BLOOD CELL (RBC) LOSS OR DILUTION ANEMIA

There are many potential sources of RBC loss. These sources include occult GI bleeding, urologic bleeding, menstruation, pulmonary bleeding, and phlebotomies (eg, blood donation, laboratory testing). Blood loss must be addressed as a potential cause for all anemias because identification of an early-stage malignancy such as colon cancer can be potentially life saving. Indolent blood loss over a period of time often results in iron deficiency and loss of the ability of the bone marrow to properly increase RBC production. Anemia secondary to blood loss and IDA should prompt a complete workup in men, regardless of age, and in postmenopausal women for a source of bleeding. In menstruating women, an initial trial of iron is warranted, but with further evaluation if there is no response to therapy. Occasionally, anemia is secondary to an increased plasma volume rather than a decrease in RBC mass. The only common clinical situations in which this situation occurs are pregnancy and iatrogenic fluid overload from intravenous fluids.[1] Hemoglobin concentration in pregnancy is typically reduced to 11 to 12 g/dL.

Clinical History

Careful questioning about blood loss is important. Unless there is evidence of an overdose, blood loss on anticoagulant and antithrombotic medications is not physiologic and the source must be identified rather than attributed to anticoagulation.

GI blood losses are one of the most common sources of blood loss. Past history of medications that can cause GI ulceration or inflammation such as nonsteroidal antiinflammatory agents, aspirin, and bisphosphonates may help the practitioner narrow down potential sources. A history of gastric reflux symptoms or use of gastric reflux medications may indicate the potential for GI blood loss secondary to chronic gastritis. Patients may report hematemesis with either bright red blood or emesis described as like coffee grounds in appearance. Questioning about bright red blood with bowel movements, dark tarry stools or melena, known diverticular disease, or previous diverticular bleeding are important to identify possible GI losses. Occasionally, swallowed blood from the upper respiratory tract can present as apparent GI blood loss. Confirmation of colorectal cancer screening is crucial.

In women, a careful menstrual history is mandatory, including the amount of blood loss, the frequency of periods, and the duration of menstruation. The prevalence of IDA in menstruating women is reported to be between 25% and 47.5%.[20,21] Women with decreases in iron intake or even small increases in blood loss as seen in menorrhagia or metrorrhagia can further deplete iron stores, contributing to worsened anemia.

Urinary blood loss is often underappreciated. Changes in urine color, with variations of a pink tint to deep red, can point to a urinary source. Microscopic hematuria may represent underlying urinary disease, including benign prostatic hypertrophy, renal calculi, polycystic kidney disease, or more concerning causes such as bladder, prostate, or kidney cancer. Intrinsic renal disease represents another potential for microscopic hematuria that can result in IDA.[22]

Pulmonary and upper airway bleeding often present as varying degrees of hemoptysis. Patients may ascribe to a chronic cough with hemoptysis described as either obvious blood-colored or rust-colored sputum, raising suspicion of a pulmonary lesion. Patients may not recognize hemoptysis because most sputum is swallowed and never visualized.

There are several potential spaces within the body that can sequester large amounts of blood and be relatively asymptomatic: the pleural space, the retroperitoneal space, and the thigh. Trauma, even minor, especially in the setting of antithrombotic or anticoagulant medications can result in significant blood loss. Intracranial, retinal, or joint space hemorrhages are small in volume and are unlikely to present as anemia. Hip or flank pain, vague abdominal complaints, and lower extremity paresis can be symptoms associated with retroperitoneal hemorrage.[23]

A careful history of blood donation, frequency of phlebotomy for laboratory examinations, and potential surreptitious phlebotomy should be obtained. Iron deficiency from blood donation is a reported cause of anemia.[24] Repetitive phlebotomy during hospitalization can result in a meaningful decline in hemoglobin.[25] Rarely, Munchausen syndrome has been associated with anemia in patients seeking unneeded therapy by bloodletting or intentional diet modifications.[26]

Physical Examination

The focus of the physical examination depends largely on the acuity of the blood loss. Orthostatic vital signs are important in acute blood loss because a patient at rest can seem hemodynamically stable and become profoundly hypotensive with standing. GI blood loss may be evident on nasogastric lavage or digital rectal examination. Inspection of the urine color may reveal hematuria. Suspicion of gynecologic bleeding requires a complete pelvic examination. Trauma, lacerations, or venous puncture sites may be visible. A complete musculoskeletal examination may reveal focal pain or swelling, suggesting a hematoma or internal blood loss.

Laboratory Findings

The severity of anemia varies depending on the amount and chronicity of blood loss. Typically, anemia of acute blood loss remains normocytic and as iron stores are depleted the RDW increases and the mean corpuscular volume (MCV) decreases. Initial screening tests include stool for occult blood, urinalysis, or sputum analysis, as directed by the clinical history. Localized complaints of pain or swelling may represent collections of blood and can direct imaging studies. If a patient history and workup are consistent with blood loss, a negative screen for bleeding does not eliminate the need for direct imaging of likely sites by procedures such as colonoscopy, esophagogastroduodenoscopy, or visualization of the upper aerodigestive tract by endoscopy.

Red Blood Cell (RBC) Destruction

RBC destruction is a challenging cause of anemia because of the large number of conditions in the differential diagnosis. The normal erythrocyte has a life span of approximately 100 to 140 days.[1] The processes through which the body identifies older or damaged RBC for clearance are not fully understood; hypotheses include decreased deformability or alterations in the RBC membrane. There are two main sites for the body to destroy RBC: within the blood vessels (intravascular hemolysis) and ingestion of RBC by macrophages in the spleen and liver (extravascular hemolysis).[1,27]

Intravascular

Under normal circumstances, only some RBC are destroyed in the vascular space. Circulating haptoglobin binds to free hemoglobin, and haptoglobin-hemoglobin complexes are cleared by the liver, with the hemoglobin converted to iron and biliverdin (further converted to bilirubin).[1,19]

Extravascular

Macrophages in the spleen and liver engulf RBC and heme is cleaved into iron and biliverdin, which is later converted into bilirubin. This is the main route for normal RBC catabolism. Haptoglobin is decreased in extravascular hemolysis as well from hemoglobin spilling from macrophages.[1,19]

It is possible to divide hemolytic anemias into intravascular and extravascular processes; however, the cause often overlaps between these 2 processes. Further, chronic RBC destruction can lead to nutritional deficiencies such as iron deficiency from urinary losses and folate deficiency from increased nucleic acid turnover.[1] A reasonable clinical approach is to divide hemolysis into mechanical, immune-mediated, and intrinsic RBC abnormalities and recognize that the destruction can occur at multiple sites.

Mechanical

Within blood vessels, RBC can be destroyed by physical trauma such as from prosthetic cardiac valves and by repetitive trauma of vascular beds, as is seen in march hemoglobinuria. Pathologic processes such as systemic infections, thrombotic thrombocytopenic purpura (TTP), and vasculitis sheer RBC passing through obstructed small vessels. Injury from toxins and heat as well as injury from parasites such as malaria and *Babesia* and bacteria such as *Clostridium* species are other possible means of RBC destruction.

Immune-mediated
Immune-mediated destruction or RBC can be from autoreactive antibodies or alloreactive antibodies. Autologous antibodies can result from neoplastic, infectious, drug-associated, and idiopathic processes, whereas alloreactive antibodies are not apparent unless there is sensitization and exposure to allergenic RBC. Depending on the antibody, immune-mediated hemolysis can occur in the intravascular space, extravascular space, or both.

Hereditary syndromes
Hereditary syndromes can present as chronic hemolysis throughout the lifetime of the individual or as paroxysms of hemolysis with an environmental trigger. A full discussion of hemoglobin variants (ie, sickle cell anemia, thalassemias) is beyond the scope of this review but should be considered in the appropriate clinical setting. Carriers of hemoglobin S, C, and E rarely have obvious hematologic abnormalities, but carriers of thalassemia minor (both α and β) may be microcytic and mildly anemic. An important group of patients are those with RBC enzyme deficiencies because these can present in adulthood as specific episodes of hemolysis caused by an environmental trigger.

Clinical History and Physical Examination

A clinical history suggestive of RBC destruction includes the normal signs and symptoms of anemia (eg, fatigue, pallor). Hemolysis should be strongly suspected with a history of jaundice and changes in urine color. A careful history of recent illnesses and medications is important in the diagnosis of immune-mediated hemolysis or drug-induced hemolysis. Review of travel history, sick contacts, and sexual history may be clues of underlying infections. Hemolysis can be associated with a hypercoagulable state and patients may present with venous thromboembolic disease.

The physical examination is useful in assessing the stability of the patient. Most patients with hemolysis have jaundice. If there is an underlying infectious or neoplastic disorder, lymphadenopathy or splenomegaly may be apparent. Patients with vasculitis may present with neurologic complaints and skin lesions. Patients with TTP or hemolytic uremic syndrome (HUS) may have accompanying symptoms, including fevers and neurologic complaints. Occasionally, patients present with cholelithisis or cholecystitis from pigmented gallstones.

Laboratory Findings

The degree of anemia is variable in hemolytic anemias and can range from mild to severe. Markers of hemolysis such as LDH, indirect bilirubin, and urinary urobilinogen are increased, and haptoglobin is suppressed. A reticulocyte count is usually increased except in acute hemolysis in which the bone marrow has not had a chance to increase RBC production or in chronic hemolysis if individuals have developed concurrent nutritional deficiencies.

Review of the peripheral blood smear is important. In nonimmune-mediated hemolysis, the peripheral blood smear may reveal characteristic burr cells, schistocytes, helmet cells, and microspherocytes from physical destruction of the RBC (see **Fig. 2**B). In immune-mediated hemolysis, the peripheral smear may reveal spherocytes, fragmented red cells, acanthocytes, bite or blister cells, or RBC clumping (see **Fig. 2**D).

Mechanical hemolysis

Mechanical breakdown of RBC is the result of physical trauma, microangiopathic hemolysis, infections associated with destruction, and several other miscellaneous processes.

- Physical trauma: repetitive trauma to vascular beds can cause destruction of erythrocytes, as seen in runners or in soldiers forced to march long distances, resulting in march hemoglobinuria. Individuals present with discrete episodes of hemolysis, which may include dark urine or muscle aches/pains. Laboratory and physical examination findings are usually negative but occasionally jaundice and hepatosplenomegaly are present. Malfunctioning prosthetic cardiac valves or abnormalities of native valves can cause shearing of RBC and hemolysis. Hemolysis is seen in many prosthetic valves, with a higher risk in mitral versus aortic valve replacement and mechanical versus bioprosthetic valves.[28] Review of the peripheral smear shows red cell fragments (see **Fig. 2B**).
- Microangiopathic hemolytic anemia: the underlying process is destruction or shearing of the RBC in the microcirculation and leads to the classic finding of schistocytes or helmet cells on review of the peripheral blood smear (see **Fig. 2B**). Schistocytes are seen in most individuals; however, in pathologic conditions, the percentage of schistocytes usually exceeds 1%.[29] Signs and symptoms of anemia are often secondary to signs and symptoms of the underlying disorder. The clinical setting varies, but markers of hemolysis (increased LDH, decreased haptoglobin) are almost universally present. Disorders that can cause a microangiopathic hemolytic anemia include TTP, HUS, systemic infections (with or without diffuse intravascular coagulation), systemic malignancy, malignant hypertension, and preeclampsia/HELLP syndrome in pregnant women. In general, coagulation studies are normal and the diagnosis is made with clinical criteria in the setting of a microangiopathic hemolytic anemia on peripheral blood smear. The diagnosis and treatment of microangiopathic hemolytic anemias is complex and an accurate diagnosis is important. Classic TTP can be diagnosed with low levels of the ADAMTS13 protease and an excess of high-molecular-weight Von Willebrand multimers.[30] The diagnosis of other microangiopathic hemolytic anemias has recently been reviewed.[1,30]
- Infections: malaria and *Babesia* are parasites that reside within the RBC. Intravascular hemolysis occurs as a result of reproduction of the parasites within the RBC. Severe malarial infections can mimic the signs and symptoms of TTP; however, review of the peripheral smear reveals parasites within RBC.[31,32] Toxins produced by infections such as *E coli* O157:H7 and *Clostridium* species result in direct RBC destruction; diagnosis is made by the clinical history and isolation of bacterial toxins from stool or bacteria from the blood (**Table 3**).[1]
- Miscellaneous: snake, spider, and insect toxins can cause hemolysis. The clinical picture is usually dominated by the particular toxin to which the patient is exposed. Accidental infusion of hypotonic solutions can cause rupture of RBC. A careful review of all clinical events surrounding hemolysis and review of all infusions can help make the diagnosis.

Immune-mediated hemolysis

Autoimmune hemolytic anemias are divided into primary and secondary processes.[1,27] Patients have variable degrees of anemia and typical laboratory findings of hemolysis (increased LDH, depressed haptoglobin, increased indirect bilirubin) and anemia. The diagnosis of autoimmune hemolytic anemia is made by showing binding of antibodies

Table 3
Infections associated with anemia

Type	Organism	Pathophysiology
Bacterial	*Clostridium perfringens*	Toxin-mediated direct RBC lysis
	E coli (O157:H7)	Toxin-mediated direct RBC lysis
	Helicobacter pylori	B_{12} deficiency secondary to gastritis
	Mycoplasma pneumoniae	Cold autoimmune hemolysis
	Streptococcus pneumoniae	Mechanical hemolysis with bacterial endocarditis or DIC
Fungal	*Histoplasma capsulatum*	Bone marrow infiltration typically associated with HIV
	Mycobacterium tuberculosis and *M avium*	Bone marrow infiltration typically associated with HIV
Parasitic	*Babesia microti* and *B divergens*	Direct RBC lysis and RBC membrane fragility
	Plasmodium falciparum, *P malariae,* and *P vivax*	Direct RBC lysis and RBC membrane fragility
Viral	Cytomegalovirus	Cold autoimmune hemolysis
	Epstein-Barr virus	Cold autoimmune hemolysis
	Hepatitis B and C	Bone marrow suppression
	HIV	Bone marrow suppression or infiltration, chronic inflammation
	Parvovirus B19	Bone marrow suppression or failure (pure red cell aplasia)

Abbreviation: DIC, disseminated intravascular coagulation.

or complement to RBC as assessed with the direct antiglobulin (DAT or Coombs) test. The indirect antiglobulin test measures the ability of patients' sera to bind to allogenic RBC. In general, the indirect antiglobulin test is less helpful than the DAT, except for the rare occasions when the patient has a low-affinity antigen. Autoimmune hemolytic anemia is divided into warm and cold autoimmune hemolytic anemia depending on the reactivity of the antibody at body temperature.

- Warm autoimmune hemolytic anemias: in general, warm autoimmune hemolytic anemias are caused by immunoglobulins of IgG subclasses and react to RBC at body temperature (37°C). The DAT are positive for IgG with or without C3d. Most IgG subclasses fix complement poorly and the predominant site of RBC destruction is the spleen. Review of the peripheral smear reveals an increase in the number of reticulocytes, spherocytes, and some bite cells (see **Fig. 2**D). Secondary causes of warm autoimmune hemolytic anemia include viral infections (usually in children), autoimmune and connective tissues disorders, lymphomas and lymphoproliferative disorders, and drugs.[27,33]
- Cold autoimmune hemolytic anemias: cold autoimmune hemolytic anemias are a group of disorders in which the red cells are bound by antibodies with a thermal amplitude less than body temperature, but greater than temperatures in the peripheral circulation (approximately 30°C).[1,27] Most cold autoimmune hemolytic anemias are secondary to another process. The IgM multimers (pentamers and hexamers) are large enough to bind more than 1 RBC, causing agglutination of RBC. Exposure to cold in the periphery can result in agglutination of RBC in small vessels and acrocyanosis. Review of the peripheral blood smear may reveal RBC clumps. The IgM antibodies fix complement on the RBC membrane and can

cause direct lysis of the RBC as well as macrophage-mediated RBC ingestion in the spleen and liver. The DAT is characterized by binding of C3d to RBC. Occasionally, IgM is seen on the RBC surface if the thermal amplitude is sufficiently high. The titer of the cold antibody is reported as the minimum concentration at which the patient's serum agglutinates allogenic RBC. The thermal amplitude is the maximum temperature at which the antibody causes RBC agglutination. The degree of hemolysis is related to the amount and reactivity of the antibody and the ability of the antibody to bind complement. In some individuals, hemolysis is minimal or absent and the only presenting symptom is acrocyanosis.

There are several naming conventions for cold autoimmune hemolytic anemia, but understanding the pathophysiology helps overcome this limitation. Antibody specificity is occasionally helpful in determining the cause of the hemolytic anemia; anti-I specificity is associated with primary cold autoimmune hemolytic anemia, as well as *Mycoplasma pneumoniae* and lymphoma. Anti-i is associated with hemolysis caused by mononucleosis or lymphoma.

○ Primary cold agglutinin disease: patients have a chronic hemolysis and usually have a monoclonal IgM autoantibody detected on serum electrophoresis. Malignancies such as lymphoma and Waldenstrom macroglobulinemia should be ruled out with imaging and bone marrow examination in most cases. Antibody specificity is usually anti-I.

○ Secondary cold agglutinin disease: secondary cold agglutinin disease is caused by hematologic malignancies (chronic lymphocytic leukemia, lymphomas), nonhematologic malignancies, and infections. Infections commonly associated with cold autoimmune hemolytic anemia are mononucleosis and *Mycoplasma pneumoniae.* Hemolysis occurs several weeks after the infection and usually lasts 2 to 4 weeks. Antibody specificity is Anti-i. Neoplastic processes can have anti-I or anti-i; however, finding an anti-i in the absence of an infectious cause is suspicious for lymphoma.

• Drug-mediated: drugs can induce immune-mediated RBC injury through several mechanisms (**Table 4**).

○ Hapten: the combination of drug bound to RBC membrane proteins elicits an immune response. Classically, this response is associated with high-dose penicillin. Hemolysis usually begins 7 to 10 days after exposure, and resolves days to weeks after the drug is withdrawn.[1]

○ Ternary complex: drug-antibody complexes form and bind weakly to RBC membranes and fix complement, causing destruction of RBC. Hemolysis can occur quickly after exposure to drug.

○ Autoantibody: in the presence of drug, nondrug-dependent autoantibodies form; α-methyldopa is the classic representation of this effect.

• Alloimmune: transfused RBC invoke an immune response. Reactions are either immediate or delayed. Immediate hemolytic transfusion reactions are usually related to ABO incompatibility or with preformed alloantibodies (with previous exposure either through blood products or pregnancy). Delayed transfusion reactions usually require formation of alloantibodies. Diagnosis is based on an indirect antiglobulin test (antibody screen) and discovery of an antibody reactive to allogenic RBC only.

Table 4
Medications associated with anemia

Category	Class/Medication	Pathophysiology
Autoimmune hemolysis	α-Methyldopa	Autoimmune RBC binding with splenic sequestration
	Penicillins	Hapten/drug absorption with splenic sequestration
	Sulfonamides	Neoantigen formation with autoimmune RBC destruction
	Quinidine	Ternary complex formation with direct RBC lysis
Bone marrow suppression	ACE inhibitors	Suppress erythropoietin
	Alkylating agents	Direct marrow toxicity
	Anthracyclines	Direct marrow toxicity
	Antiandrogens	Decreased testosterone
	Antimetabolites	Direct marrow toxicity
	Chloramphenicol	Direct toxicity to cell mitochondria
	Colchicine	Direct marrow toxicity
	Zidovudine (AZT)	Megaloblastic anemia by inhibition of nucleic acid synthesis
Decreased RBC production	Anticonvulsants	Megaloblastosis associated with folic acid deficiency
	Hydroxyurea	Megaloblastic anemia by inhibition of nucleic acid synthesis
	Metformin	Decreased folic acid intestinal absorption
	Methotrexate	Dihydrofolate reductase inhibitor causing folic acid deficiency
	Proton pump inhibitors	Decreases vitamin B_{12} levels with long-term use

Abbreviation: ACE, angiotensin-converting enzyme.

Enzyme deficiencies, abnormal hemoglobins, and red blood cell (RBC) membrane abnormalities

Abnormalities in RBC metabolism, structural proteins, or hemoglobin result in fragile RBC predisposed to destruction. The number of abnormalities is vast and can be either acquired or hereditary.

- Acquired
  - Medications and toxins: a variety of drugs and toxins can bind and damage RBC membranes. Toxins include arsenic hydride, lead, and copper. There are case reports of many medications causing RBC membrane abnormalities.[1] Evaluation is based on exposure (see **Table 4**).
  - Paroxysmal nocturnal hemoglobinuria (PNH): PNH is an acquired clonal disorder in which mutations in the PIG-A gene cause defects in glycosylphosphatidylinositol (GPI) anchor synthesis and absence of many proteins from the surface of circulating RBC. Laboratory and clinical workup reveals hemolysis, no evidence of immune-mediated hemolysis, and perhaps a history of aplastic anemia or thrombosis. Diagnosis is made by measuring the presence of GPI-anchored proteins on circulating cells.
- Inherited: the number of inherited RBC disorders resulting in increased RBC destruction and anemia is vast, reflecting the complex nature of the RBC. Disorders range from defects in hemoglobin (ie, thalassemias and sickle cell anemias),

RBC membrane proteins (hereditary spherocytosis), and RBC enzyme deficiencies (eg, glucose-6-phosphate dehydrogenase [G6PD] deficiency). Many of these defects are detected at birth, although thalassemia minor/trait may not be diagnosed until adulthood. A full discussion of these defects is beyond the scope of this review, but should be suspected if abnormally shaped RBC are present on peripheral smear without evidence for another cause. G6PD deficiency and other RBC enzyme deficiencies are relatively common and affect RBC survival, especially after exposure to certain foods and drugs. Hemoglobin electrophoresis and specific enzyme assays can make these diagnoses in the nonacute setting. Bite cells (degmacytes) are seen with G6PD deficiency, and a special test for Heinz bodies (denatured hemoglobin clumps in RBCs) may be helpful in making a diagnosis.

RED BLOOD CELL (RBC) PRODUCTION

The ability to maintain a stable hemoglobin concentration depends on the ability of the bone marrow to produce RBC to balance losses from bleeding, natural aging of RBC, and RBC destruction. Failure of the bone marrow to produce RBC results in anemia. RBC have a life span of 100 to 140 days in the circulation under normal circumstances.[1] Abrupt cessation of hematopoiesis seldom results in abrupt decreases in hemoglobin concentration in the absence of increased blood loss or decreased life span of the RBC. Nutrient deficiencies, organ dysfunction, bone marrow dysfunction from primary marrow processes, and hemoglobin synthesis errors can result in decreased RBC production.

Clinical History

The symptoms of anemia are often less apparent than the primary pathologic process such as thyroid dysfunction, malignant processes, or infection. A careful nutritional history is essential because various dietary restrictions predispose individuals to deficiencies in iron, vitamin B_{12}, and folic acid. History of bowel resection or bariatric procedures may prevent proper nutrient absorption. A drug and alcohol history is also important. More obscure are nonfood substances such as lead, which may result from use of improperly manufactured cookware or work in various occupations.[34]

Physical Examination

Decreased RBC production is usually not discernable on physical examination; however, a physical examination may help guide the diagnosis by focusing on potential sites of organ dysfunction or malignancy.

Laboratory Findings

The size of the RBC is varied in anemia associated with decreased production. In general, the reticulocyte count is inappropriately low for the hemoglobin, and other blood cell lines may be suppressed. Review of the peripheral blood smear is important, with a variety of morphologic findings possible depending on the underlying cause.

Causes for Alterations in RBC Production

The causes of decreased RBC production are best divided into 3 main categories: nutrient deficiencies, organ dysfunction, and bone marrow dysfunction.

Nutrient deficiencies

IDA is the most common cause of anemia worldwide and accounts for more than half of cases of anemia. Other common nutrient deficiencies are vitamin B_{12} (cobalamin) and vitamin B$_9$ (folic acid). In general, vitamin B$_{12}$, folic acid, and iron status should be evaluated in anyone with an anemia associated with decreased RBC production because these conditions are not rare and multiple deficiencies can present in the same patient.

- IDA: IDA is the most common cause of anemia worldwide, affecting as many as 20% of the world's population.[35] Iron absorption occurs mostly in the jejunum, and altered uptake, nutrition, digestion, and poor absorption can result in iron deficiency. Microcytosis is a marker of iron-deficient hematopoiesis but usually occurs when the hemoglobin decreases below normal. An increased RDW is often an early marker of iron deficiency, indicating developing anisocytosis. A serum ferritin level is a simple, inexpensive test. A serum ferritin level of 30 ng/mL or lower is diagnostic for IDA. Ferritin is an acute-phase reactant, thus making levels difficult to interpret in the setting of acute inflammation. Previously, a serum ferritin level of 70 ng/mL or lower in the setting of acute inflammation was considered diagnostic of IDA; however, what constitutes acute inflammation is unclear.[36] Given changes associated with acute inflammation, the serum ferritin level that effectively excludes IDA in the setting of inflammation is not established. Review of the peripheral blood smear reveals numerous hypochromic RBC with central pallor in patients with severe IDA (see **Fig. 2**C). **Table 5** reviews the laboratory findings in IDA. A therapeutic trial of iron can also aid in the diagnosis. The provider must determine the cause of iron deficiency because malignancy is not uncommon. The gold standard for the diagnosis of IDA is a bone marrow biopsy, revealing absence of iron stores.[1]
- Cobalamin (vitamin B$_{12}$) deficiency: the gastric parietal cells produce intrinsic factor, which binds to dietary vitamin B$_{12}$, allowing absorption in the ileum. Severe vitamin B$_{12}$ deficiency results in megaloblastic macrocytosis, although only if there is inadequate folic acid. In addition to large RBC, the peripheral blood smear may reveal hypersegmented neutrophils (see **Fig. 2**E). In severe cases, total white cell count and platelet count are decreased. Vitamin B$_{12}$ deficiency can result from poor oral intake or poor absorption. A vitamin B$_{12}$ level greater than 300 pg/mL effectively excludes vitamin B$_{12}$ deficiency and a vitamin B$_{12}$

Table 5
Diagnosis of IDA

	Normal	Iron Deficiency Without Anemia	Mild IDA	Severe IDA
Hemoglobin (g/dL)	Normal	Normal	9–12	6–8
Ferritin (ng/mL)	40–200	<40	<20	<10
Serum iron (μg/dL)	60–180	60–180	<60	<40
TIBC (μg/dL)	250–450	>450	>450	>450
Transferrin saturation (%)	20–50	30	<15	<10
Transferrin (μg/dL)	300–360	300–390	350–400	>410
MCHC	27–31	Normal	<27	<27
MCV	82–96	Normal	Normal	<82
RDW	11.5–14.5	Normal	Normal	>14.5
Red cell morphology	Normal	Normal	Slightly hypochromic	Hypochromic and microcytosis

Abbreviations: MCHC, mean corpuscular hemoglobin concentration; TIBC, total iron-binding capacity.

Table 6
Diagnosis of vitamin B$_{12}$ (cobalamin) and vitamin B$_9$ (folic acid) deficiency

	Deficiency Excluded	Vitamin B$_{12}$ Deficiency	Deficiency Excluded	Vitamin B$_{12}$ Deficiency ± Folate Deficiency	Folic Acid Deficiency
Vitamin B$_{12}$ (pg/mL)	>300	<140	≤300	≤300	≤300
Serum folic acid (ng/mL)	>4	>4	≤4	≤4	≤4
Erythrocyte folate (μg/L)	>140	NA	NA	NA	<140
Homocysteine (mmol/L)	NA	NA	5–14	5–14; >14	>14
MMA[a] (nmol/L)	NA	NA	70–270	>270	70–270

Abbreviation: NA, not applicable.
[a] MMA can be increased in kidney failure.

level less than 140 pg/mL is diagnostic of vitamin B$_{12}$ deficiency. For vitamin B$_{12}$ levels between 140 and 300 pg/mL, increased methylmalonic acid (MMA) and homocysteine levels support the diagnosis (**Table 6**). A diagnosis of pernicious anemia resulting from autoimmune destruction of the gastric parietal cells was historically made using a Schilling test, but presence of intrinsic factor or antiparietal cell antibodies are now most often used.

- Folic acid (vitamin B$_9$) deficiency: folic acid deficiency results in a macrocytic anemia. Causes of folic acid deficiency include poor nutritional intake and malabsorption. In addition, folic acid deficiency can result from several medications used to treat seizure disorders (phenytoin), autoimmune diseases (methotrexate), infection (pentamidine, trimethoprim), and malignancy (hydroxyurea, methotrexate). Metformin and cholestyramine can decrease folate absorption, and patients may require supplementation. Disorders of increased red cell turnover (such as hemolysis) may result in increased folate requirements and folate deficiency. Serum folate levels fluctuate daily depending on diet so measurements are not useful. Red cell folate levels should be ordered if folic acid deficiency is suspected. A normal MMA level and an increased homocysteine level strongly support the diagnosis of folic acid deficiency (see **Table 6**).
- Other nutritional deficiencies: deficiencies in vitamin A, vitamin B$_6$, copper, and dietary protein are rare causes of anemia.[1]

Organ dysfunction

- Thyroid: the cause of anemia from hypothyroidism is unclear but may be from decreased stimulation of erythropoiesis by thyroid hormone.[37] Red cell size is variable and workup depends on other signs and symptoms of hypothyroidism.[38] Evaluation should include testing serum thyroid-stimulating hormone and free T4 level.
- Liver: liver dysfunction from any cause is associated with anemia.[39] Physical examination may reveal jaundice, ascites, caput medusa, spider angiomas, or hepatomegaly, prompting an evaluation of underlying liver disease.

- Kidney: chronic kidney disease causes normocytic anemia secondary to a decrease in erythropoietin production.[40] Erythropoietin is a humoral factor produced by the kidney that regulates RBC production. Anemia varies in severity and most patients present with mild to moderate reductions in hemoglobin. Even mild decreases in the glomerular filtration rate are associated with increased rates of anemia.[9,41–43]
- Hypogonadism: testosterone increases hemoglobin in men beginning at the time of puberty and is likely the cause of increased hemoglobin levels in men compared with women.[15] A decreased level of testosterone in both elderly men and women has been shown to be a risk factor for anemia.[16] Gonadotropin-releasing hormone analogues such as leuprolide used in treatment of prostate cancer decrease erythropoiesis by suppression of testosterone production.[17] Symptoms associated with hypogonadism include diminished libido, decreased body hair, truncal obesity, decreased energy, and generalized weakness. The anemia is usually mild.
- Heart failure: anemia is common in individuals with heart failure. Causes may be varied and include decreased renal perfusion, hepatic congestion, or decreased absorption of vital nutrients from the gut.[44]

Bone marrow dysfunction

Bone marrow disorders can be divided into primary marrow disorders and secondary marrow disorders. In primary marrow disorders, abnormalities within the bone marrow result in the inability to produce RBC. In secondary bone marrow disorders, a systemic process from outside the marrow space invades the bone marrow or suppresses production of RBC.

- Primary bone marrow disorders: these disorders reflect processes that are intrinsic to the bone marrow. Review of the peripheral blood smear and bone marrow biopsy are important in identifying these processes.
  - Myelodysplastic syndromes (MDS) and myeloproliferative disorders (MPD): MDS/MPD occasionally result in isolated marrow dysfunction of the erythroid cell lines and present with anemia and decreased reticulocyte count.[19] Patients may have additional cell lineages involved with abnormal numbers of WBC or platelets. Diagnosis is typically made with bone marrow biopsy with aspiration. The evaluation of peripheral blood for the JAK V617F can help with the diagnosis MPD.
  - Leukemia: acute leukemias often present abruptly with obvious manifestations and circulating immature WBC. Rarely, acute leukemia may present with isolated anemia. Chronic leukemias can be more subtle in presentation. Review of the peripheral blood smear and bone marrow examination are crucial in diagnosis. Flow cytometry of peripheral blood may assist in the diagnosis of chronic lymphocytic leukemia and evaluation of the peripheral blood for the BCR/ABL transcript may assist in the diagnosis of chronic myeloid leukemia.
  - Multiple myeloma: multiple myeloma is on the differential for decreased red cell production, especially in the setting of concurrent renal failure, hypercalcemia, or pathologic bone fractures. Serum protein electrophoresis, urine protein electrophoresis, evaluation of serum free light chain ratio, skeletal survey, and a bone marrow biopsy are helpful diagnostic tests.
  - Bone marrow failure syndromes: failure of marrow progenitor cells results in varying conditions. Pure red cell aplasia results in normocytic anemia with absent reticulocytosis. It is associated with T-cell–mediated attack of erythroid progenitors.[45] Aplastic anemia typically presents as pancytopenia from T-cell–

mediated attack. Bone marrow cellularity is markedly reduced on bone marrow biopsy.[46] PNH, although more commonly thought of as an increased RBC destructive process, lies on a continuum with aplastic anemia and also can have diminished erythropoeisis.[47]

- Secondary bone marrow dysfunction: several causes of infiltrative processes disrupt the ability of the bone marrow to produce RBC, resulting in anemia. Leukemia, lymphoma, fibrosis, infectious agents, and metastatic solid tumors to the bone marrow can result in a normocytic anemia with pancytopenia.[19] Infiltrative processes can result in displacement of the hemopoietic bone marrow tissue to the peripheral blood, resulting in myelophthisis or leukoerythroblastic reaction. The peripheral blood smear reveals tear-drop cells (dacrocytes) and nucleated RBC, and occasionally immature WBC (see **Fig. 2**F). Often, patients are older and present with signs and symptoms consistent with the underlying malignancy. Splenomegaly, hepatomegaly, and adenopathy may be present on physical examination. Diagnosis is confirmed with a bone marrow biopsy.
  - ○ Infiltration by malignancies: most malignancies have the potential to invade the bone marrow, the more common malignancies to metastasize to the bone marrow include solid tumors including lung, breast, GI, and prostate.[48]
  - ○ Infiltration by infectious processes: *Mycobacterium avium* complex, *Mycobacterium tuberculosis*, and *Histoplasma capsulatum* infections can result in anemia by bone marrow infiltration and are more often seen in patients with AIDS (see **Table 3**).[49]
  - ○ Infiltration by other disorders: the bone marrow can rarely be infiltrated by other systemic processes such as sarcoidosis or amyloidosis.[50,51]
- Bone marrow suppression: the bone marrow can be suppressed, resulting in an inability to produce RBC. The broad categories of bone marrow suppression include inflammation, infection, autoimmune, and toxicity. Anemia of inflammation and autoimmune causes are discussed in a separate section.
  - ○ Infection: parvovirus B19, human immunodeficiency virus (HIV), and viral hepatitis are known to have immune-mediated effects on bone marrow with the potential to cause isolated anemia to pancytopenia. Parvovirus B19, a single-stranded DNA virus, can cause anemia by direct RBC destruction but also arrest of erythroid maturation in the bone marrow.[52] Parvovirus B19 polymerase chain reaction assays are the most sensitive test for diagnosis. Most patients with HIV have anemia at some point in their disease course; anemia is associated with increased mortality independent of the severity of their infection.[49] The anemia associated with HIV has a complex pathogenesis and is related to direct marrow suppression by the virus, invasion of the marrow by malignancies, and increased destruction of RBC.[53]
  - ○ Medications: toxicity from drugs, chemotherapy, and irradiation destroys the pluripotent stem cells of the bone marrow and can result in anemia or pancytopenia. The most commonly associated drugs and chemotherapeutic agents associated with bone marrow suppression include alkylating agents, topoisomerase inhibitors, and antimetabolites (see **Table 4**). Anemia associated with the treatment of malignancy is an often-anticipated side effect. Most medications have been linked to bone marrow suppression. **Table 4** lists a few common medications. Antiandrogens such as spironolactone and bicalutamide can result in decreased erythropoiesis by decreasing testosterone activity.
  - ○ Alcohol: alcohol is a commonly overlooked bone marrow suppressant. Chronic alcohol consumption suppresses bone marrow function and has a direct effect

on heme synthesis.[54] Alcoholism is the most common cause of macrocytic anemia (which may not be related to B_{12} or folate deficiencies) and accounts for 15% to 65% of cases depending on the population.[55] Testing γ-glutamyl-transferase levels can confirm suspicion of alcohol consumption in patients who report abstinence. Once a patient is abstinent from alcohol, the macrocytic anemia corrects over 1 to 2 months. Patients with alcoholism are at risk of underlying vitamin B_{12} or folate deficiencies.

o Environmental toxins: some chemical exposures can cause bone marrow suppression. Benzene, used in industrial dyes, detergents, explosives, pesticides, synthetic rubber, plastics, and pharmaceuticals, can have toxic effects on the bone marrow. Radiation exposure also has toxic effects on bone marrow. Occupational history may reveal a potential environmental exposure.

o Heavy metal toxicity: patients exposed to toxic levels of heavy metals can develop anemia. Potential heavy metal toxins include lead and zinc. Toxic levels of lead result in alterations of hemoglobin synthesis, altering RBC production. Sources of heavy metal exposure in adults include drinking water, faulty cookware, and metal working. The Agency for Toxic Substances and Disease Registry, an agency within the US Department of Health and Human Services, releases a detailed report on lead toxicity that lists all potential exposures.[34] Associated symptoms include abdominal pain and behavioral changes. Patients with a potential exposure history and microcytic anemia should have their serum lead level checked. If the result is positive, the entire household should be screened. A peripheral blood smear may reveal basophilic stippling.

ANEMIA OF INFLAMMATION

Anemia of inflammation (or anemia of chronic disease) is a well-known but poorly defined entity. The pathophysiology is complex and involves both decreased RBC production and increased RBC destruction. At times, the source of the inflammation is evident such as inflammatory bowel disease, a rheumatologic disease, cancer, or chronic infection such as osteomyelitis. At other times, the source of inflammation is not apparent. Anemia of inflammation is the second most common cause of anemia worldwide. In older adults, anemia of inflammation represents the cause of nearly one-fifth of anemias.[56]

Pathophysiology

Initially a diagnosis of exclusion, anemia of inflammation was believed to represent a broad process of inflammation affecting erythropoiesis. Research has revealed an increasingly complicated pathogenesis that results in changes of iron homeostasis, altered proliferation of erythoid progenitor cells, decreased production of erythropoietin, and shortened life span of the RBC.[57] Iron metabolism is altered by diversion of iron to within cells of the reticuloendothelial system. Removal of circulating iron restricts the ability to produce RBC, creating a pseudoiron-deficient state. Sequestration of iron in inflammatory states is believed to be an adaptive process because previous evidence has shown that iron increases microbial growth and increases proliferation of malignant cells.[58] Alteration in proliferation of erythroid progenitor cells is not clearly understood but seems most associated with increases of interferon-γ.[59] In vitro studies of erythropoietin have shown decreased production in inflammatory states associated with increases in interleukin-1 and tumor-necrosing factor α.[60] In addition, inflammatory states increase circulating cytokines, which damage RBC membranes, and induce free radicals, resulting in increased erythrophagocytosis.[57]

Together these processes inhibit normal RBC production and turnover, resulting in refractory anemia.

Multiple causes of anemia of inflammation have been implicated, including autoimmune diseases, chronic kidney disease, chronic transplant rejection, infections, and malignancy. Autoimmune diseases most often associated with anemia of inflammation include rheumatoid arthritis, systemic lupus erythematosus, vasculitis, inflammatory bowel disease, and sarcoidosis. Multiple infectious processes have been implicated in anemia of inflammation, but evaluation of HIV represents a chronic and often indolent process that must be considered.[57]

Patient History

The inflammatory illness can be obvious or occult. Review of the past medical history and any presenting symptoms may provide some clues. Common illnesses include infections, rheumatologic diseases, inflammatory bowel disease, and malignancies. Often a careful history and physical examination can guide the workup. Sometimes no cause is evident, or the inflammation is transient and the findings resolve. Following the patient over time may provide an answer.

Physical Examination

Examination of a patient should focus on potential findings to suggest an underlying inflammatory disease. The examination should be directed toward identifying the inflammatory illness. A lymph node examination, abdominal examination for masses, cardiac examination for a new murmur, and examination of the joints and the skin may reveal the underlying condition.

Laboratory Findings

Anemia varies in severity, and most patients present with mild to moderate reductions in hemoglobin. Laboratory workup typically reveals a normochromic normocytic anemia, although hypochromic microcytic anemia is occasionally seen.[61] Reticulocyte count is low, consistent with suppression of RBC production. In anemia of inflammation, serum iron and total iron-binding capacity is low, whereas ferritin levels remain normal or increased. It is important to evaluate for IDA, although both conditions can exist concurrently. Increases of the C-reactive protein level and the erythrocyte sedimentation rate and low albumin are nonspecific markers of inflammation that can be helpful in supporting the diagnosis of anemia of inflammation. The soluble transferin receptor serum test is not increased in the anemia of inflammation but is increased in IDA, but the clinical utility is not established.

SUMMARY

Anemia is a common clinical condition. The workup and evaluation are difficult because there is not a precise definition of what is normal and abnormal. A careful clinical assessment with initial laboratory studies helps determine the mechanism of anemia in most cases as being from increased RBC loss, increased RBC destruction, or from decreased RBC production. The evaluation and assessment of anemia requires a detailed knowledge of hematopoiesis as well as an overall understanding of the interconnections within the human body.

This review does not discuss the treatment of anemia. Treatment must be tailored for each individual. There is little to lose and much to gain in identifying and stopping a bleeding source, supplementing a nutritional deficiency, or improving organ function. The difficulty arises as to whether we should treat anemia as a disease. Does a mild anemia associated with diabetes and mild chronic kidney disease require any other treatment than to maximize diabetes treatment and prevent further damage to the kidneys?

Regardless of whether an anemia is treated or not, it is important to determine why the patient is anemic. This strategy often leads to insights into the patient's overall health or catches diseases at early or curable stages. A systematic and logical approach, often over many visits, may be required to diagnose and treat anemia.

REFERENCES

1. Lichtman MA, Beutler E, Kipps TJ, et al, editors. Williams hematology. 7th edition. New York (NY): The McGraw-Hill Companies, Inc.; 2006.
2. Nissenson AR, Goodnough LT, Dubois RW. Anemia: not just an innocent bystander? Arch Intern Med 2003;163(12):1400–4.
3. Zakai NA, Katz R, Hirsch C, et al. A prospective study of anemia status, hemoglobin concentration, and mortality in an elderly cohort: the Cardiovascular Health Study. Arch Intern Med 2005;165(19):2214–20.
4. Nutritional anaemias. Report of a WHO scientific group. World Health Organ Tech Rep Ser 1968;405:5–37.
5. Beutler E, Waalen J. The definition of anemia: what is the lower limit of normal of the blood hemoglobin concentration? Blood 2006;107(5):1747–50.
6. Ganesh SK, Zakai NA, van Rooij FJ, et al. Multiple loci influence erythrocyte phenotypes in the CHARGE Consortium. Nat Genet 2009;41(11):1191–8.
7. den Elzen WP, Gussekloo J. Anaemia in older persons. Neth J Med 2011;69(6). 260–7.
8. Kuk JL, Saunders TJ, Davidson LE, et al. Age-related changes in total and regional fat distribution. Ageing Res Rev 2009;8(4):339–48.
9. Zakai NA, McClure LA, Prineas R, et al. Correlates of anemia in American blacks and whites: the REGARDS Renal Ancillary Study. Am J Epidemiol 2009;169(3):355–64.
10. Culleton BF, Manns BJ, Zhang J, et al. Impact of anemia on hospitalization and mortality in older adults. Blood 2006;107(10):3841–6.
11. Zakai NA, French B, Arnold A, et al. Hemoglobin decline and health outcomes in the elderly: the cardiovascular health study. ASH Annual Meeting Abstracts 2008; 112(11):3448.
12. Beutler E, West C. Hematologic differences between African-Americans and whites: the roles of iron deficiency and alpha-thalassemia on hemoglobin levels and mean corpuscular volume. Blood 2005;106(2):740–5.
13. Dill DB, Terman JW, Hall FG. Hemoglobin at high altitude as related to age. Clin Chem 1963;12:710–6.
14. Beall CM, Brittenham GM, Strohl KP, et al. Hemoglobin concentration of high-altitude Tibetans and Bolivian Aymara. Am J Phys Anthropol 1998;106(3): 385–400.
15. Shahidi NT. Androgens and erythropoiesis. N Engl J Med 1973;289(2):72–80.
16. Ferrucci L, Maggio M, Bandinelli S, et al. Low testosterone levels and the risk of anemia in older men and women. Arch Intern Med 2006;166(13):1380–8.
17. Curtis KK, Adam TJ, Chen SC, et al. Anaemia following initiation of androgen deprivation therapy for metastatic prostate cancer: a retrospective chart review. Aging Male 2008;11(4):157–61.
18. Pratt MC, Lewis-Barned NJ, Walker RJ, et al. Effect of angiotensin converting enzyme inhibitors on erythropoietin concentrations in healthy volunteers. Br J Clin Pharmacol 1992;34(4):363–5.

19. Adamson J, Longo D. Anemia and Polycythemia. In: Fauci A, Braunwald E, Kasper D, et al, editors. Harrison's Principles of Internal Medicine. 17th edition. New York: McGraw-Hill; 2008. p. 337. Chapter 57.
20. Hallberg L, Hulthén L, Bengtsson C, et al. Iron balance in menstruating women. Eur J Clin Nutr 1995;49(3):200–7.
21. Bermejo B, Olona M, Serra M, et al. Prevalence of iron deficiency in the female working population in the reproductive age. Rev Clin Esp 1996;196(7):446–50 [in Spanish].
22. Yun EJ, Meng MV, Carroll PR. Evaluation of the patient with hematuria. Med Clin North Am 2004;88(2):329–43.
23. González C, Penado S, Llata L, et al. The clinical spectrum of retroperitoneal hematoma in anticoagulated patients. Medicine (Baltimore) 2003;82(4):257–62.
24. Skikne B, Lynch S, Borek D, et al. Iron and blood donation. Clin Haematol 1984; 13(1):271–87.
25. Salisbury AC, Reid KJ, Alexander KP, et al. Diagnostic blood loss from phlebotomy and hospital-acquired anemia during acute myocardial infarction. Arch Intern Med 2011;171(18):1646–53.
26. Zahner J, Schneider W. Munchausen syndrome in hematology: case reports of three variants and review of the literature. Ann Hematol 1994;68(6):303–6.
27. Lechner K, Jager U. How I treat autoimmune hemolytic anemias in adults. Blood 2010;116(11):1831–8.
28. Mecozzi G, Milano AD, Carlo MD, et al. Intravascular hemolysis in patients with new-generation prosthetic heart valves: a prospective study. J Thorac Cardiovasc Surg 2002;123(3):550–6.
29. Burns ER, Lou Y, Pathak A. Morphologic diagnosis of thrombotic thrombocytopenic purpura. Am J Hematol 2004;75(1):18–21.
30. George JN. How I treat patients with thrombotic thrombocytopenic purpura: 2010. Blood 2010;116(20):4060–9.
31. White NJ. The treatment of malaria. N Engl J Med 1996;335(11):800–6.
32. Hatcher JC, Greenberg PD, Antique J, et al. Severe babesiosis in Long Island: review of 34 cases and their complications. Clin Infect Dis 2001;32(8): 1117–25.
33. Crowther M, Chan YLT, Garbett IK, et al. Evidence-based focused review of the treatment of idiopathic warm immune hemolytic anemia in adults. Blood 2011; 118(15):4036–40.
34. Toxicological profile for lead. Atlanta (GA): US Department of Health & Human Services, Public Health Service, Agency for Toxic Substances and Disease Registry; 2007. Available at: http://www.atsdr.cdc.gov/toxprofiles/tp.asp?id=96&tid=22. Accessed November 01, 2011.
35. Stoltzfus R. Defining iron-deficiency anemia in public health terms: a time for reflection. J Nutr 2001;131(2S-2):565S–7S.
36. Cook JD. Diagnosis and management of iron-deficiency anaemia. Best Pract Res Clin Haematol 2005;18(2):319–32.
37. Das KC, Mukherjee M, Sarkar TK, et al. Erythropoiesis and erythropoietin in hypo- and hyperthyroidism. J Clin Endocrinol Metab 1975;40(2):211–20.
38. Colon-Otero G, Menke D, Hook CC. A practical approach to the differential diagnosis and evaluation of the adult patient with macrocytic anemia. Med Clin North Am 1992;76(3):581–97.
39. Qamar AA, Grace ND. Abnormal hematological indices in cirrhosis. Can J Gastroenterol 2009;23(6):441–5.

40. Humphries JE. Anemia of renal failure. Use of erythropoietin. Med Clin North Am 1992;76(3):711–25.
41. Peralta CA, Shlipak MG, Judd S, et al. Detection of chronic kidney disease with creatinine, cystatin C, and urine albumin-to-creatinine ratio and association with progression to end-stage renal disease and mortality. JAMA 2011;305(15): 1545–52.
42. Astor BC, Muntner P, Levin A, et al. Association of kidney function with anemia: the Third National Health and Nutrition Examination Survey (1988-1994). Arch Intern Med 2002;162(12):1401–8.
43. Ble A, Fink JC, Woodman RC, et al. Renal function, erythropoietin, and anemia of older persons: the InCHIANTI study. Arch Intern Med 2005;165(19): 2222–7.
44. Kosiborod M, Curtis JP, Wang Y, et al. Anemia and outcomes in patients with heart failure: a study from the National Heart Care Project. Arch Intern Med 2005;165(19):2237–44.
45. Fisch P, Handgretinger R, Schaefer HE. Pure red cell aplasia. Br J Haematol 2000;111(4):1010–22.
46. Young NS. Acquired aplastic anemia. Ann Intern Med 2002;136(7):534–46.
47. Bacigalupo A, Passweg J. Diagnosis and treatment of acquired aplastic anemia. Hematol Oncol Clin North Am 2009;23(2):159–70.
48. Makoni SN, Laber DA. Clinical spectrum of myelophthisis in cancer patients. Am J Hematol 2004;76(1):92–3.
49. Volberding PA, Baker KR, Levine AM. Human immunodeficiency virus hematology. Hematology Am Soc Hematol Educ Program 2003;294–313. Available at: http://asheducationbook.hematologylibrary.org/content/2003/1.toc. Accessed February 21, 2012.
50. Browne PM, Sharma OP, Salkin D. Bone marrow sarcoidosis. JAMA 1978; 240(24):2654–5.
51. Licci S. Extensive bone marrow amyloidosis. Ann Hematol 2011.
52. Leguit RJ, van den Tweel JG. The pathology of bone marrow failure. Histopathology 2010;57(5):655–70.
53. Semba RD, Martin BK, Kempen JH, et al. The impact of anemia on energy and physical functioning in individuals with AIDS. Arch Intern Med 2005;165(19): 2229–36.
54. Hourihane DO, Weir DG. Suppression of erythropoiesis by alcohol. Br Med J 1970;1(5688):86–9.
55. Kaferle J, Strzoda CE. Evaluation of macrocytosis. Am Fam Physician 2009;79(3): 203–8.
56. Patel KV. Epidemiology of anemia in older adults. Semin Hematol 2008;45(4): 210–7.
57. Weiss G, Goodnough LT. Anemia of chronic disease. N Engl J Med 2005;352(10): 1011–23.
58. Zarychanski R, Houston DS. Anemia of chronic disease: a harmful disorder or an adaptive, beneficial response? CMAJ 2008;179(4):333–7.
59. Wang CQ, Udupa KB, Lipschitz DA. Interferon-gamma exerts its negative regulatory effect primarily on the earliest stages of murine erythroid progenitor cell development. J Cell Physiol 1995;162(1):134–8.
60. Jelkmann W. Proinflammatory cytokines lowering erythropoietin production. J Interferon Cytokine Res 1998;18(8):555–9.
61. Sears DA. Anemia of chronic disease. Med Clin North Am 1992;76(3):567–79.

62. Kratz A, Ferraro M, Sluss PM, et al. Case records of the Massachusetts General Hospital. Weekly clinicopathological exercises. Laboratory reference values. N Engl J Med 2004;351(15):1548–63.
63. Kueviakoe I, Segbena AY, Jouault H, et al. Hematological reference values for health adults in Togo. ISRN Hematol 2011;2011:1–5.
64. Saathoff E, Schneider P, Kleinfeldt V, et al. Laboratory reference values for healthy adults from southern Tanzania. Trop Med Int Health 2008;13(5):612–25.
65. Tsegaye A, Messele T, Tilahun T, et al. Immunohematological reference ranges for adult Ethiopians. Clin Diagn Lab Immunol 1999;6(3):410–4.

Why Does My Patient Have Thrombocytopenia?

Ellice Y. Wong, MD, Michal G. Rose, MD*

KEYWORDS

- Thrombocytopenia • Immune thrombocytopenic purpura • Platelet destruction
- Drug-induced thrombocytopenia

Thrombocytopenia, usually defined as a platelet count of less than 150,000/μL, is a common reason for a hematology consult in both the inpatient and outpatient setting. In most patients, the cause of the thrombocytopenia can be identified and treated. This article reviews the clinical approach to the patient with thrombocytopenia, the mechanisms that underlie it, and the laboratory tests available to investigate it. A practical approach to the investigation and management of thrombocytopenia in the clinical settings commonly encountered by the hematology consultant is then described.

PERTINENT HISTORY IN THE PATIENT WITH THROMBOCYTOPENIA

Thrombocytopenia classically causes mucosal-type bleeding, and patients should be asked about epistaxis, gingival bleeding, and menorrhagia in women. Other bleeding manifestations may include petechiae, bruising, hematochezia, and melenic stools. A history of bleeding associated with past hemostatic challenges must be obtained, including surgeries, dental procedures, trauma, and child birth. The patient's past and present alcohol use should be documented, and the patient should be asked about a history of liver disease, cirrhosis, jaundice, and risk factors for human immunodeficiency virus (HIV) and hepatitis infections. The medication history must also include questions about over-the-counter medications, herbal supplements, and the consumption of tonic water, which contains quinine, a cause of immune thrombocytopenia. Specific questions about the presence of a family history of bleeding are important, as congenital thrombocytopenia and Von Willebrand disease (VWD) can be diagnosed in young adults (reviewed in Ref.[1]) (**Table 1**).

PHYSICAL EXAMINATION

The physical examination in a patient with thrombocytopenia must establish first and foremost if there is evidence of bleeding associated with the thrombocytopenia, and

Yale University School of Medicine and Cancer Center, Veterans Affairs Connecticut Healthcare System, 950 Campbell Avenue (III-d), West Haven, CT 06516, USA
* Corresponding author.
E-mail address: michal.rose@yale.edu

Hematol Oncol Clin N Am 26 (2012) 231–252
doi:10.1016/j.hoc.2012.02.006
0889-8588/12/$ – see front matter Published by Elsevier Inc.

hemonc.theclinics.com

Table 1 Pertinent items in history taking and physical examination in a patient with thrombocytopenia	
History	Bleeding symptoms
	Epistaxis
	Gingival bleeding
	Menorrhagia
	Petechiae
	Bruising
	Hematochezia
	Melena
	Hemostatic challenges
	Surgeries
	Dental
	Trauma
	Childbirth
	Alcohol use
	Liver disease, hepatitis
	HIV risk factors
	Medication history
	Platelet function inhibitors
	Over-the counter medications/herbal supplements
	Tonic water (quinine)
	Family history of bleeding
Physical examination	General
	Pallor
	Tachycardia
	Skin
	Petechiae
	Purpura
	Splinter hemorrhages
	Ecchymosis
	Mucous membranes
	Blood blisters
	Lymphadenopathy
	Splenomegaly
	Heart murmur

Abbreviation: HIV, human immunodeficiency virus.

whether the bleeding is in proportion to the degree of thrombocytopenia. Patients with platelet counts greater than 50,000/μL do not exhibit spontaneous bleeding unless a coagulopathy is also present, the platelets are dysfunctional, and/or the patient is on a platelet inhibitor. The first sign of spontaneous bleeding from thrombocytopenia is usually petechiae on dependent areas such as the lower legs, or in areas of pressure (eg, at the site of a blood pressure cuff). Other signs of bleeding associated with more severe thrombocytopenia include ecchymosis and blood-filled blisters on the oral mucosa. The physical examination may also establish the underlying condition causing the thrombocytopenia, such as enlarged lymph nodes and spleen in lymphoma, and splenomegaly, telangiectasias, palmar erythema, jaundice, and other stigmata of chronic liver disease in patients with cirrhosis (reviewed in Ref.[1]; see **Table 1**).

ANCILLARY TESTS

A complete blood count with a white blood cell differential is the first step in the workup of thrombocytopenia, and establishes whether the patient has other cytopenias and/or abnormal circulating cells. A review of the peripheral blood smear is essential, as it will rule out pseudothrombocytopenia (see later discussion), and enable the evaluation of all 3 cell lines for morphologic abnormalities. More specialized tests are ordered based on the initial clinical and laboratory evaluations, and are listed in **Table 2**. Platelet-associated antibodies and reticulated platelet counts, although widely available, lack standardization and, in the authors' opinion, are rarely helpful in establishing the cause of the thrombocytopenia.

Table 2
Ancillary tests for the workup of patients with thrombocytopenia

Test	Use
Complete blood count	Establish presence of other cytopenias Establish presence of lymphocytosis
Peripheral blood smear	Rule out pseudothrombocytopenia Morphology of platelets (large platelets suggest ITP, giant platelets suggest congenital disorders) Red blood cell fragments suggest microangiopathic process Toxic granulation suggests sepsis Abnormal lymphocytes suggest viral infection or lymphoproliferative disorder Neutrophil inclusions (Döhle bodies) suggest congenital thrombocytopenias Malaria, ehrlichiosis, and babesiosis can be diagnosed by demonstrating intracellular organisms on peripheral blood/buffy coat
PT and PTT Fibrinogen, D-dimer	Disseminated intravascular coagulation Evidence for Von Willebrand disease
Reticulated platelet count and antiplatelet antibodies	Lack standardization, usually not useful
Heparin-associated antiplatelet factor 4 and serotonin release assay	Heparin-induced thrombocytopenia
HIV and hepatitis C serology	Common causes for ITP
ANA, anti–double-stranded DNA	Systemic lupus erythematosus
Anticardiolipin antibody, lupus anticoagulant, anti-β2 glycoprotein 1	Antiphospholipid antibody syndrome
Drug-associated increase in antiplatelet IgG	Drug-induced ITP
Flow cytometry of peripheral blood	Lymphoproliferative disorders
Serum protein electrophoresis	Myeloma, lymphoma
Bone marrow aspirate and biopsy	Myelophthisic processes Hematologic malignancies Storage disease (eg, Gaucher disease)
Ultrasonogram of liver and spleen	Establish spleen size when not palpable Evaluate liver for cirrhosis
Liver/spleen scan	Establish spleen size Determine presence of accessory spleen Colloid shift indicates portal hypertension

Abbreviations: ANA, antineutrophil antibody; HIV, human immunodeficiency virus; IgG, immunoglobulin G; ITP, immune thrombocytopenic purpura; PT, prothrombin time; PTT, partial thromboplastin time.

MECHANISMS OF THROMBOCYTOPENIA

Platelets are produced from proplatelets, which are long, branching processes that extend from the cytoplasm of mature megakaryocytes. Their production is regulated by cytokines, especially thrombopoietin (TPO), and by close interactions with the bone marrow stroma. Approximately 4 to 7 days are required for the megakaryocyte progenitor cell to mature, at which point it produces 1000 to 3000 platelets before its residual nuclear material is engulfed by macrophages. Platelets normally circulate for approximately 10 days, although this life span is decreased to 5 to 7 days in patients with thrombocytopenia.[2,3] Disruption of any part of this process, when severe enough, can lead to thrombocytopenia.

When evaluating a patient with thrombocytopenia, the first step is to rule out pseudothrombocytopenia, a laboratory artifact with no clinical significance. True thrombocytopenia can be secondary to increased destruction of platelets, decreased production, sequestration (usually in the spleen), and hemodilution (**Table 3**). Although in most clinical situations a predominant mechanism can be identified, in many patients more than one pathway contributes to the thrombocytopenia.

Table 3
Mechanisms of thrombocytopenia

Mechanism	Examples

Increased destruction (immune mediated)	Primary ITP
	Secondary ITP
	   Infections (HIV, hepatitis C, *Helicobacter pylori*)
	   Lymphoproliferative disorders
	   Medications (eg, quinine, quinidine, gold)
	Medications: nonclassic ITP (eg, heparin, glycoprotein IIb/IIIa inhibitors)
	Posttransfusion thrombocytopenia

Increased destruction (non–immune mediated)	DIC Thrombotic microangiopathies (TTP, HUS, disseminated cancer, eclampsia, HELLP syndrome) Cardiopulmonary bypass, intra-aortic balloon pump, ventricular assist devices Abnormal vascular surfaces (aneurysms, heart valves, Merritt-Kasabach syndrome) Hemophagocytosis
Decreased production	Congenital B_{12} and folate deficiency Medications (valproic acid, chemotherapy) Radiation Toxins (alcohol) Infections (parvovirus, CMV, erlichiosis) Liver disease (TPO deficiency) Primary marrow disorders (myelodysplasia, myelofibrosis, acute and chronic leukemias, lymphoproliferative disorders) Marrow replaced by solid tumors Granulomatous diseases of the marrow
Sequestration	Splenomegaly
Dilutional	Massive transfusion

Abbreviations: CMV, cytomegalovirus; DIC, disseminated intravascular coagulation; HIV, human immunodeficiency virus; HELLP, hemolysis, elevated liver enzymes, low platelets; HUS, hemolytic uremic syndrome; ITP, immune thrombocytopenic purpura; TTP, thrombotic thrombocytopenic purpura; TPO, thrombopoietin.

Pseudothrombocytopenia

Pseudothrombocytopenia, also called spurious thrombocytopenia, is an ex vivo phenomenon occurring in 0.09% to 0.29% of the population, in which platelets clump when blood is anticoagulated with a calcium chelator such as ethylenediaminetetraacetic acid (EDTA). Automated counters do not correctly identify the clumps as platelets, and as a result the platelet count is reported as low. Furthermore, the platelet clumps are sometimes misrecognized as neutrophils, causing pseudoleukocytosis. Review of a peripheral blood smear (**Fig. 1**) demonstrates the clumps, and the automated platelet count is usually higher when blood is collected into an alternative anticoagulant such as citrate or heparin. Pseudothrombocytopenia is caused by circulating antiplatelet antibodies against platelet membrane glycoproteins that are modified by the exposure to anticoagulants.[4–6] Platelet satellitism is a less common form of pseudothrombocytopenia in which EDTA causes antibodies against glycoprotein (GP) IIb/IIIa to attach platelets to neutrophils and monocytes via the leukocyte Fcγ receptor III. The peripheral blood smear (**Fig. 2**) demonstrates platelets forming rosettes around the neutrophils and/or monocytes.[7]

There are no known pathologic effects of the presence of the antiplatelet antibodies associated with pseudothrombocytopenia, and it is important to establish and document the diagnosis so that patients are not subjected to unnecessary testing and treatment.

Thrombocytopenia from Increased Platelet Destruction

The normal platelet life span of 7 to 10 days can be shortened by both immune-mediated and non–immune-mediated processes, and, when the destructive process overwhelms the bone marrow's ability to increase platelet production, the result will be thrombocytopenia.

Immune Destruction of Platelets

In patients with immune-mediated thrombocytopenia, antibodies attach to platelets and promote their destruction by the reticuloendothelial system. These antibodies can be either autoantibodies or alloantibodies. The most common cause of autoimmune platelet destruction is immune thrombocytopenic purpura (ITP), which is usually caused by antibodies of the immunoglobulin G subtype directed against platelet membrane glycoproteins.[8] In heparin-induced immune platelet destruction, autoantibodies target a heparin-platelet factor 4 complex and cause thrombocytopenia by binding to the membrane Fc receptor and activating the platelets (see **Table 3**).

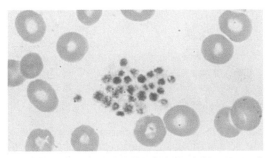

Fig. 1. Peripheral blood smear showing platelet clumping. (*Courtesy of* Dr Henry M. Rinder, Yale School of Medicine.)

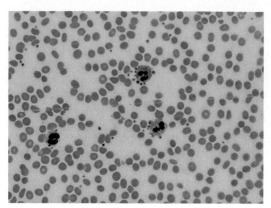

Fig. 2. Peripheral blood smear showing platelet satellitism. (*Courtesy of* Dr Richard Torres, VA Connecticut and Yale School of Medicine.)

Alloimmune destruction is a rare but severe cause of thrombocytopenia, in which platelets are destroyed by alloantibodies usually targeting the platelet antigen HPA-1a (PlA1) that have been transmitted through a transfusion (see discussion of post-transfusion purpura).

Nonimmune Destruction of Platelets

Nonimmune destruction of platelets occurs in patients with thrombotic microangiopathies such as thrombotic thrombocytopenic purpura, hemolytic uremic syndrome, and the elevated liver enzymes, low-platelet (HELLP) syndrome of pregnancy. In these patients thrombocytopenia results from the shearing of platelets in a damaged microvasculature filled with thrombi. Microangiopathic hemolytic anemia is also present, and coagulation parameters are normal or near normal (see **Table 3**).

Disseminated intravascular coagulation (DIC) is a common cause of thrombocytopenia in acutely ill patients, and here the platelet destruction is secondary to their activation by thrombin and proinflammatory cytokines (see **Table 3**). Patients who have undergone cardiopulmonary bypass, insertion of an intra-aortic balloon pump, or insertion of a ventricular assist device develop thrombocytopenia as a result of the activation and destruction of platelets exposed to the artificial surfaces (see later discussion). Patients with a severely abnormal endovascular surface such as a damaged, malfunctioning heart valve, aortic aneurysm, or a vascular malformation may also develop thrombocytopenia secondary to activation of platelets on the abnormal surface.

Decreased Production of Platelets

Multiple processes affecting megakaryocyte maturation and differentiation, either directly or through a more global effect on hematopoiesis, may result in thrombocytopenia, often accompanied by anemia and/or leukopenia (see **Table 3**).

Sequestration of Platelets

Hypersplenism is defined as anemia, leukopenia, and/or thrombocytopenia that are caused by abnormal splenic-mediated destruction often associated with splenomegaly. Normally, approximately 30% of the platelet mass resides in the spleen. This percentage increases with increased spleen size, and most patients with splenomegaly will have thrombocytopenia. When the cause of the thrombocytopenia is hypersplenism, the platelet count will rarely drop below 20,000/μL, and the low platelet count is not usually associated with bleeding unless other hemostatic abnormalities are present (see also **Table 1**).[9,10] Thrombocytopenia is usually the first manifestation of hypersplenism in patients with liver disease, and the hematologist sometimes establishes the diagnosis of otherwise clinically occult cirrhosis during the workup of a low platelet count.[11]

Dilutional Thrombocytopenia

Thrombocytopenia develops in patients receiving infusions of large amounts of non–platelet-containing fluids. A rapid transfusion of 10 to 12 units of packed red blood cells will result in a platelet drop of approximately 50%.[12,13]

THROMBOCYTOPENIA IN THE INTERNAL MEDICINE PATIENT

This section focuses on the different causes of thrombocytopenia that the clinician may encounter in either the outpatient or inpatient medical setting.

Nutritional Deficiencies

Vitamin B_{12} and folate deficiency cause megaloblastosis and pancytopenia through inhibition of purine synthesis. Thrombocytopenia may be the predominant cytopenia, and can be severe (reviewed in Ref.[14]). Because these are common, readily treatable conditions, all patients with thrombocytopenia should have documentation of normal levels of vitamin B_{12} and folic acid as part of their workup. Repletion of the deficient vitamin will rapidly correct the thrombocytopenia, and it is the authors' practice to offer repletion to all patients with low or borderline levels. Folate deficiency is commonly associated with ethanol abuse, and the etiology of thrombocytopenia may be multifactorial in these patients (see later discussion).

Iron Deficiency

Iron deficiency is usually associated with thrombocytosis. In rare cases, however, thrombocytopenia may be present,[15] and in these patients both increased and decreased numbers of megakaryocytes in the bone marrow have been reported. Although the exact mechanism remains unclear, the observation of increased megakaryocytes in the marrow accompanied by a rapid increase in platelets after iron administration suggests the involvement of iron in late-stage thrombopoiesis.[16]

Alcohol Abuse and Thrombocytopenia

Thrombocytopenia is the most common hematologic abnormality in patients who abuse alcohol.[17] Alcohol ingestion may lead to acute thrombocytopenia, and a common scenario is a falling platelet count in a patient admitted after binge drinking. With alcohol cessation and adequate folate and vitamin B_{12} repletion, recovery of platelet counts occurs within 1 to 2 weeks and may even be associated with a rebound thrombocytosis.

Heavy alcohol consumption has direct toxic effects on the bone marrow and causes a reversible suppression of platelet production.[18] Peripheral blood smear examination reveals thrombocytopenia, and may also show macrocytosis and stomatocytes. Marrow examination usually reveals a normal megakaryocyte count, but their number can also be significantly reduced.[19] Because alcohol inhibits heme biosynthesis, ringed sideroblasts are common.[18,20]

Liver Disease and Thrombocytopenia

Thrombocytopenia in patients with liver disease is multifactorial. Chronic thrombocytopenia in a patient with liver cirrhosis is usually a result of portal hypertension and splenomegaly, leading to splenic sequestration. Splenomegaly can be associated with any combination of cytopenia(s), including isolated thrombocytopenia.[20] There may also be direct marrow-suppressive effects from the cause of the liver damage, whether from alcoholism or viral or immune hepatitis. Hepatitis C and autoimmune hepatitis are associated with immune-mediated thrombocytopenia.[21,22] Chronic liver disease can also lead to deficiency of thrombopoietin, the hematopoietic growth factor responsible for platelet production.[23] In addition, DIC leading to platelet consumption is seen in severe liver disease.[24] Indeed, the combined hematologic effects of ongoing alcohol abuse in patients with cirrhosis who have pancytopenia and coagulopathy are particularly severe, with bleeding complications often necessitating significant transfusion support.

The Congenital Thrombocytopenias

Although congenital thrombocytopenias are rare, this is an essential diagnosis to establish, because patients are often misdiagnosed as having ITP, and subjected to unnecessary and potentially harmful treatments.[25] Some important considerations for diagnosing congenital thrombocytopenias are the age of onset and chronicity of symptoms.[26] Patients with inherited conditions associated with severe thrombocytopenia are generally recognized shortly after birth. Patients with milder forms of thrombocytopenia may present later in life, particularly during times of hemostatic challenge (eg, onset of menses, childbirth, trauma, surgery). Many other patients with mild to moderate thrombocytopenia, however, may be clinically asymptomatic and present only after routine blood tests.

If congenital thrombocytopenia is suspected, further evaluation is guided by platelet size. When a male patient presents with small platelets, an X-linked thrombocytopenia such as Wiskott-Aldrich syndrome should be considered. For patients presenting with normal-sized platelets, the differential includes neonatal conditions such as congenital amegakaryocytic thrombocytopenia, thrombocytopenia with absent radii, and a familial platelet disorder with predisposition to acute myeloid leukemia. Large platelets are seen in several inherited disorders of platelets including VWD 2B, MYH9-related diseases such as the May-Hegglin anomaly, Bernard-Soulier syndrome, and the gray platelet syndrome.

Von Willebrand Disease 2B

VWD 2B, also known as platelet-type VWD, deserves special mention as patients may present for the first time in adulthood. This rare autosomal dominant disorder is characterized by the presence of ultralarge multimers of Von Willebrand factor (VWF), which bind preferentially to platelets, leading to clumping and mild, fluctuating thrombocytopenia. VWD 2B, like other forms of VWD, presents clinically with excessive mucous membrane, menstrual, and/or postpartum hemorrhage.

Review of a peripheral blood smear may show pseudothrombocytopenia (see earlier discussion), and the platelet size is normal or large. Laboratory tests show a disproportionate reduction in VWF activity assays relative to VWF antigen, and absence of high molecular weight multimers. Desmopressin should be avoided, as it may lead to worsening thrombocytopenia caused by the increase in VWF multimers and increased platelet agglutination and clearance.

MYH9-related diseases

The MYH9-related diseases are associated with macrothrombocytopenia and involve myosin IIA mutations. The May-Hegglin anomaly is the most common form. The peripheral smear shows giant platelets and Döhle-like bodies in neutrophils (**Fig. 3**). Associated features include cataracts, hearing loss, and renal failure. Automated counters often underestimate the true platelet count because of limitations from preset size restrictions. Although the platelet count is variable and sometimes less than 20,000/μL, platelet function is normal and patients are usually asymptomatic.

Bernard-Soulier syndrome

Bernard-Soulier syndrome, caused by an absent GP Ib-V-IX complex on the platelet surface, leads to bleeding out of proportion to the platelet count. Similar to the MYH9-related diseases, the peripheral smear demonstrates giant platelets. In homozygous patients the diagnosis is made by platelet aggregation studies showing lack of aggregation to ristocetin and a negative VWD workup. Flow cytometry to quantify platelet glycoproteins is particularly helpful in identifying heterozygote patients.

DRUG-INDUCED THROMBOCYTOPENIA

Drug-induced thrombocytopenia (DITP) is an important entity to consider in all patients presenting with thrombocytopenia, and included in this discussion is thrombocytopenia caused by over-the-counter supplements and food items. The onset may be sudden and severe (platelet count nadirs are often <20,000/μL), leading to significant morbidity and even mortality[27,28] if the offending agent is not promptly removed. DITP can be misdiagnosed as idiopathic ITP, and the underlying etiology may be missed if patients are not specifically asked about foods, beverages, and/or herbal supplements.

DITP can be caused by nonimmune (eg, valproic acid or chemotherapy resulting in myelosuppression) or, more commonly, immune-mediated processes.[28,29] The immunologic mechanisms include autoantibody production (eg, gold [Ridaura; Solganal, others]), drug glycoprotein complex(es) (eg, quinine [Quinamm; Quindan, others]), ligand-induced binding (eg, eptifibatide [Integrilin]), and hapten-dependent binding (eg, penicillin) (reviewed in Ref.[30]). The mechanism for heparin-induced thrombocytopenia (HIT) is unique, as antibodies against platelet factor 4–heparin complexes cause platelet activation, thrombocytopenia, and thrombosis, rather than bleeding (see **Table 3**).

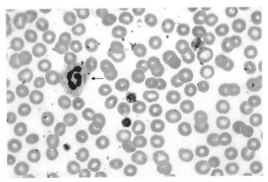

Fig. 3. Peripheral blood smear in a patient with the May-Hegglin anomaly. Giant platelets are present along with a Döhle body in a granulocyte (*arrow*). (*Courtesy of* Dr Henry M. Rinder, Yale School of Medicine.)

Drug-dependent antiplatelet antibodies usually occur within 1 to 2 weeks of exposure to the offending drug, but in some instances may develop after chronic, intermittent exposure (reviewed in Refs.[27,28]). On rare occasions acute immune-mediated thrombocytopenia may develop within several hours of exposure, as in the case of GP IIb/IIIa inhibitors used in cardiac procedures (see the section on thrombocytopenia in the cardiac care unit).[31] Regardless of the specific mechanism, DITP occurs only in the presence of the offending agent, and removal of the drug should lead to improvement within 1 to 2 days, with resolution of the platelet count within 1 to 2 weeks. Indefinite avoidance of the offending agent is recommended. If ITP was initially suspected and corticosteroids were initiated, therapy may be stopped once the offending agent has been removed and the platelet count normalizes.

DITP should be suspected when a patient presents with severe thrombocytopenia of unclear etiology, particularly in patients with repeated episodes and prompt resolution. In a cohort of 343 patients diagnosed as ITP, 8% were subsequently diagnosed with DITP, with quinine (including tonic water) being the most common cause.[32] The 2 most common causes of thrombocytopenia in one case-controlled study were trimethoprim/sulfamethoxazole (Bactrim; Septra) and quinine, in 38 and 26 cases/10^6 users/week, respectively.[33]

A systematic review of all published reports of DITP as of October 2010 is available online at www.ouhsc.edu/platelets. A causal relationship between a drug and thrombocytopenia is defined in that database if there is a single report with definite evidence or at least 2 reports with probable evidence.[34] A modified list of the most common drugs causing thrombocytopenia is also provided in **Table 4**. There is currently no published comprehensive list of foods or herbal remedies associated with thrombocytopenia, but convincing case reports suggest that tahini (pulped sesame seeds),[35] *Lupinus termis* beans,[36] *Jui* Chinese herbal tea,[37] cow's milk,[38] and cranberry juice[39] can cause thrombocytopenia.

The diagnosis of DITP is usually made clinically by identifying potential offending agents and withholding them to see whether thrombocytopenia resolves. The Blood Center of Wisconsin offers drug-dependent platelet-reactive antibody testing (http://www.bcw.edu/bcw.) If a drug is confirmed as the cause of a patient's thrombocytopenia, the authors recommend the clinician alert the Food and Drug Administration Adverse Event Reporting System via www.fda.gov/medwatch/. A case report should be published if available literature is lacking.

Primary Immune Thrombocytopenia

ITP is a relatively common clinical entity encountered in hematology practice. ITP is characterized by autoimmune-mediated platelet destruction and suppression of megakaryocyte platelet production, leading to an increased risk of bleeding.[40,41] The exact etiology of autoantibody production leading to ITP remains unclear.

ITP is a diagnosis of exclusion. The definition of primary ITP by the International Working Group is a platelet count less than 100,000/μL without other reasons to explain the thrombocytopenia.[42] The goal of the history taking and physical examination in these patients is to identify evidence of bleeding and to exclude other causes of thrombocytopenia. Laboratory investigation should include a complete blood count and peripheral blood smear review. Abnormalities in the peripheral smear other than isolated thrombocytopenia should lead to further investigation, for example, schistocytes in thrombotic microangiopathies, significantly increased giant or small platelets suggesting an inherited thrombocytopenia, and pseudothrombocytopenia resulting from EDTA-dependent platelet agglutination. All patients should be offered HIV and hepatitis C serologic testing, and *Helicobacter pylori* testing can be considered (see

Table 4
Drugs commonly associated with thrombocytopenia

Drug	Number of Reports (Definite or Probable)	Antibody Testing
Quinidine (Quinaglute; Cardioquin, others)	58	Yes
Quinine (Quinamm; Quindan, others)	24	Yes
Trimethoprim/sulfamethoxazole (Bactrim; Septra)	15	Yes
Abciximab (ReoPro)	13	Yes
Gold (Ridaura; Solganal, others)	11	Yes
Rifampin (Rifadin; Rimactane)	10	Yes
Carbamazepine (Tegretol)	10	Yes
Eptifibatide (Integrilin)	9	Yes
Tirofiban (Aggrestat)	8	Yes
Vancomycin (Vancoled)	7	Yes
Acetaminophen (Tylenol; Panadol, others)	7	Yes
Danazol (Danocrine)	7	No
Interferon-α (Roferon-A; Intron A)	7	No
Methyldopa (Aldomet)	6	Yes
Cimetidine (Tagamet)	6	Yes
Nalidixic acid (NegGram)	6	No
Efalizumab (Raptiva)	6	No
Diclofenac (Cataflam; Voltaren)	5	Yes
Hydrochlorthiazide (Aquazide-H; Esidrex, others)	5	Yes
Ranitidine (Zantac)	5	Yes
Chlorpropamide (Diabinese)	5	Yes

Each listed drug is associated with 5 or more published reports (individual and/or group data) with definite or probable evidence for drug-induced thrombocytopenia. The reference database is from www.ouhsc.edu/platelets. Specific antibody testing is available from the Blood Center of Wisconsin.

later discussion). A routine bone marrow evaluation is not necessary unless the initial workup points to a marrow disorder (see also the American Society of Hematology 2011 evidence-based practice guidelines for immune thrombocytopenia).[43]

Treatment of ITP is generally recommended when the platelet count falls below 30,000/μL. The standard first-line therapy is corticosteroids, and immunoglobulins are used when a more rapid response is needed or when steroids are contraindicated. Splenectomy, rituximab (Rituxan),[44] and the thrombopoietin receptor agonists romiplostim (Nplate)[45] and eltrombopag (Promacta)[46,47] are used in refractory or relapsing patients.

Secondary Immune Thrombocytopenic Purpura (ITP)

Systemic lupus erythematosus

Secondary immune-mediated thrombocytopenia may occur in many rheumatologic conditions, but is by far the most common in systemic lupus erythematosus (SLE). Most patients with SLE will exhibit a chronic thrombocytopenia, and acute, severe thrombocytopenia in the setting of a multiorgan lupus flare[48] is also common. A bleeding tendency out of proportion to the thrombocytopenia because of platelet dysfunction has been described in these patients.[49]

Treatment of the thrombocytopenia associated with SLE is analogous to that of ITP,[49] and corticosteroids remain the standard first-line therapy. An area of ongoing controversy is whether splenectomy is effective for refractory patients.[50]

Antiphospholipid antibody syndrome

Thrombocytopenia is seen in up to 50% of patients with antiphospholipid antibody syndrome, and tends to be mild and sporadic.[51,52] Similar to ITP, the mechanism is thought to be due, at least in part, to platelet glycoprotein-reactive autoantibodies.[53] However, in contrast to ITP, these patients are at increased risk for thrombosis, and therapy for the thrombocytopenia is usually not necessary.

Thrombocytopenia and HIV infection

Thrombocytopenia is the first sign of HIV infection in 10% of patients, is found in about 40% of patients overall, and correlates with a shorter survival.[54,55] Risk factors for thrombocytopenia include uncontrolled HIV replication, concurrent hepatitis C virus (HCV) infection, and cirrhosis.[56]

The most common cause of thrombocytopenia in HIV-infected patients is immune destruction through molecular mimicry between glycoproteins on the platelet surface and the outer membrane of the HIV. The antibody-coated platelets are then destroyed by splenic macrophages and by complement-mediated mechanisms. HIV also causes decreased platelet production by direct infection of megakaryocytes, as these cells can bind and internalize the virus through their CD4 receptor.[57,58] Other causes of thrombocytopenia in an HIV-infected patient include bone marrow infiltration by malignancy, opportunistic infections, side effects of drugs (eg, trimethoprim/sulfamethoxazole), and HIV-related thrombocytic microangiopathy. For patients found to have ITP secondary to HIV, initial management is antiviral therapy, which results in improvement of the thrombocytopenia in more than 75% of patients.[59]

Hepatitis C and Immune Thrombocytopenic Purpura (ITP)

Thrombocytopenia is reported in as many as 45% of patients with HCV infection, and it usually improves when the infection responds to interferon and ribavirin.[59] However, because interferon is a common cause of thrombocytopenia, it is relatively contraindicated in patients with platelet counts of less than 75,000/μL. An acute drop in platelet count in a patient with HCV usually indicates ITP, and should be treated with steroids and/or high-dose immunoglobulins.[60,61] A trial investigating the use of the TPO mimetic eltrombopag in HCV-associated thrombocytopenia was terminated early, however, because of increased rates of portal venous thrombosis.

Helicobacter pylori and Immune Thrombocytopenic Purpura (ITP)

H pylori has been reported to be associated with ITP, and the detection of an infection by urea breath test, stool antigen test, or endoscopic biopsy should prompt treatment for eradication when associated with otherwise unexplained thrombocytopenia.[43,62] However, the data showing improvement in platelet count after H pylori eradication have been variable. One meta-analysis showed an overall response rate (platelet count at least 30,000/μL and doubling of baseline) in 50% of patients after H pylori treatment.[62]

POSTTRANSFUSION PURPURA

Posttransfusion purpura (PTP) is a rare thrombocytopenia that should be suspected if a patient presents with an acute drop in platelet count 1 to 14 days after a transfusion. The classic presentation is an older, multiparous woman who presents with bleeding and severe thrombocytopenia 1 week after receiving a blood product containing platelets.[63] Rarely, thrombocytopenia may develop within hours of exposure.[63,64] The diagnosis is made by the demonstration of platelet-specific alloantibodies targeting antigens not found on the patient's platelets. Despite the fact that the patient's platelets do not display the targeted antigen, they are destroyed as "innocent bystanders" by a poorly understood mechanism, resulting in severe thrombocytopenia that is relatively refractory to platelet transfusions.[65] Most alloantibodies are HPA-1a, with HPA-1b, HPA-5/5b, and other platelet antigens much less common.[63]

Treatment with high-dose immunoglobulins should begin as soon as PTP is suspected, and response within 2 to 3 days occurs in more than 90% of patients.[63,65–67] If left untreated, patients may have a protracted course with severe bleeding lasting a mean of 10 days, and mortality of up to 10%.[63]

THROMBOCYTOPENIA ASSOCIATED WITH INFECTIONS

Thrombocytopenia is commonly associated with both acute and chronic infections, and can be caused by multiple mechanisms (**Table 5**).[71] Unexplained thrombocytopenia in a patient with fever and other infectious symptoms should prompt a search for pathogens with a review of the peripheral blood smear for intracellular organisms, blood and other cultures, and appropriate serologic and molecular tests.

THROMBOCYTOPENIA IN THE INTENSIVE CARE UNIT

Thrombocytopenia is very common in patients admitted to the intensive care unit (ICU).[72–75] In a review of 24 studies that included 6894 patients from medical, surgical, mixed, and trauma ICUs, thrombocytopenia on admission was found in 8% to 68% of patients, and thrombocytopenia developed during the ICU stay in 13% to 44% of patients.[72] Many of the studies demonstrated that high illness severity, sepsis, and organ dysfunction correlated with thrombocytopenia. Most studies have found that thrombocytopenia in the ICU is associated with an increased risk of death.[72,74,75]

The main causes of thrombocytopenia in the ICU include sepsis and DIC, dilution secondary to massive fluid and/or transfusion resuscitation, and/or medications (**Table 6**).

Heparin-Induced Thrombocytopenia in the ICU

HIT deserves special mention, as most ICU patients are exposed to heparin, and those who develop HIT suffer high rates of morbidity and mortality.[76,77] However, the clinical diagnosis of HIT in the ICU is difficult to make, as thrombocytopenia and thrombosis are common in these patients and most have alternative explanations for their thrombocytopenia. There are limited data on the utility of the 4 Ts scoring system, a clinical tool that classifies patients into low, moderate, and high pretest probability for HIT (see **Table 3**), in critically ill patients.[78,79] Furthermore, whereas in all comers approximately 50% of patients with a positive platelet factor 4–dependent enzyme-linked immunosorbent assay will have a positive serotonin release assay and likely HIT, in the ICU setting that percentage is only 10% to 20%.[80]

Sakr and colleagues[76] reviewed records of 13,948 patients admitted to a surgical ICU in a German hospital, and found that the incidence of HIT was only 0.63%. Thus, the consultant should bear in mind that HIT explains fewer than 1% of cases of thrombocytopenia in the ICU (reviewed in Ref.[81]), and overdiagnosis of HIT results in the unnecessary use of more expensive anticoagulants, which have an increased bleeding risk, especially in critically ill patients.[82,83]

Table 5
Infectious causes of thrombocytopenia

Pathogen Group	Specific Organism and Proposed Mechanisms
All	DIC SIRS Marrow suppression Medication effect Hemophagocytosis Splenomegaly

Viruses	HIV
	    ITP
	    Medications (SMZ/TMP)
	    Opportunistic infections (CMV, MAI)
	    Marrow suppression (megakaryocyte infection)
	    Thrombotic microangiopathies
	Acute EBV
	    Hemophagocytosis
	    Splenomegaly
	Hepatitis C
	    ITP
	    Splenomegaly/portal hypertension
	    Medications (interferon)
	CMV
	    Marrow suppression
	    Medications (ganciclovir)
	Parvovirus B19
	    Marrow suppression

Bacteria	*H pylori*
	    ITP
	E coli (Shiga toxin producing)
	    HUS

Parasites	*Babesia* species[68]
	    DIC?
	Ehrlichia species[69]
	    DIC
	    Hemophagocytosis
	    Marrow granulomas
	Malaria[70]
	    DIC
	    Hypersplenism

Abbreviations: CMV, cytomegalovirus; DIC, disseminated intravascular coagulation; EBV, Epstein-Barr virus; HIV, human immunodeficiency virus; HUS, hemolytic uremic syndrome; ITP, immune thrombocytopenic purpura; MAI, mycobacterium avium intracellulare; SIRS, systemic inflammatory response syndrome; SMZ/TMP, sulfamethoxazole/trimethoprim.

Thrombocytopenia in the Cardiac Care Unit

Rapid development of severe thrombocytopenia after treatment with anti-GP IIb/IIIa inhibitors such as abciximab, eptifibatide, and tirofiban occurs in 0.4% to 2% of patients, with the highest incident reported with abciximab.[84] Thrombocytopenia is usually severe, with platelet counts dropping to around 5000 to 10,000/μL, and is often associated with bleeding because most patients are also on other antiplatelet agents. The pathogenesis is thought to be immune mediated, and the incidence is higher among patients previously exposed to GP IIb/IIIa inhibitors. The incidence of

Table 6	
Thrombocytopenia in the intensive care unit (ICU)	
Unit	**Etiology**
All ICUs	Dilution (massive fluid or blood resuscitation)
	Sepsis
	Heparin
	Other medications
Surgical ICU	Post–cardiopulmonary bypass
	Ventricular assist devices
	Heparin
Cardiac ICU	Glycoprotein IIb/IIIa inhibitors
	Intra-aortic balloon pump
	Heparin
	Thrombotic microangiopathy (clopidogrel)

pseudothrombocytopenia with these drugs is also high, so the diagnosis of thrombocytopenia must be confirmed with smear review. Bleeding patients should receive urgent platelet transfusions. Delayed-onset thrombocytopenia (48 hours to 2 weeks after administration) has also been reported with GP IIb/IIIa inhibitors.

Rapid-onset HIT must also be considered in these patients if they have been exposed recently to heparin.[85] The intra-aortic balloon pump causes thrombocytopenia in approximately 50% of patients, with a nadir 3 days after placement. The thrombocytopenia is usually in the range of 50% from baseline, and a drop below this level should prompt further workup for alternative causes.[84]

Thrombocytopenia and cardiopulmonary bypass

Both thrombocytopenia and significant prolongation of the bleeding time occur in all patients undergoing cardiopulmonary bypass, with severities that are in proportion to the period of time that the patient is exposed to the extracorporeal oxygenator. The causes of the platelet abnormalities are dilution by the priming solution, and the activation and destruction of platelets on the membrane. The abnormal platelet function normalizes within an hour after the exposure to the membrane ends. The platelet count drops by approximately 50% and usually recovers by the fourth postoperative day.[86]

One of the more challenging consults in the surgical ICU is the post–bypass surgery patient with prolonged thrombocytopenia, because the vast majority of these patients are exposed to heparin and the available assays for HIT are unreliable in this setting. In the first 10 days after cardiac surgery, 25% to 70% of patients develop a positive immunoassay for antiplatelet factor 4–heparin antibodies, and 4% to 20% have an abnormal serotonin release assay.[87] Pouplard and colleagues[88] described 2 patterns of thrombocytopenia in these patients: profile 1, in which the platelet count recovers and then drops again between postoperative days 5 and 10; and profile 2, in which thrombocytopenia does not resolve after surgery and persists beyond day 5. In a prospective study of 581 cardiac surgery patients, HIT was found only in 3 (0.5%), but all 3 patients had a profile-1 thrombocytopenia.[89]

Thrombocytopenia is almost universal in patients after ventricular assist device implantation, and is caused by the preceding cardiopulmonary bypass use, infections, and exposure to heparin. The incidence of clinical HIT is estimated at 10% with a high risk of cerebrovascular infarcts, leading some experts to recommend alternative anticoagulation in these patients.[90]

THROMBOCYTOPENIA IN THE PATIENT WITH A HEMATOLOGIC MALIGNANCY

ITP is often associated with lymphoproliferative disorders, with the highest incidence seen in chronic lymphocytic leukemia[91] (incidence 2%–5%). Patients with other types of lymphoma have a 0.2% to 1% incidence of ITP.[92,93] In all these patients the differential diagnosis must include marrow infiltration, splenomegaly, and/or chemotherapy and biological therapy. In approximately 50% of patients with ITP associated with non-Hodgkin lymphoma, the diagnosis of ITP precedes the lymphoma diagnosis, whereas ITP associated with Hodgkin lymphoma usually occurs after the lymphoma has been diagnosed. ITP associated with active lymphoproliferative disease usually responds to antilymphoma therapy. Patients with large granular lymphocyte disorders often have mild thrombocytopenia, but in approximately 1% of patients platelets are severely reduced secondary to suppression of megakaryocytes by the malignant T cells.[92]

Virtually all patients with acute leukemia have thrombocytopenia at diagnosis. Patients with promyelocytic leukemia usually present dramatically with bleeding, thrombocytopenia, and coagulopathy, which reverse rapidly with all-*trans* retinoic acid and/or arsenic trioxide.

THROMBOCYTOPENIA IN THE SOLID TUMOR PATIENT

In most patients with solid tumors, thrombocytopenia can be explained by chemotherapy and/or radiation therapy. The incidence of chemotherapy-induced thrombocytopenia (platelet count <100,000/μL) is 21.8%, with the highest frequency seen in patients receiving carboplatin alone or in combination.[94] Drug-induced immune-mediated thrombocytopenia is also associated with chemotherapy agents, and has been described most commonly with oxaliplatin, fludarabine, and rituximab.[95,96]

In patients with advanced bone marrow metastasis, thrombocytopenia as part of the pancytopenia of a myelophthisic process can be readily diagnosed by demonstrating a leukoerythroblastic picture in the peripheral blood. However, less common causes of thrombocytopenia should not be overlooked. Patients may have thrombocytopenia as part of a consumptive coagulopathy (especially common in patients with widespread adenocarcinoma of the prostate, stomach, lung, and breast), which may also be associated with venous or arterial thrombosis and a Trousseau syndrome. In these patients low fibrinogen and other markers of DIC will be present, and they may respond to heparin therapy.

Thrombotic microangiopathy (TMA) mimicking thrombotic thrombocytopenic purpura or hemolytic uremic syndrome is an uncommon but well described complication of solid tumors, especially gastric and breast cancer, and other mucin-producing adenocarcinomas. Patients usually have widely disseminated cancer and do not respond to plasmapheresis.[97] Chemotherapy agents, mainly mitomycin (incidence 2%–15%) and gemcitabine (incidence 0.25%–0.4%), cause TMA likely through direct endothelial cell damage.[98] Data are now emerging that some of the newer, targeted antineoplastic agents are also associated with TMA, especially bevacizumab and sunitinib, drugs that target the vascular endothelial growth factor pathway.[99]

ITP is rare and potentially treatable complication of solid tumors, and should be suspected when the platelet count is lower than what would be expected by the antineoplastic therapy or the myelophthisic processes alone. In these patients a high index of suspicion is required and, as in other ITP patients, the diagnosis can often only be confirmed when response to treatment with steroids and/or immunoglobulins is demonstrated.[100]

THROMBOCYTOPENIA IN THE STEM CELL AND SOLID ORGAN TRANSPLANT PATIENT

Thrombocytopenia in the patient who has undergone a stem cell or organ transplant has a broad differential and is often a poor prognostic feature. Posttransplant TMA occurs in 9% to 15% of allogeneic stem cell transplants and in 5% of renal transplants. It is associated with the calcineurin inhibitors tacrolimus and cyclosporine, infections (*Aspergillus*, cytomegalovirus, adenovirus), and acute graft-versus-host disease. Renal damage is prominent, and overall prognosis is poor.[101,102] Other causes of thrombocytopenia in these patients include medications (methotrexate, ganciclovir, trimethoprim/sulfamethoxazole), ITP, splenomegaly, and infections, especially cytomegalovirus, which is associated with both stem cell graft failure and isolated thrombocytopenia.

SUMMARY

Thrombocytopenia is a common laboratory finding and is a frequent reason for a hematology consult. Once pseudothrombocytopenia has been ruled out, the differential diagnosis of thrombocytopenia includes platelet destruction, reduced platelet production, splenic sequestration, and hemodilution. The causes, severity, and acuity of thrombocytopenia vary widely depending on the clinical scenario. Infection, hemodilution, and DIC are common causes in the ICU. ITP and congenital causes are usually encountered in the outpatient setting. Alcohol consumption and medications are common causes in both the outpatient and inpatient setting. A thorough history, physical examination, and examination of the peripheral blood smear will reveal the cause in most patients. This review describes the mechanisms causing thrombocytopenia, and discusses the causes and management of a low platelet count in the different clinical settings likely encountered by the hematologist.

REFERENCES

1. Coller BS, Schneiderman PI. Clinical evaluation of hemorrhagic disorders: the bleeding history and differential diagnosis of purpura. In: Hoffman R, editor. Hematology: basic principles and practice. 8th edition. Philadelphia: Churchill Livingstone Elsevier; 2008. p. 1851–76.
2. Kaushansky K. Megakaryopoiesis and thrombopoiesis. In: Lichtman MA, Kipps TJ, Seligsohn U, et al, editors. Williams hematology. 8th edition. New York: McGraw-Hill; 2010. Chapter 113. Available at: http://www.accessmedicine.com/content.aspx?aID=6230972. Accessed December 17, 2011.
3. Thon JN, Italiano JE. Platelet formation. Semin Hematol 2010;47:220–6.
4. Froom P, Barak M. Prevalence and course of pseudothrombocytopenia in outpatients. Clin Chem Lab Med 2011;49:111–4.
5. Onder O, Weinstein A, Hoyer LW. Pseudothrombocytopenia caused by platelet agglutinins that are reactive in blood anticoagulated with chelating agents. Blood 1980;56:177–82.
6. Bizzaro N. EDTA-dependent pseudothrombocytopenia: a clinical and epidemiological study of 112 cases, with 10-year follow-up. Am J Hematol 1995;50:103–9.
7. Morselli M, Longo G, Bonacorsi G, et al. Anticoagulant pseudothrombocytopenia with platelet satellitism. Haematologica 1999;84:655.
8. McMillan R. Autoantibodies and autoantigens in chronic immune thrombocytopenic purpura. Semin Hematol 2000;37:239–48.

9. Aster RH. Pooling of platelets in the spleen: role in the pathogenesis of "hypersplenic" thrombocytopenia. J Clin Invest 1966;45:645–57.

10. Jandl JH, Aster RH. Increased splenic pooling and the pathogenesis of hyprsplenism. Am J Med Sci 1967;253:383–98.

11. Qamar AA, Grace ND, Groszmann RJ, et al. Incidence, prevalence and clinical significance of abnormal hematologic indices in compensated cirrhosis. Clin Gastroenterol Hepatol 2009;7:689–95.

12. Hess JR. Blood and coagulation support in trauma care. Hematology Am Soc Hematol Educ Program 2007;187–91.

13. Levy JH. Massive transfusion coagulopathy. Semin Hematol 2006;43(Suppl 1): S59–63.

14. Gerwitz AM. Thrombocytopenia due to decreased platelet production. In: Hoffman R, editor. Hematology: basic principles and practice. 8th edition. Philadelphia: Churchill Livingstone Elsevier; 2008. p. 421–2.

15. Lopas H, Rabiner SF. Thrombocytopenia associated with iron deficiency anemia. A report of five cases. Clin Pediatr (Phila) 1966;5:609–16.

16. Perlman MK, Schwab JG, Nachman JB, et al. Thrombocytopenia in children with severe iron deficiency. J Pediatr Hematol Oncol 2002;24:380–4.

17. Cowan D. Effect of alcoholism on hemostasis. Semin Hematol 1980;17:137–47.

18. Colman N, Herbert V. Hematologic complications of alcoholism. Semin Hematol 1980;17:164–76.

19. Gewirtz AM, Hoffman R. Transitory hypomegakaryocytic thrombocytopenia: aetiological association with ethanol abuse and implications regarding regulation of human megakaryocytopoiesis. Br J Haematol 1986;62:333–44.

20. Lindenbaum J. Hematologic complications of alcohol abuse. Semin Liver Dis 1987;7:169–81.

21. Stasi R, Willis F, Shannon MS, et al. Infectious causes of chronic immune thrombocytopenia. Hematol Oncol Clin North Am 2009;23:1275–97.

22. Kurihara Y, Shishido T, Oku K, et al. Polymyositis associated with autoimmune hepatitis, primary biliary cirrhosis, and autoimmune thrombocytopenia purpura. Mod Rheumatol 2011;21:325–9.

23. Afdhal N, McHutchison J, Brown R, et al. Thrombocytopenia associated with chronic liver disease. J Hepatol 2008;48:1000–7.

24. Mammen EF. Coagulation abnormalities in liver disease. Hematol Oncol Clin North Am 1992;6:1247–57.

25. Cines DB, Bussel JB, McMillan RB, et al. Congenital and acquired thrombocytopenia. Hematology Am Soc Hematol Educ Program 2004;390–406.

26. Drachman JG. Inherited thrombocytopenia: when a low platelet count does not mean ITP. Blood 2004;103:390–8.

27. George J, Raskob GE, Shah SR, et al. Drug-induced thrombocytopenia: a systemic review of published case reports. Ann Intern Med 1998;129:886–90.

28. Aster RH, Curtis BR, McFarland JG, et al. Drug-induced immune thrombocytopenia: pathogenesis, diagnosis and management. J Thromb Haemost 2009;7:911–8.

29. Delgado MR, Riela AR, Mills J, et al. Thrombocytopenia secondary to high valproate levels in children with epilepsy. J Child Neurol 1994;9:311.

30. Wartenkin TE. Thrombocytopenia due to platelet destruction and hypersplenism. In: Hoffman R, editor. Hematology: basic principles and practice. 8th edition. Philadelphia: Churchill Livingstone Elsevier; 2008. p. 2117–8.

31. Gao C, Boylan B, Bougie D, et al. Eptifibatide-induced thrombocytopenia and thrombosis in humans require FcgammaRIIa and the integrin b3 cytoplasmic domain. J Clin Invest 2009;119:504–11.

32. Neylon AJ, Saunders PW, Howard MR, et al. Clinically significant newly presenting autoimmune thrombocytopenic purpura in adults: a prospective study of a population-based cohort of 245 patients. Br J Haematol 2003;122:966–74.
33. Kaufman DW, Kelly JP, Johannes CB, et al. Acute thrombocytopenic purpura in relation to the use of drugs. Blood 1993;82:2714–8.
34. George J, Aster R. Drug-induced thrombocytopenia: pathogenesis, evaluation, and management. Hematology Am Soc Hematol Educ Program 2009;153–8.
35. Arnold J, Ouwehand WH, Smith GA, et al. A young woman with petechiae. Lancet 1998;352:618.
36. Lavy R. Thrombocytopenic purpura due to *Lupinus termis* bean. J Allergy Clin Immunol 1964;35:386–8.
37. Azuno Y, Yaga K, Sasayama T, et al. Thrombocytopenia induced by Jui, a traditional Chinese herbal medicine. Lancet 1999;354:304–5.
38. Caffrey EA, Sladen GE, Isaacs PE, et al. Thrombocytopenia caused by cow's milk. Lancet 1981;2:316.
39. Davies JK, Ahktar N, Ranasinge E. A juicy problem. Lancet 2001;358:2126.
40. Cines D, Bussel J, Liebman H, et al. The ITP syndrome: pathogenic and clinical diversity. Blood 2009;113:6511–21.
41. Bromberg ME. Immune thrombocytopenic purpura—the changing therapeutic landscape. N Engl J Med 2006;355:1643–5.
42. Rodeghiero F, Stasi R, Gernsheimer T, et al. Standardization of terminology, definitions, and outcome criteria in immune thrombocytopenic purpura of adults and children: report from an international working group. Blood 2009;113: 2386–93.
43. Neunert C, Lim W, Crowther M, et al. The American Society of Hematology 2011 evidence-based practice guideline for immune thrombocytopenia. Blood 2011; 117:4190–207.
44. Zaja F, Baccarani M, Mazza P, et al. Dexamethasone plus rituximab yields higher sustained response rates than dexamethasone monotherapy in adults with primary immune thrombocytopenia. Blood 2010;115(14):2755–62.
45. Kuter DJ, Bussel JB, Lyons RM, et al. Efficacy of romiplostim in patients with chronic immune thrombocytopenic purpura: a double-blind randomized controlled trial. Lancet 2008;371:395–403.
46. Bussel JB, Provan D, Shamsi T, et al. Effect of eltrombopag on platelet counts and bleeding during treatment of chronic idiopathic thrombocytopenic purpura: a randomised, double-blind, placebo-controlled trial. Lancet 2009;373:641–8.
47. Bussel JB, Cheng G, Saleh MN, et al. Eltrombopag for the treatment of chronic idiopathic thrombocytopenic purpura. N Engl J Med 2007;357:2237–47.
48. Miller MH, Urowitz MB, Gladman DD. The significance of thrombocytopenia in systemic lupus erythematosus. Arthritis Rheum 1983;26:1181–6.
49. Arnal C, Piette JC, Leone J, et al. Treatment of severe immune thrombocytopenia associated with systemic lupus erythematosus: 59 cases. J Rheumatol 2002;29:75–83.
50. Yu YN, Tefferi A, Nagorney DM. Outcome of splenectomy for thrombocytopenia associated with systemic lupus erythematosus. Ann Surg 2004;240:286–92.
51. Mader R, Ziporen L, Mader R, et al. Antiphospholipid antibodies in a heterogeneous group of patients: experience from a central laboratory. Clin Rheumatol 2002;21:386–90.
52. Krause I, Blank M, Fraser A, et al. The association of thrombocytopenia with systemic manifestations in the antiphospholipid syndrome. Immunobiology 2005;210:749–54.

53. Galli M, Daldossi M, Barbui T. Anti-glycoprotein Ib/IX and IIb/IIIa antibodies in patients with antiphospholipid antibodies. Thromb Haemost 1994;71:571–5.
54. Pechere M, Samii K, Hirschel B. HIV related thrombocytopenia. N Engl J Med 1993;328:1785–6.
55. Sullivan PS, Hanson DL, Chu SY, et al. Surveillance for thrombocytopenia in persons infected with HIV: results from the multistate adult and adolescent spectrum of disease project. J Acquir Immune Defic Syndr Hum Retrovirol 1997;14:374–9.
56. Marks KM, Clarke RM, Bussel JB, et al. Risk factors for thrombocytopenia in HIV patients in the era of potent antiretroviral therapy. J Acquir Immune Defic Syndr 2009;52:595–9.
57. Kouri Y, Borkowsky W, Nardi M, et al. Human megakaryocytes have a CD4+ molecule capable of binding human immunodeficiency virus-1. Blood 1993; 81:2664–70.
58. Zucker-Franklin D, Seremetis S, Heng ZY. Internalization of human immunodeficiency virus type I and other retroviruses by megakaryocytes and platelets. Blood 1990;75:1920–3.
59. Vannappagari V, Nkhoma ET, Atashili J, et al. Prevalence, severity, and duration of thrombocytopenia among HIV patients in the era of highly active antiretroviral therapy. Platelets 2011;22:611–8.
60. Louie KS, Micallef JM, Pimenta JM, et al. Prevalence of thrombocytopenia among patients with chronic hepatitis C: a systematic review. J Viral Hepat 2011;18:1–7.
61. Hernadez F, Blanquer A, Linares M, et al. Autoimmune thrombocytopenia associated with hepatitis C infection. Acta Hematologica 1998;99:217–20.
62. Stasi R, Sarpatwari A, Segal JB, et al. Effects of eradication of Helicobacter pylori infection in patients with immune thrombocytopenic purpura: a systemic review. Blood 2009;113:1231–40.
63. Mueller-Eckhardt C, Kroll H, Kiefel V, et al. Posttransfusion purpura. In: Kaplan-Gouet C, Schlegel N, Salmon C, editors. Platelet immunology: fundamental and clinical aspects. London: Colloque INSERM/John Libbey Eurotext Ltd; 1991. p. 249.
64. Ballem PJ, Buskard NA, Decary F, et al. Post-transfusion purpura secondary to passive transfer of anti-PlA1 by blood transfusion. Br J Haematol 1987;66:113–4.
65. Warkentin TE, Smith JW, Hayward CP, et al. Thrombocytopenia caused by passive transfusion of anti-glycoprotein Ia/IIa alloantibody (anti-HPA-5b). Blood 1992;79:2480–4.
66. Shulman NR, Jordan JV. Platelet immunology. Philadelphia: JB Lippincott; 1982.
67. Mueller-Eckhardt C, Kiefel V. High-dose IgG for post-transfusion purpura—revisited. Blut 1988;570:163–7.
68. Krause PJ. Babesiosis diagnosis and treatment. Vector Borne Zoonotic Dis 2003;3:45–51.
69. Dumler J, Madigan J, Pusteria N, et al. Ehrlichioses in humans: epidemiology, clinical presentation, diagnosis, and treatment. Clin Infect Dis 2007;45:S45–51.
70. Patel U, Gandhi G, Friedman S, et al. Thrombocytopenia in malaria. J Natl Med Assoc 2004;96:1212–4.
71. Wilson JJ, Neame PB, Kelton JG. Infection-induced thrombocytopenia. Semin Thromb Hemost 1982;8:217–33.
72. Hui P, Cook D, Lim W, et al. The frequency and clinical significance of thrombocytopenia complicating critical illness: a systematic review. Chest 2011;139: 271–8.

73. Rice TW, Wheeler AP. Coagulopathy in critically ill patients. Part 1: platelet disorders. Chest 2009;136:1622–30.
74. Moreau D, Timsit JF, Vesin A, et al. Platelet count decline. An early prognostic marker in critically ill patients with prolonged ICU stays. Chest 2007;131:1735–41.
75. Brogly N, Devos P, Boussekey N, et al. Impact of thrombocytopenia on outcome of patients admitted to ICU for severe community-acquired pneumonia. J Infect 2007;55:136–40.
76. Sakr Y, Haetscher F, Gosalves MD, et al. Heparin-induced thrombocytopenia type II in a surgical intensive care unit. J Crit Care 2011. Available at: http://dx.doi.org/10.1016/j.jcrc.2011.06.016. Accessed February 13, 2012.
77. Kuitenen A, Suojaranta-Ylinen R, Raivio P, et al. Heparin-induced thrombocytopenia following cardiac surgery is associated with poor outcome. J Cardiothorac Vasc Anesth 2007;21:18–22.
78. Crowther MA, Cook DJ, Albert M, et al. The 4Ts scoring system for heparin-induced thrombocytopenia in medical-surgical intensive care unit patients. J Crit Care 2010;25:287–93.
79. Berry C, Tcherniantchouk O, Ley EJ, et al. Overdiagnosis of heparin-induced thrombocytopenia in surgical ICU patients. J Am Coll Surg 2011;213:10–8.
80. Levine RI, Hergenroeder GW, Francis JL, et al. Heparin-platelet factor 4 antibodies in intensive care unit patients: an observational seroprevalence study. J Thromb Thrombolysis 2010;30:142–8.
81. Warkentin TE. Heparin-induced thrombocytopenia in critically ill patients. Crit Care Clin 2011;27:805–23.
82. Tschudi M, Lammle B, Alberio I. Dosing lepirudin in patients with heparin-induced thrombocytopenia and normal or impaired renal function: a single-center experience with 68 patients. Blood 2009;113:2402–9.
83. Hoffman WD, Czyz Y, McCollum DA, et al. Reduced argatroban doses after coronary artery bypass graft surgery. Ann Pharmacother 2008;42:309–16.
84. Matthai WH. Evaluation of thrombocytopenia in the acute coronary syndrome. Curr Opin Hematol 2010;17:398–404.
85. Hochtl T, Pachinger L, Unger G, et al. antiplatelet drug induced isolated profound thrombocytopenia in interventional cardiology: a review based on individual case reports. J Thromb Thrombolysis 2007;24:59–64.
86. Harker LA, Malpass TW, Branson HE, et al. Mechanism of abnormal bleeding in patients undergoing cardiopulmonary bypass: acquired transient platelet dysfunction associated with selective alpha-granule release. Blood 1980;56:824–34.
87. Warkentin TE, Greinacher A. Heparin-induced thrombocytopenia and cardiac surgery. Ann Thorac Surg 2003;76:2121–31.
88. Pouplard C, May MA, Regina S, et al. Changes in platelet count after cardiac surgery can effectively predict the development of pathogenic heparin-dependent antibodies. Br J Haematol 2005;128:837–41.
89. Selleng S, Malowsky B, Strobel U, et al. Early-onset and persisting thrombocytopenia in post-cardiac surgery patients is rarely due to heparin-induced thrombocytopenia, even when antibody tests are positive. J Thromb Haemost 2010;8:30–6.
90. Warkentin TE, Greinacher A, Koster A. Heparin-induced thrombocytopenia in patients with ventricular assist devices: are new prevention strategies required? Ann Thorac Surg 2009;87:1633–40.
91. Hodgson K, Ferrer G, Pereira A, et al. Autoimmune cytopenia in chronic lymphocytic leukaemia: diagnosis and treatment. Br J Haematol 2011;154:14–22.

92. Liebman HA. Recognizing and treating secondary immune thrombocytopenic purpura associated with lymphoproliferative disorders. Semin Hematol 2009; 46(1 Suppl 2):S33–6.
93. Hauswirth AW, Skrabs C, Schutzinger C, et al. Autoimmune thrombocytopenia in non-Hodgkin's lymphomas. Haematologica 2008;93:447–50.
94. Ten Berg MJ, van den Bernt PM, Shantakumar S, et al. Thrombocytopenia in adult cancer patients receiving cytotoxic chemotherapy: results from a retrospective hospital-based cohort study. Drug Saf 2011;34:1151–60.
95. Aster RH, Bougie DW. Drug-induced immune thrombocytopenia. N Engl J Med 2007;357:580–7.
96. Bautista MA, Stevens WT, Chen CS, et al. Hypersensitivity reaction and acute immune-mediated thrombocytopenia from oxaliplatin: two case reports and a review of the literature. J Hematol Oncol 2010;3:12.
97. Elliott MA, Letendre L, Gastineau DA, et al. Cancer-associated microangiopathic hemolytic anemia with thrombocytopenia: an important diagnostic consideration. Eur J Haematol 2010;85:43–50.
98. Zakarija A, Bennett C. Drug-induced thrombotic microangiopathy. Semin Thromb Hemost 2005;31:681–90.
99. Blake-Haskins JA, Lechleider RJ, Kreitman RJ. Thrombotic microangiopathy with targeted cancer agents. Clin Cancer Res 2011;17:5858–66.
100. Krauth MT, Puthenparambil J, Lechner K. Paraneoplastic autoimmune thrombocytopenia in solid tumors. Crit Rev Oncol Hematol 2012;81:75–81.
101. Laskin BL, Goebel J, Davies SM, et al. Small vessels, big trouble in the kidneys and beyond: hematopoietic stem cell transplantation-associated thrombotic microangiopathy. Blood 2011;118:1452–62.
102. Pulanic D, Lozier JN, Pavletic SZ. Thrombocytopenia and hemostatic disorders in chronic graft versus host disease. Bone Marrow Transplant 2009;44:393–403.

Why is My Patient Neutropenic?

John L. Reagan, MD*, Jorge J. Castillo, MD

KEYWORDS

- Neutrophil • Neutropenia • Differential diagnosis
- Consultative hematology

NEUTROPHIL OVERVIEW

Neutrophils (also called granulocytes) are produced exclusively in the bone marrow during normal conditions. Approximately 10^{12} neutrophils are produced per day in the bone marrow and then stored in the marrow until prompted for release by chemokines, cytokines, microbial products, or other mediators of inflammation. Once released into the bloodstream the average half-life of neutrophils is 6 to 8 hours. Circulating neutrophils, the ones reported in a standard complete blood count (CBC), account for only 2% to 3% of all neutrophils. Clearance occurs in the liver, spleen, or bone marrow and occurs through macrophage phagocytosis of aged or apoptotic neutrophils. The local production of inflammatory cytokines and chemokines leads to neutrophil attachment to the vascular endothelium and the subsequent transmigration of neutrophils into tissue. The migration of neutrophils into tissue is a key component of the innate immune system, as evident by the increased risk of infections seen in the setting of neutropenia.

NEUTROPENIA

Neutropenia is defined as an absolute neutrophil count (ANC) less than 1500 cells/μL; it may be mild (ANC 1000–1500 cells/μL), moderate (500–1000 cells/μL), or severe (<500 cells/μL) (**Table 1**). In general, infection risk increases with ANC less than 1000 cells/μL; however, the risk for infections varies depending on the cause of neutropenia. For example, patients with neutropenia and acute leukemia seem to have a high risk for overwhelming infection in the setting of neutropenia, particularly in cases with ANC less than 500 cells/μL.[1] Therefore, the context in which neutropenia occurs must be considered because some causes of neutropenia, namely ethnic neutropenia and chronic idiopathic neutropenia (CIN), have few overall infection risks.

Disclosures: The authors have no conflict of interest to disclose.
Division of Hematology and Oncology, The Miriam Hospital, The Warren Alpert Medical School of brown university, 164 Summit Avenue, Providence, RI 02906, USA
* Corresponding author.
E-mail address: jreagan@lifespan.org

Hematol Oncol Clin N Am 26 (2012) 253–266
doi:10.1016/j.hoc.2012.02.003
0889-8588/12/$ – see front matter © 2012 Elsevier Inc. All rights reserved.

Table 1 Severity of neutropenia		
	ANC	Risk of Infection
Mild neutropenia	ANC <1500 but >1000	Mild
Moderate neutropenia	ANC <1000 but >500	Moderate
Severe neutropenia	ANC <500 but >200	Severe
Agranulocytosis	ANC <200	Severe

DIAGNOSTIC WORKUP

Initial workup consists of a CBC, with a differential count to evaluate the severity of the neutropenia. A full history is also essential to determine race, ethnicity, new medications (including over-the-counter and complementary medications), and potential infectious exposures. Review of systems should focus on fevers, chills, night sweats, weight loss, excess bleeding or bruising, or recurrent infections. A comprehensive physical examination should be performed, with a focus on an examination for signs of infection, hepatosplenomegaly, and lymphadenopathy. After this examination, a detailed review of the peripheral smear should follow, to look for neutrophil abnormalities such as Döhle bodies (infection), immature neutrophil precursors (infection, myelodysplasia, myelopthisis), hypoplastic changes in the neutrophils (myelodysplasia), hyperlobulation (nutritional deficiencies), and white cell inclusions (eg, anaplasmosis (**Fig. 1**), bartonellosis). Review of red cell morphology on peripheral smear may also offer clues to the cause of neutropenia because dacrocytes (teardrop cells) and nucleated red cells (myelodysplasia, fibrosis, myelopthisis) in addition to red cell inclusions (eg, babesiosis, malaria) may all be seen in disease states associated with neutropenia.

Additional routine blood work should include:

- Reticulocyte count
- Lactate dehydrogenase
- Erythrocyte sedimentation rate
- Rheumatoid factor/anticyclic citrullinated protein antibody
- Antinuclear antibodies
- Thyroid-stimulating hormone

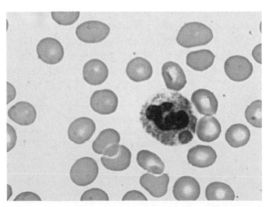

Fig. 1. Neutrophil with an intracellular morula in a patient with anaplasmosis.

- Human immunodeficiency virus (HIV) enzyme-linked immunosorbent assay (ELISA) test with confirmation by Western blot
- Vitamin B_{12} levels
- Folate levels.

In cases in which diarrhea is present, stool samples should be checked for the presence of fecal leukocytes and cultured for *Shigella* and *Salmonella*. If tick-borne illnesses are part of the differential diagnosis, then an ELISA for *Borrelia burgdorferi*, the causative agent of Lyme disease, should be ordered and, if positive, the result should be confirmed by Western blot. If babesiosis is suspected, *Babesia* immunofluorescent antibody (IFA) and polymerase chain reaction (PCR) tests should be ordered. *Anaplasma* infection should be evaluated, if needed, by IFA, ELISA, or PCR tests. The granulocyte agglutination test or granulocyte immunofluorescence test for antigranulocyte antibodies to evaluate potential autoimmune neutropenic syndromes may be considered. Bone marrow aspirate and biopsy should be reserved for those cases in which there is a high suspicion for malignancy, either hematologic or metastatic solid tumor.

CAUSES

The most common causes of neutropenia are shown in **Boxes 1–3**.

ETHNIC VARIATION

Ethnic neutropenia has been described in persons of African, African American, Yemenite Jewish, West Indian, and Arab Jordanian ancestry.[2,3] In the United States, the prevalence of neutropenia (ANC <1500 cells/µL) amongst African Americans is 4.5%, whereas it has been reported at 0.79% and 0.38% in whites and Mexican-Americans, respectively.[2] The pathophysiology in ethnic neutropenia seems to be a decrease in the number of neutrophil precursors within the bone marrow. However, there is no decrease in the functionality of the neutrophils.[4] Ethnic neutropenia is a benign process that carries no increased risks for infections but should be considered early in the initial diagnostic workup to prevent unnecessary testing. Recently, the role of ethnic neutropenia has been addressed in patients receiving chemotherapy, because most clinical trials withhold chemotherapy in the setting of an ANC less than 1500 cells/µL. Hsieh and colleagues[2] make the case that chemotherapy can be administered with granulocyte colony-stimulating factor (G-CSF) support, if appropriate, in patients with ethnic neutropenia at ANC of 500 to 1500 cells/µL.

CONGENITAL NEUTROPENIA

The hematologist who treats adults should also be familiar with congenital forms of neutropenia (see **Box 2**). Cases can be mild and therefore not diagnosed until patients reach their adult years and have more regular blood work performed. Moreover, patients with severe forms of congenital neutropenia are living longer and require transitions from pediatric hematologists to their adult counterparts. The 2 most common forms of congenital neutropenia, cyclic neutropenia and severe congenital neutropenia (SCN, or Kostmann syndrome), are reviewed here with other causes of congenital neutropenia.

Cyclic Neutropenia

Typically, in cyclic neutropenia a family history is important because the condition occurs through autosomal-dominant inheritance, although sporadic cases have

---

Box 1
Causes of neutropenia

1. Ethnic variations
2. Immune-related
   a. Primary immune neutropenia
   b. Secondary immune neutropenia
      i. Felty syndrome (FS)
      ii. Systemic lupus erythematosus (SLE)
      iii. Rheumatoid arthritis (RA)
3. Infectious
   a. Sepsis
   b. Parasitic
   c. Viral
   d. Bacterial
4. Malignancy
   a. Acute leukemia
   b. Myelodysplastic syndrome (MDS)
   c. Myelophthisis
   d. Large granulocytic lymphocytic leukemia
5. Medication
   a. Antibiotics
   b. Cardiac
   c. Anticonvulsants
   d. Psychiatric
   e. Antiinflammatory
   f. Hypoglycemics
   g. Antineoplastic agents
6. Mechanical
   a. Splenomegaly
7. Nutritional deficiencies
   a. Vitamin B_{12} (cobalamin)
   b. Folic acid
   c. Copper
8. Other
   a. Hypothyroidism/hyperthyroidism

---

been reported. The neutrophil count cycles over an approximately 21-day period. Patients commonly develop oral ulcerations, fevers, cervical lymphadenopathy, and skin infections during neutrophil nadir periods, but severe infections are usually not seen. The disorder is secondary to a mutation in the neutrophil elastase gene that leads to increased apoptosis in neutrophil precursors.[5] Treatment, if required, is

Box 2
Causes of congenital neutropenia
1. Severe congenital neutropenia (SCN)
2. Cyclic neutropenia
3. WHIM (warts, hypogammaglobulinemia, infections, and myelokathexis) syndrome
4. Shwachman-Diamond syndrome
5. Barth syndrome
6. Pearson syndrome
7. Glycogen storage disease type 1B
8. Cartilage-hair hypoplasia
9. Dyskeratosis congenita

centered on G-CSF with good overall results. The level of neutropenia sometimes improves with age.[6]

Severe Congenital Neutropenia (Kostmann Syndrome)

Initially described by the Swedish physician Rolf Kostmann in 1956 in a cohort of children who presented with agranulocytosis and severe infections. SCN was, at first, believed to occur through autosomal-recessive inheritance. However, autosomal-dominant inheritance and sporadic cases of SCN have also been reported. Like cyclic neutropenia, mutations in the neutrophil elastase gene have been found in patients with SCN, although bone marrow biopsy shows maturation arrest at the promyelocyte stage. However, the role of these mutations remains unclear because they were found in a subgroup of patients with SCN but were also found in phenotypically normal family members.[5] HAX1 gene mutations have been associated with autosomal-recessive forms of SCN,[7] whereas ELA2 mutations are commonly found in autosomal-dominant and sporadic cases of the disease.[8] More recently, a mutation in the G6PC3 gene has also been shown to result in SCN.[9] More than 90% of the patients respond to G-CSF administration. Long-term complications include a risk for transformation to myelodysplasia or leukemia in 22% of patients. This transformation has been unmasked now that patients live longer because of G-CSF therapy.[10] Vasculitis, splenomegaly, and osteoporosis frequently occur in this patient population.[11]

IMMUNE-RELATED NEUTROPENIA

Immune causes of neutropenia are secondary to circulating antibodies binding to and destroying peripheral neutrophils. Autoimmune neutropenia (AIN) can be either primary, when no clear underlying cause is present, or secondary, when it is associated with an underlying autoimmune condition. Disease states seen with secondary AIN are typically RA and SLE, although other autoimmune diseases, malignancies, infection, and drugs may also be associated.

Primary AIN

The diagnosis of primary AIN is based on the presence of antigranuloctye antibodies and the absence of a potential underlying disease-specific cause, as outlined in the section on secondary AIN. Primary AIN is usually seen in children younger than 2 years of age, and common associated infections include skin, upper respiratory, and ear infections. Most patients with AIN have antibodies that recognize antigens on the

---

Box 3
Infectious causes of neutropenia

1. Sepsis
2. Parasitic
   a. Malaria
   b. Leishmaniasis (kala-azar)
   c. Babesiosis
3. Viral
   a. HIV
   b. Human herpesviruses
      i. Herpes simplex virus 1 and 2
      ii. Varicella zoster virus
      iii. Epstein-Barr virus
      iv. Cytomegalovirus (CMV)
      v. Roseolovirus (sixth disease)
   c. Parvovirus B19 (fifth disease)
   d. Hepatitis A, B, and C virus
   e. Measles
   f. Rubella
4. Bacterial
   a. *Shigella*
   b. *Salmonella* (typhoid fever)
   c. Zoonotic diseases (tularemia, brucellosis)
   d. Anaplasmosis
   e. Lyme disease
5. Mycobacterial
   a. *Mycobacterium tuberculosis*
   b. *M avium*

IgG Fc receptor IIIb. In terms of clinical course, primary AIN is usually self-limited. In severe cases of primary AIN in which there is persistent infection or when surgery is required, G-CSF, steroids, or intravenous immunoglobulin can be used, with response rates of 100%, 75%, and 50%, respectively.[12]

Pure White Cell Aplasia

Neutropenia in which there are no neutrophil precursors present in the bone marrow alongside normal red blood cell and platelet precursors is termed pure white cell aplasia (PWCA). PWCA is a rare cause of neutropenia, for which only case reports are available. There seems to be an association with thymoma,[13] with treatment centered on thymoma removal along with immunosuppressive therapy such as rituximab and cyclosporine.[14,15] The mechanism of action is immune mediated by antibody development to neutrophil progenitor cells that spares pluripotent stem cells, erythroid precursors, and mature neutrophils.[16]

Secondary AIN

Systemic lupus erythematosus

Neutropenia has been reported in approximately 20% to 50% of patients with SLE.[17–19] The incidence of moderate to severe neutropenia is less; 1% to 5% of patients with SLE had ANCs less than 1000 cells/μL.[18] Associated findings in patients with SLE and moderate to severe neutropenia are use of medications known to cause neutropenia (ie, cotrimoxazole, phenytoin, and amoxicillin/clavulanic acid), immuno-suppressive drugs, thrombocytopenia, and central nervous system involvement of SLE.[20] The mechanism by which neutropenia occurs in SLE is through antineutrophil antibody production, increased apoptosis of circulating neutrophils,[21] and a direct myelosuppressive effect by SLE on the bone marrow.[22,23] In terms of antibody production, 1 hypothesis is that anti-SSA (Ro) and anti-SSB antibodies either cross-react with neutrophil epitopes or bind directly to neutrophil antigens. In the case of anti-SSA, antibody binds neutrophils, activating complement fixation and neutrophil destruction.[24] Anti-SSB antibodies have been detected in the sera of patients with neutropenia and have been shown to increase neutrophil apoptosis.[25] The first step in treating SLE-associated neutropenia is to treat the SLE itself. Persistent moderate to severe neutropenia in a patient with well-controlled SLE warrants a closer look at potential offending medications as well as possible infectious causes, particularly when immunosuppression is present. G-CSF should be used in caution in patients with SLE because mild to severe disease flares have been described, including cases of irreversibly damaged renal function.[26]

Rheumatoid arthritis and felty syndrome

FS is a variant of RA associated with leukopenia, most often manifesting as neutrope-nia, splenomegaly, severe arthralgias, rheumatoid nodules, pulmonary fibrosis, and vasculitis. Laboratory findings associated with FS are increased levels of RF, hyper-gammaglobulinemia, and immune complexes in the blood.[27] Almost 90% of patients with FS are HLA-DR4+. This same high percentage is seen in patients with RA and large granular lymphocytic (LGL) leukemia, suggesting that these 2 diseases may represent 1 entity.[28] The primary treatment of FS is immunosuppression; however, care must be taken given the high rate of overwhelming sepsis in this patient popula-tion. Methotrexate, hydroxychloroquine, and intravenous immunoglobulin have been used with varying success. Rituximab does not have activity in FS. In cases of severe neutropenia, G-CSF can be used with the goal of an ANC greater than 1000 cells/μL but as in SLE-induced neutropenia the use of G-CSF has been associated with vascu-litic flares and worsening arthralgias.[29]

Hyperthyroidism (Graves disease)

Hyperthyroidism has been shown to cause neutropenia, with improvement in neutro-phil levels with correction of excess thyroid hormone production.[30] Both cell-bound and circulating antineutrophil antibodies have been found in the serum of patients with Graves disease, suggesting an underlying autoimmune process.[31]

Chronic idiopathic neutropenia

Patients without another clear cause for their neutropenia are frequently labeled with CIN. The clinical hallmarks of CIN are an acquired neutropenia with a relatively stable, suppressed neutrophil count without recurrent infections.

Full diagnostic criteria are as follows:

- ANC less than 1800 cells/μL in whites or less than 1500 cells/μL in individuals of African ancestry for greater than 3 months

- No clinical, serologic, or imaging evidence for another cause of neutropenia
- Absence of radiation exposures, chemical compound use, or drug intake associated with neutropenia
- Normal bone marrow karyotype
- No antineutrophil antibodies detected in the serum (a minimum of 2 methods such as the granulocyte agglutination and granulocyte immunofluorescence test should be used for confirmatory purposes).

Historically, this diagnosis served as one of exclusion, with no clear underlying pathophysiologic mechanism. Recently, however, new data have described CIN as a failure of the bone marrow microenvironment. Patients with CIN have increased inflammatory changes within the bone marrow through the presence of activated T cells as well as interferon γ, tumor necrosis factor α, Fas-ligand, and transforming growth factor β1 (TGF-β1).[8] Mesenchymal stem cells seem to play a role in the formation of the bone marrow microenvironment through the increasing production of TGF-β1.[32] The overproduction of TGF-β1 in turn suppresses interleukin 10, an antiinflammatory cytokine.[33] These changes lead to increased apoptosis within neutrophil progenitor cells.

DRUGS

Drug-induced neutropenia is a rare condition, with reports of 2 to 15 cases per million per year. However, it remains a common cause for neutropenia and should be considered at the outset in any patient presenting with neutropenia. The incidence increases with age, likely because older patients are exposed to more drugs than younger individuals. Almost all medication classes have been implicated; however, the major causes of drug-induced neutropenia include β-lactam antibiotics, cotrimoxazole, antithyroid medications, ticlodipine, neuroleptics such as clozaril, antiepileptics, and nonsteroidal antiinflammatory medications.[34] The onset of neutropenia and time to resolution of neutropenia are dependent on the drug involved.[35] Ten common causes of drug-induced neutropenia are outlined in **Table 2**.

Neutropenia secondary to medications is typically caused by either repeated exposure to the drug, resulting in myelosuppression, or through intermittent exposure, causing an immunologic phenomenon. Immune-mediated drug-induced neutropenia is most commonly seen in β-lactam antibiotics and antithyroid medications and is directly secondary to antibody production and subsequent neutrophil or neutrophil progenitor destruction. A bone marrow biopsy can be informative to define the duration of neutropenia. In scenarios in which no neutrophil precursors are present, recovery of neutrophils can take up to 14 days. However, in other settings, there is a picture of myeloid maturation arrest in which precursors are still present but mature neutrophils are absent. In this case, recovery takes 5 to 7 days.[34]

In a recent systemic review by Andersohn and colleagues that compiled all case reports of drug-induced neutropenia,[35] those with an ANC less than 100 cells/μL experienced higher rates of fatal complications than patients with ANC greater than 100 cells/μL. With regard to treatment, the first intervention is discontinuation of the suspected medication. The investigators also include data about the typical length of time culprit medications are taken before neutropenia occurs and the expected time for recovery once culprit medications are discontinued. Careful assessment of the risks for infection is necessary, with action taken if fevers develop. The role of growth factor support is less clear. Andersohn and colleagues show no statistically significant difference in the percentage of deaths in patients with drug-induced thrombocytopenia who were given growth factor support (5%) versus those who were not (6%). Therefore, in

Table 2
The 10 most common medications that cause drug-induced neutropenia as adapted from Andersohn et al.[35] All medications have at least 1 definite case report as a causative agent for neutropenia

Drug	Class	Definite Cases	Probable Cases	Duration of Exposure Before Neutropenia Onset (d)	Time to Neutrophil Recovery (d)
Dipyrone	Nonsteroidal antiinflammatory	6	5	2	10
Procainamide	Antiarrythmic	3	19	47	8
Quinidine	Antiarrythmic	3	4	35	4
Nafcillin	Antibiotic	1	4	22	8
Oxacillin	Antibiotic	2	4	22	4
Penicillin G	Antibiotic	4	7	25	4
Levamisole	Antirheumatic	2	6	60	10
Propylthiouracil	Antithyroid	1	10	36	10
Chlorpromazine	Antipsychotic	2	6	45	11
Clozapine	Antipsychotic	4	49	56	12

the setting of fevers and drug-induced neutropenia, broad-spectrum antibiotic coverage is warranted and growth factor support can be considered.[34,35]

Rituximab

Rituximab (Rituxan) is a chimeric anti-CD20 monoclonal antibody commonly used for the treatment of B-cell lymphomas and autoimmune conditions. Late-onset neutropenia (LON) has been described in which neutrophil counts decrease 3 to 4 weeks after the last rituximab infusion. The incidence has been reported as between 3% and 27% of patients, with those most at risk for LON being patients after autologous stem cell transplant, HIV-positive patients, and those patients who have received purine analogues such as fludarabine. The infection rate is close to 17%, and no clear mechanism of action has been defined.[36]

INFECTIONS
HIV

When evaluating the HIV-positive patient for neutropenia, it is paramount to first exclude indirect effects of HIV infection, such as medication effect from antiretroviral medications, opportunistic infections like CMV, or malignancy, before focusing on the role that HIV has on neutropenia (see **Box 3**). In terms of medications, the myelosuppressive effect of zidovudine (AZT) on the bone marrow was recognized in the late 1980s. The use of AZT has declined in the United States, although it continues to be one of the most common agents used in developing countries. In terms of frequency of drug-induced neutropenia in HIV, the primary culprit is AZT followed by trimethoprim/sulfamethoxazole and ganciclovir. In this patient population, chemotherapy- induced neutropenia was more likely to result in infection than other drug causes of neutropenia.[37] Opportunistic infections such as M avium complex (MAC), M tuberculosis, and Histoplasma capsulatum should be considered in the HIV patient with neutropenia in addition to the more common infections associated in neutropenia outlined later.

In terms of neutropenia frequency, the Women's Interagency HIV Study involving 1729 women found 44% of those with HIV with an ANC less than 2000 cells/μL, whereas 7% had an ANC less than 1000 cells/μL. During the 7.5-year follow-up period, 31% had at least 1 ANC less than 1000 cells/μL. Factors associated with neutropenia were a low CD4 count (<200 cells/μL) and high HIV viral load (>100,000 copies/mL). Conversely, an increased CD4 count (>500 cells/μL) and HAART (highly active antiretroviral therapy) were associated with correction of underlying neutropenia. No link between neutropenia and survival was found.[38] Another multinational study conducted in Africa, Asia, South America, the Caribbean, and the United States in which neutropenia was defined as an ANC less than 1300 cells/μL also found lower CD4 counts in addition to thrombocytopenia associated with neutropenia in newly diagnosed HIV-positive patients.[39] Low CD4 counts and the link to neutropenia have been described elsewhere.[40] The duration of neutropenia in patients with HIV is typically less than 2 weeks, with most individuals not developing infections.[41] The exact mechanism by which neutropenia occurs in patients with HIV is unclear. Studies have suggested direct effects of HIV causing increased apoptosis in neutrophils[42] as well as premature phagocytosis of bone marrow cells, which may account for the observed neutropenia. In addition, G-CSF levels in patients with HIV are lower than those without HIV.[43] In a randomized controlled trial, daily or intermittent filgastrim to keep the ANC greater than 2000 cells/μL was shown to decrease the number of episodes of severe neutropenia (ANC <500 cells/μL) or death in a statistically significant manner compared with the control population who received G-CSF only for severe neutropenia.[44]

Other Viruses

A great deal of literature discusses the role of HIV in neutropenia. However, other notable viruses can be the cause of neutropenia. Many of these viruses such as human herpesvirus 6 and measles are typically seen in children. Others, like CMV, are typically seen in immunocompromised individuals but can occasionally be present in immunocompetent patients.

Bacterial

Sepsis is one of the most common bacterial causes of neutropenia and may be secondary to any bacteria type. Sepsis-induced neutropenia is caused by the consumption of neutrophils from the overwhelming infection. *Shigella* and *Salmonella* are potential causes, particularly in patients with a history of diarrhea. Typhoid fever secondary to *Salmonella* should be considered in patients with neutropenia and abdominal pain, particularly those who have recently traveled outside the United States to endemic areas. Zoonotic diseases such as tularemia and brucellosis may also present with neutropenia in patients with recent animal exposures.[45] In areas where tick-borne illnesses are abundant, anaplasmosis should be considered in the differential for patients who present with fevers and neutropenia. The neutropenia seen in anaplasmosis is through the direct infection of neutrophils with the gram-negative bacteria *Anaplasma phagocytophilum*.[45]

Parasites

Parasitic infections typically cause neutropenia via an indirect mechanism. In cases of malaria or visceral leishmaniasis, the resulting splenomegaly that develops through hemolysis leads to neutropenia.[45] Careful attention should be paid in the initial assessment to travel to areas where these diseases are endemic.

MALIGNANCY
LGL Leukemia

LGL leukemia can be either T-cell–mediated (T-LGL) (85%) or NK-cell–mediated (NK-LGL) (15%). LGL leukemia is most frequently seen in older patients, with an average age at diagnosis of 60 years. Neutropenia is seen in both T-LGL and NK-LGL leukemia, with case series reporting rates of 48% to 84% of patients with ANC less than 1500 cells/μL and 7% to 48% with ANC less than 500 cells/μL. Diagnosis is based on flow cytometry.[46] Clinical findings include splenomegaly in 25% to 50% of patients. Approximately half of patients require treatment because of either persistent neutropenia or anemia. No standard treatment modality exists, but immunosuppressive medications such as steroids, methotrexate, cyclophosphamide, and cyclosporine are commonly used. In observational data, cyclophosphamide seems to have the highest response rates.[47]

MDS

MDSs are a heterogeneous group of disorders characterized by ineffective hematopoiesis. Amongst types of MDS there is a variable rate of progression to acute myeloid leukemia. The hallmark of the disease is cytopenia, which typically manifests as isolated anemia, anemia in combination with neutropenia or thrombocytopenia, or pancytopenia. Cases in which neutropenia is present are more likely to be caused by refractory anemia with excess blasts than refractory anemia with ringed sideroblasts.[48] Clues to the diagnosis are seen in the peripheral smear in the form of a macrocytic anemia and dysplastic changes in the neutrophils such as Pelger-Huet-like cells and hypogranulation. Diagnosis is confirmed through bone marrow biopsy and reveals a hyperplastic marrow with dysplastic findings in 1 or all lineages.

SUMMARY

Neutropenia is a common reason for a hematology consultation in the outpatient and the inpatient settings. The hematology consultant needs to obtain a full patient history, which includes details about the recent period during which neutropenia occurs, the patient's own history of neutrophil counts, recent changes in medications, and symptoms suggesting potential infections, rheumatologic disorders, or malignancies. Next, the hematology consultant should perform a complete physical examination, which can frequently yield important clues to the cause of the neutropenia. The hematologist provides the critical expertise in assessment of blood morphology through a careful analysis or the peripheral blood smear. Determination of the underlying cause for neutropenia is essential, because some causes such as ethnic neutropenia and CIN carry little risk for infection, whereas others, such as SCN, LGL leukemia, and MDS, are more likely to result in infections. However, data on the management of neutropenia remain scant and additional studies are needed.

REFERENCES

1. Bodey GP, Rodriguez V, Chang HY, et al. Fever and infection in leukemic patients: a study of 494 consecutive patients. Cancer 1978;41:1610–22.
2. Hsieh MM, Everhart JE, Byrd-Holt DD, et al. Prevalence of neutropenia in the U.S. population: age, sex, smoking status, and ethnic differences. Ann Intern Med 2007;146:486–92.
3. Shoenfeld Y, Alkan ML, Asaly A, et al. Benign familial leukopenia and neutropenia in different ethnic groups. Eur J Haematol 1988;41:273–7.
4. Rezvani K, Flanagan AM, Sarma U, et al. Investigation of ethnic neutropenia by assessment of bone marrow colony-forming cells. Acta Haematol 2001;105: 32–7.
5. Horwitz MS, Duan Z, Korkmaz B, et al. Neutrophil elastase in cyclic and severe congenital neutropenia. Blood 2007;109:1817–24.
6. James RM, Kinsey SE. The investigation and management of chronic neutropenia in children. Arch Dis Child 2006;91:852–8.
7. Klein C, Grudzien M, Appaswamy G, et al. HAX1 deficiency causes autosomal recessive severe congenital neutropenia (Kostmann disease). Nat Genet 2007; 39:86–92.
8. Palmblad J, Papadaki HA. Chronic idiopathic neutropenias and severe congenital neutropenia. Curr Opin Hematol 2008;15:8–14.
9. Boztug K, Appaswamy G, Ashikov A, et al. A syndrome with congenital neutropenia and mutations in G6PC3. N Engl J Med 2009;360:32–43.
10. Rosenberg PS, Zeidler C, Bolyard AA, et al. Stable long-term risk of leukaemia in patients with severe congenital neutropenia maintained on G-CSF therapy. Br J Haematol 2010;150:196–9.
11. Welte K, Zeidler C, Dale DC. Severe congenital neutropenia. Semin Hematol 2006;43:189–95.
12. Bux J, Behrens G, Jaeger G, et al. Diagnosis and clinical course of autoimmune neutropenia in infancy: analysis of 240 cases. Blood 1998;91:181–6.

13. Degos L, Faille A, Housset M, et al. Syndrome of neutrophil agranulocytosis, hypogammaglobulinemia, and thymoma. Blood 1982;60:968–72.
14. Chakupurakal G, Murrin RJA, Neilson JR. Prolonged remission of pure white cell aplasia (PWCA), in a patient with CLL, induced by rituximab and maintained by continuous oral cyclosporin. Eur J Haematol 2007;79:271–3.
15. Fumeaux Z, Beris P, Borisch B, et al. Complete remission of pure white cell aplasia associated with thymoma, autoimmune thyroiditis and type 1 diabetes. Eur J Haematol 2003;70:186–9.
16. Levitt LJ, Ries CA, Greenberg PL. Pure white-cell aplasia. N Engl J Med 1983; 308:1141–6.
17. Beyan E, Beyan CG, Turan M. Hematological presentation in systemic lupus erythematosus and its relationship with disease activity. Hematology 2007;12:257–61.
18. Dias AM, Do Couto MC, Duarte CC, et al. White blood cell count abnormalities and infections in one-year follow-up of 124 patients with SLE. Ann N Y Acad Sci 2009;1173:103–7.
19. Nossent J, Swaak A. Prevalence and significance of haematological abnormalities in patients with systemic lupus erythematosus. QJM 1991;80:605–12.
20. Martínez-Baños D, Crispín JC, Lazo-Langner A, et al. Moderate and severe neutropenia in patients with systemic lupus erythematosus. Rheumatology (Oxford) 2006;45:994–8.
21. Courtney PA, Crockard AD, Williamson K, et al. Increased apoptotic peripheral blood neutrophils in systemic lupus erythematosus: relations with disease activity, antibodies to double stranded DNA, and neutropenia. Ann Rheum Dis 1999;58: 309–14.
22. Lorand-Metze I, Carvalho MA, Costallat LT. Morphology of bone marrow in systemic lupus erythematosus. Pathologe 1994;15:292–6.
23. Pereira RM, Velloso ER, Menezes Y, et al. Bone marrow findings in systemic lupus erythematosus patients with peripheral cytopenias. Clin Rheumatol 1998;17: 219–22.
24. Kurien BT, Newland J, Paczkowski C, et al. Association of neutropenia in systemic lupus erythematosus (SLE) with anti-Ro and binding of an immunologically cross-reactive neutrophil membrane antigen. Clin Exp Immunol 2000;120:209–17.
25. Hsieh SC, Yu HS, Lin WW, et al. Anti-SSB/La is one of the antineutrophil autoantibodies responsible for neutropenia and functional impairment of polymorphonuclear neutrophils in patients with systemic lupus erythematosus. Clin Exp Immunol 2003;131:506–16.
26. Vasiliu IM, Petri MA, Baer AN. Therapy with granulocyte colony-stimulating factor in systemic lupus erythematosus may be associated with severe flares. J Rheumatol 2006;33:1878–80.
27. Berliner N, Horwitz M, Loughran TP. Congenital and acquired neutropenia. Hematology Am Soc Hematol Educ Program 2004;63–79.
28. Starkebaum G, Loughran TP, Gaur LK, et al. Immunogenetic similarities between patients with Felty's syndrome and those with clonal expansions of large granular lymphocytes in rheumatoid arthritis. Arthritis Rheum 1997;40:624–6.
29. Newman KA, Akhtari M. Management of autoimmune neutropenia in Felty's syndrome and systemic lupus erythematosus. Autoimmun Rev 2011;10:432–7.
30. Eakin DL, Peake RL, Weiss GB. Effect of therapy on the neutropenia of hyperthyroidism. South Med J 1983;76:335–7, 340.
31. Weitzman SA, Stossel TP, Harmon DC, et al. Antineutrophil autoantibodies in Graves' disease. Implications of thyrotropin binding to neutrophils. J Clin Invest 1985;75:119–23.

32. Stouvroulaki E, Kastranaki M, Pontikoglou C, et al. Mesenchymal stem cells contribute to the abnormal bone marrow microenvironment in patients with chronic idiopathic neutropenia by overproduction of transforming growth factor-β1. Stem Cells Dev 2011;20(8):1309–18.

33. Pyrovolaki K, Mavroudi I, Papadantonakis N, et al. Transforming growth factor-beta1 affects interleukin-10 production in the bone marrow of patients with chronic idiopathic neutropenia. Eur J Haematol 2007;79:531–8.

34. Andres E, Kurtz J, Maloisel F. Nonchemotherapy drug-induced agranulocytosis: experience of the Strasbourg teaching hospital (1985-2000) and review of the literature. Clin Lab Haematol 2002;24:99–106.

35. Andersohn F, Konzen C, Garbe E. Systematic review: agranulocytosis induced by nonchemotherapy drugs. Ann Intern Med 2007;146:657–65.

36. Wolach O, Bairey O, Lahav M. Late-onset neutropenia after rituximab treatment: case series and comprehensive review of the literature. Medicine 2010;89: 308–18.

37. Meynard J, Guiguet M, Arsac S, et al. Frequency and risk factors of infectious complications in neutropenic patients infected with HIV. AIDS 1997;11(8):995–8.

38. Levine AM, Karim R, Mack W, et al. Neutropenia in human immunodeficiency virus infection: data from the women's interagency HIV study. Arch Intern Med 2006;166:405–10.

39. Firnhaber C, Smeaton L, Saukila N, et al. Comparisons of anemia, thrombocytopenia, and neutropenia at initiation of HIV antiretroviral therapy in Africa, Asia, and the Americas. Int J Infect Dis 2010;14:e1088–92.

40. Babadoko AA, Aminu SM, Suleiman AN. Neutropenia and human immunodeficiency virus-1 infection: analysis of 43 cases. Niger J Med 2008;17:57–60.

41. Moore DAJ, Benepal T, Portsmouth S, et al. Etiology and natural history of neutropenia in human immunodeficiency virus disease: a prospective study. Clin Infect Dis 2001;32:469–75.

42. Salmen S, Montes H, Soyano A, et al. Mechanisms of neutrophil death in human immunodeficiency virus-infected patients: role of reactive oxygen species, caspases and map kinase pathways. Clin Exp Immunol 2007;150:539–45.

43. Mauss S, Steinmetz HT, Willers R, et al. Induction of granulocyte colony-stimulating factor by acute febrile infection but not by neutropenia in HIV-seropositive individuals. J Acquir Immune Defic Syndr 1997;14(5):430–4.

44. Kuritzkes DR, Parenti D, Ward DJ, et al. Filgrastim prevents severe neutropenia and reduces infective morbidity in patients with advanced HIV infection: results of a randomized, multicenter, controlled trial. AIDS 1998;12(1):65–74.

45. Dale DC. Neutropenia. In: Encyclopedia of life sciences (eLS). John Wiley; 2001.

46. Bareau B, Rey J, Hamidou M, et al. Analysis of a French cohort of patients with large granular lymphocyte leukemia: a report on 229 cases. Haematologica 2010;95:1534–41.

47. O'Malley DP. T-cell large granular leukemia and related proliferations. Am J Clin Pathol 2007;127:850–9.

48. Juneja SK, Imbert M, Jouault H, et al. Haematological features of primary myelodysplastic syndromes (PMDS) at initial presentation: a study of 118 cases. J Clin Pathol 1983;36:1129–35.

Why Does My Patient Have Erythrocytosis?

Marina Kremyanskaya, MD, PhD[a],*, John Mascarenhas, MD[a],
Ronald Hoffman, MD[b]

KEYWORDS

- Erythrocytosis • Congenital polycythemia • Polycythemia vera
- JAK2^{V617F} • Myeloproliferative neoplasms

The term polycythemia comes from the Greek, meaning too many cells in the blood, and refers to an increase in the red cell mass; it is frequently used interchangeably with the term erythrocytosis. Polycythemia may have several causes, and can be classified as relative or absolute.[1] Relative polycythemia occurs when the patient has a modest increase of the hematocrit level without an increased red cell mass caused by contraction of the plasma volume. Absolute polycythemia is accompanied by an increase in the circulating red cell mass. Red cell production can be influenced by numerous factors including nutrients, growth factors, numbers, and function of marrow progenitor and precursor cells, as well as cellular receptors and transcription factors.[2] The hematopoietic growth factor erythropoietin (EPO) is considered to be the physiologic regulator of the terminal phases of erythropoiesis.[3] Alterations in its production are followed by adjustments in the rate of formation of red blood cells.

Hematocrit values more than 52% in men and more than 48% in women are abnormal and require further investigation into their causes. Polycythemic states can also be divided into primary or secondary polycythemias (**Box 1**). Primary polycythemias are the result of intrinsic abnormalities of the hematopoietic progenitors and stem cells that lead to constitutive overproduction of red cells accompanied by low EPO levels. Secondary polycythemias can be a result of several conditions causing increased EPO production, which acts on normal progenitors to increase the red cell production. These conditions can usually be distinguished by in vitro assays of erythroid progenitor cells, measurement of serum EPO levels, and detection of somatic JAK2 mutations. In a small number of patients, the cause of erythrocytosis cannot be determined, and these patients are classified as having idiopathic erythrocytosis.

Disclosures: None.
[a] Department of Hematology/Oncology, Tisch Cancer Institute, Mount Sinai School of Medicine, One Gustave L. Levy Place, Box 1079, New York, NY 10029, USA
[b] Myeloproliferative Disorders Research Program, Tisch Cancer Institute, Mount Sinai School of Medicine, One Gustave L. Levy Place, Box 1079, New York, NY 10029, USA
* Corresponding author.
E-mail address: marina.kremyanskaya@mountsinai.org

Hematol Oncol Clin N Am 26 (2012) 267–283
doi:10.1016/j.hoc.2012.02.011
0889-8588/12/$ – see front matter © 2012 Elsevier Inc. All rights reserved.

> **Box 1**
> **Differential diagnosis of erythrocytosis**
>
> Secondary polycythemias
>
> > Appropriately increased EPO
> >
> > > Cyanotic heart disease
> > >
> > > Pulmonary disease
> > >
> > > Obstructive sleep apnea
> > >
> > > Pickwickian syndrome
> > >
> > > Smokers' polycythemia, hookah polycythemia
> > >
> > > High altitude
> >
> > Inappropriately Increased EPO
> >
> > > Renal cell carcinoma
> > >
> > > Hepatocellular carcinoma
> > >
> > > Uterine fibroma
> > >
> > > Hemangioblastoma
> > >
> > > Renal lesions (cysts, hydronephrosis)
> > >
> > > Following renal transplantation
> >
> > Drug induced polycythemia
> >
> > Congenital polycythemias
> >
> > > Chuvash polycythemia and abnormalities of O_2 sensing
> > >
> > > Methemoglobinemia
> > >
> > > 2,3-bisphosphoglycerate (BPG) deficiency
>
> Primary polycythemias
>
> > Polycythemia vera (PV)
> >
> > Primary familial and congenital polycythemias (activating mutations of EPO receptor [EPOR] and mutations yet to be determined)

REGULATION OF ERYTHROPOIESIS

The interaction of EPO with EPOR on erythroid progenitor cells leads to its homodimerization, which results in initiation of cell division, differentiation, and prevention of apoptosis of erythroid progenitors and precursors.[4] The cytoplasmic portion of the EPOR contains a positive regulatory domain that interacts with JAK2.[5] On EPO binding, JAK2 phosphorylates itself, EPOR, and other cytoplasmic molecules including STAT5.[6] The JAK2/STAT5 signaling pathway plays an important role in EPOR-mediated regulation of erythropoiesis.

Under normal conditions, EPO production is regulated by the decreased oxygen content of hemoglobin within red cells, resulting in decreased oxygen delivery to the tissues.[7] In response to chronic hypoxia, multiple compensatory mechanisms take place over several days in the kidneys, which is the major site of EPO production.[8] Hypoxia results in the production of hypoxia-inducible factor (HIF) 1, the major factor responsible for transcriptional activation of the EPO gene.[9] HIF-1 is a heterodimeric protein consisting of HIF-1α and HIF-1β. The levels of HIF-1α increase exponentially as the oxygen concentration declines.[10] HIF-1 facilitates body oxygen delivery and responds to oxygen deprivation by regulating gene expression involved in cellular energy metabolism, pH regulation, apoptosis, erythropoiesis and iron metabolism, cell proliferation, and cell-cell and cell-matrix interactions.[11,12]

HIF-1α is constitutively expressed, but it is barely detectable in normal conditions caused by/because of rapid degradation by the ubiquitin-proteosome pathway. In conditions of hypoxia HIF-1α is rapidly accumulated because of the lack of degradation. This mechanism results in instantaneous response to hypoxia. The targeting and subsequent ubiquitination of HIF-1α requires the von Hippel-Lindau protein (VHL), oxygen, and 3 different iron-requiring proline hydroxylase (PHD) enzymes.[13] The proline hydroxylation is required for binding of HIF-1α to VHL. VHL protein is part of a multiprotein ubiquitin ligase capable of ubiquitinating HIF-1α subunits and targeting them for destruction by the proteasome.[14] As oxygen levels decrease, hydroxylation of HIF-1α decreases, and it can no longer bind VHL, thus avoiding degradation.[15] HIF-1α dimerizes with HIF-1β and activates transcription of target genes. The activity of PHDs depends on the availability of oxygen, which makes these enzymes oxygen sensors.[16]

Another protein involved in this pathway is HIF-2α which dimerizes with HIF-1β in hypoxic conditions and activates the transcription of a set of target genes that overlap with the genes targeted by HIF-1α/HIF-1β heterodimers.[17] HIF-1α is expressed by all cell types, whereas HIF-2α is expressed only in specific cell types including vascular endothelial cells, hepatocytes, cardiomyocytes, renal interstitial cells, and astrocytes.

RELATIVE POLYCYTHEMIAS

Patients with moderately increased hematocrit levels that are not necessarily accompanied by an increase in red cell mass are often erroneously assumed to be polycythemic.[18] Relative polycythemia is a term used to describe an increase of the hematocrit level due either to an acute transient state of hemoconcentration associated with intravascular volume depletion or a chronic, sustained, relative polycythemia caused by contraction of the plasma volume. Transient polycythemia may be a result of acute depletion of the plasma volume as a result of protracted vomiting or diarrhea, plasma loss from external burns, or insensible fluid loss caused by fever or diabetic ketoacidosis.

Another example of relative polycythemia is Gaisböck syndrome, which is a benign condition observed mainly in obese, hypertensive, middle-aged, male smokers. These individuals can have a chronic modest increase in their hematocrit levels without increase in their red cell mass.[19] This observation has been attributed to reduced venous compliance.

ABSOLUTE POLYCYTHEMIAS
Primary Familial and Congenital Polycythemias

Primary familial and congenital polycythemias (PFCP) is an autosomal dominant disorder.[20] Unlike patients with PV, patients with PFCP lack splenomegaly and do not progress to myelofibrosis and acute leukemia. They often present with headaches, epistaxis, exertional dyspnea, and dizziness. An increased risk of cardiovascular events and resulting premature morbidity and mortality have been reported in these patients.[21] Although clinical symptoms are resolved with reduction in red cell mass via phlebotomies, the increased risk of cardiovascular events remains. Characteristic laboratory findings are increased hematocrit without associated leukocytosis or thrombocytosis, lack of activating JAK2 mutation, low serum EPO levels, normal hemoglobin-oxygen dissociation curves, and in vitro hypersensitivity of erythroid progenitors to EPO.[22] Between 10% and 20% of patients with PFCP have mutations in EPOR. Additional disease-causing genes and their mutations have yet to be identified.[20]

Secondary Polycythemias

Secondary polycythemias can be either congenital or acquired (see **Box 1**). Conditions leading to hypoxia, such as high altitude, cyanotic heart disease, or chronic lung disease, may result in physiologic polycythemia mediated by increased levels of EPO. There are marked variations in EPO levels and the subsequent erythroid response in the face of chronic hypoxia, suggesting that some of these factors may be genetically determined.

Acquired secondary polycythemias

Polycythemias associated with cyanotic heart disease and pulmonary disease Patients with cyanotic heart disease and pulmonary disease frequently suffer from arterial hypoxemia leading to increased production of EPO and polycythemia. Excessive EPO production occurs when the Pao_2 is sustained at less than 67 mm Hg as a result of severely impaired pulmonary function.[23] Moderate increases of the hematocrit have been estimated to occur in 20% of patients with chronic obstructive pulmonary disease (COPD). Polycythemia in this setting can contribute to pulmonary hypertension, pulmonary endothelial cell dysfunction, reduced cerebral blood flow, and increased risk of venous thromboembolic disease.[24] Increased oxygen-carrying capacity may improve oxygen delivery; however, it is not obvious at what hematocrit level the resultant increase in blood viscosity impairs blood flow to the tissues, leading to a reduction in oxygen uptake.[25]

The treatment of hyperviscosity secondary to erythrocytosis in cyanotic heart disease with prophylactic phlebotomy was once a core therapeutic intervention, but is not considered so today.[26,27] Currently, experts recommend that phlebotomy should be restricted to individuals with symptoms of extreme erythrocytosis (hematocrit >65%) and before surgery to improve hemostasis.[28]

Obstructive sleep apnea–induced polycythemia Obstructive sleep apnea syndrome is characterized by repetitive episodes of partial or complete obstruction of airflow during sleep. Although the evidence is largely anecdotal, secondary polycythemia is a widely recognized complication of long-standing sleep apnea, being found in 5% to 10% of those with nocturnal apnea and hypopnea.[29] Similarly, 25% of those with unexplained polycythemia are subsequently found to have sleep apnea.[30]

Pickwickian syndrome and polycythemia Pickwickian syndrome, or obesity-hypoventilation syndrome, seen in morbidly obese individuals, is characterized by chronic hypoxemia and hypercapnia caused by alveolar hypoventilation, with a resultant increase in EPO production, polycythemia, and cor pulmonale. The 3 principal causes are the high cost of the work of respiration in morbidly obese individuals, dysfunction of the respiratory centers, and repeated episodes of nocturnal obstructive apnea.[31]

Polycythemia caused by high altitude Hypoxic conditions associated with high altitude result in adoptive hyperventilation, alkalosis, and shifting of the O_2 dissociation curve to the left, which leads to impaired oxygen release to the tissues and tissue hypoxia.[32] This hypoxia causes markedly increased EPO production leading to erythrocytosis. Residents of the Andes Mountains who live 4200 m above sea level frequently have 30% higher hematocrit levels than individuals living at sea level.[33] There is evidence of individual variation in response to hypoxia seen both in cyanotic heart and pulmonary disease and in exposure to high altitude, with not all affected individuals generating an appropriate increase in red cell mass. This individual variation suggests that there are genetic determinants underlying the erythropoietic response to hypoxia.[34]

Smokers' polycythemia or carbon monoxide–induced polycythemia Smoking is the most common cause of secondary polycythemia.[35] Those affected have a carboxyhemoglobin-induced increase in red cell mass and/or decrease in plasma volume, either of which is reversible with smoking cessation. Excessive carbon monoxide exposure can also be attributed to exposure to industrial emissions and automobile exhaust. Individuals smoking even 1 pack of cigarettes a day frequently have increased hematocrit levels. These patients characteristically have normal blood gases and increase of carboxyhemoglobin levels. The increase of the hematocrit level is reversed with cessation of smoking. Increased hematocrit levels have been observed in 3% to 5% of heavy smokers. Although these patients do develop thrombotic complications, the rate of thromboembolic events is lower compared with the rate of thromboembolic events in patients with PV.[36] Recently polycythemia was also reported with hookah use, which exposes the user to large amounts of carbon monoxide, resulting in erythrocytosis.[37]

Post–renal transplantation erythrocytosis Post–renal transplantation erythrocytosis (PTE) is defined as a persistently increased hematocrit level greater than 51% after renal transplantation without an increase of the white blood cell count or platelet count. It is found in approximately 10% to 15% of renal allograft recipients. PTE is usually seen 8 to 24 months after a successful renal transplantation. At higher hematocrit levels (usually 60%), thrombotic complications may develop.[38]

Approximately 60% of patients with PTE experience malaise, headache, plethora, lethargy, and dizziness. In addition, from 10% to 20% develop thromboembolic complications involving either arteries or veins. Retention of the native kidney is essential for the development of PTE in most cases.[39] Although the transplanted kidney produces EPO under normal regulatory mechanisms, the native kidney overproduces EPO in spite of the development of erythrocytosis.[40] The PTE frequently resolves with removal of the native kidney. Plasma EPO levels are higher (10-fold) in patients with PTE compared with nonerythrocytotic renal transplant recipients. Treatment of patients with PTE includes intermittent phlebotomy or administration of drugs. The angiotensin-converting enzyme inhibitor enalapril suppresses the renin-angiotensin pathway and virtually eliminates the need for therapeutic phlebotomy in these patients.[41] Therapy is indicated at hematocrit levels of more than 55% with the hope of maintaining hematocrit levels at less than 50% to reduce the risk of thrombosis.

Polycythemia associated with renal and liver disorders and neoplasms Polycythemia has been reported to be associated with renal cell carcinoma, Wilms tumor, polycystic kidney disease, renal artery stenosis, hydronephrosis, paragangliomas, and pituitary adenomas. Renal tumors account for one-third of cases of tumor-associated polycythemia. Tumor tissues produce excessive amounts of EPO[42] and tumor resection results in correction of erythrocytosis. Polycythemia has also been described in association with hepatocellular carcinomas in 2% to 10% of patients.[43] Cerebellar hemangioblastomas and large uterine fibromas are also associated with polycythemia.[44]

Drug-induced erythrocytosis and polycythemia in endocrine disorders The long-term administration of EPO, corticosteroids, or androgens can be associated with reversible erythrocytosis. Polycythemia can also be associated with Cushing syndrome, acromegaly, and primary aldosteronism.[45] It is also observed in older men receiving long-term androgen replacement therapy and in significant numbers of athletes taking anabolic steroids.[46,47]

Androgens have been shown to stimulate EPO production and to directly affect erythroid progenitor cells. Blood doping refers to the use of EPO to increase red cell mass in athletes, thus increasing oxygen delivery in the hope of increasing endurance.

Congenital secondary polycythemias

High-oxygen-affinity hemoglobins and bisphosphoglycerate (BPG) deficiency There are more than a 100 mutations in the hemoglobin genes leading to increased affinity for oxygen and thus decreased oxygen delivery, resulting in compensatory erythrocytosis (**Table 1**).[48] These mutations are usually well tolerated in younger patients, but older patients may develop thrombotic complications. These high-affinity hemoglobin mutations are transmitted in autosomal dominant fashion. Phlebotomy therapy for these patients has not been shown to have any clinical benefit and may be detrimental with decreased exercise tolerance and anaerobic threshold.

Table 1
Congenital polycythemias

Specific Conditions	Method of Transmission and Relevant Clinical Presentations	Specific Genes Involved
Alterations in hemoglobin oxygen affinity		
High O$_2$ affinity hemoglobin mutants	Autosomal dominant Patients usually asymptomatic	Mutations of both a and b globin genes
2,3 BPG deficiency	Unclear	Deficiency of red cell enzyme bisphosphoglyceromutase
Congenital methemoglobinemia	Autosomal recessive Most patients are asymptomatic. May have blue color of the skin and mucous membranes (cyanotic)	Deficiency of cytochrome b5 reductase Hemoglobin M disease
Alterations in hypoxia sensing		
Chuvash polycythemia mutations in VHL gene	Autosomal recessive High hemoglobin levels, increased EPO levels, varicose veins, vertebral hemangiomas, hypotension. High morbidity and mortality from thrombotic and hemorrhagic complications	Mutations in VHL gene
Proline hydroxylase 2 (PHD2) gene mutation	Autosomal dominant Increased EPO levels	PHD2 gene mutations
Hypoxia-inducible factor 2 gene mutation	Autosomal dominant	HIF-2 gene mutations
Polycythemias with undefined defects		
PFCP	Autosomal dominant	Activating mutations in EPOR only in 10%–20% of patients

A rare cause of congenital polycythemia is 2,3-BPG deficiency.[49] It is synthesized in the red blood cells and acts by reducing hemoglobin's affinity for oxygen. Its absence leads to higher oxygen affinity and results in hypoxic stimulus and erythrocytosis.

HIF pathway mutations Mutations in several proteins in the HIF pathway have been shown to lead to increased EPO production and erythrocytosis (see **Table 1**).[50] Chuvash polycythemia (CP) is one of the best-known examples. CP is an autosomal recessive disorder associated with germline mutations in VHL, and is endemic in the Chuvash population of the Russian republic.[51] A homozygous, missense mutation in the VHL gene (VHL598C → T) has been identified in patients with CP.[52] This disorder is characterized by high hemoglobin levels, usually more than 20 g/dL, increased EPO levels, varicose veins, vertebral hemangiomas, and low blood pressure.[53] The defective VHL gene product is not capable of promoting ubiquitin-mediated degradation of HIF-1α and HIF-2α, leading to their increased levels and thus increased production of EPO. Several similar types of mutations have been described in the VHL gene and have been found in a variety of other ethnic groups.[54] CP is associated with high mortality caused by thrombotic and hemorrhagic vascular complications.

A mutation in the proline hydroxylase gene PHD2 (P317R) has been described in a family with autosomal dominant erythrocytosis (see **Table 1**). The mutated protein fails to cause degradation of HIF-1α and results in increased EPO levels and erythrocytosis.[55]

A series of HIF-2α gain-of-function mutations have also been reported to lead to familial erythrocytosis. These patients present with congenital erythrocytosis and with increased or inappropriately normal EPO levels.[17]

Polycythemia vera (PV)

Introduction and epidemiology
PV is a chronic, clonal, progressive, myeloproliferative neoplasm (MPN) characterized by absolute increase in red cell mass, as well as splenomegaly, leukocytosis, and thrombocytosis. PV is the most common primary polycythemia, with reported incidences of 2.8 per 100,000 persons per year.[56,57] The prevalence of PV has been reported to be higher among Ashkenazi Jews and lower among African Americans.[58] Extremely low occurrence rates have been reported from Japan.[59] These findings suggest the importance of genetic factors in the pathogenesis of this disease. This importance is further emphasized by reports of multiple cases of MPN including PV in multiple generations of several families.[60] In a large population study reported from Sweden, it was estimated that the first-degree relatives of patients with MPN have a 5-fold to 7-fold increased risk of developing an MPN.[61] Higher incidence of PV has been reported in individuals exposed to the atomic bomb explosion in Japan, which is a notable exception to the overall low rate of PV in Japan. Increased incidence of PV has also been reported in workers in petroleum refineries and chemical plants.[62] Environmental triggers have been further implicated after a description of a cluster of patients with JAK2V617F-positive PV in an area of eastern Pennsylvania that contained numerous sources of hazardous materials.[63] Slightly more men than women develop PV, with a male/female ratio of approximately 1.2:1. The average age at diagnosis is 60 years; in several large studies, 5% of patients were younger than 40 years of age. PV has been reported to present in childhood in a small number of patients.[64]

Pathobiology
The expanded red cell mass in PV is a result of a 2-fold to 3-fold increase in the production of red cells by a hyperplastic marrow. Granulocyte and platelet production is also increased in this disorder. Various methods have been used since the

mid-1970s to show that PV is a result of clonal proliferation of neoplastic hematopoietic stem cells, and is not a consequence of excessive proliferation of normal hematopoietic stem cells.[65,66]

From the knowledge that red cell production in PV is not associated with excessive EPO production, it was hypothesized that erythroid progenitor cells in this disorder are no longer subject to physiologic regulators. PV bone marrow can form erythroid colonies termed endogenous colonies in vitro in the absence of exogenous EPO, whereas normal bone marrow is incapable of forming such colonies without the addition of EPO.[67,68]

JAK2^{V617F} mutation and other JAK2 mutations in Polycythemia vera (PV)

The genetic defect associated with PV was a focus of intense research by numerous groups. In 2005, JAK2 from hematopoietic cells of patients with PV was directly sequenced by Vainchenker and colleagues[69] in France and a single recurrent point mutation was discovered. A guanine-to-thymine mutation was observed that resulted in a substitution of valine to phenylalanine at codon 617 within the pseudokinase domain (JH2) of Janus kinase 2 (JAK2^{V617F}). These findings were rapidly confirmed by several other groups.[70–72] Analysis of germline DNA showed that JAK2^{V617F} is an acquired somatic mutation present exclusively in hematopoietic cells.[73] Using quantitative polymerase chain reaction, patients can be classed as having a low allele burden of JAK2^{V617F} (<50%) or a high allele burden of JAK2^{V617F} (>50%). A subset of patients with PV is homozygous for JAK2^{V617F}, which was shown to be the result of mitotic recombination and duplication of the mutant allele. The occurrence of this mitotic recombination event has been observed during the clinical course of individual patients, with heterozygous patients becoming homozygous over the course of their disease.

The mutational frequency of JAK2^{V617F} is more than 95% in patients with PV, and 50% to 60% in patients with essential thrombocythemia (ET) and primary myelofibrosis (PMF).[74] ET is usually associated with a low allele burden of JAK2^{V617F}.

Other mutations in JAK2 have also been shown to be associated with erythrocytosis. Several gain-of-function mutations in exon 12 of the JAK2 gene, adjacent to the pseudokinase domain, have been identified in 2.5% to 3.4% of patients with PV, and in 30% of patients who have JAK2^{V617F}-negative PV.[75] JAK2 exon 12 mutations have not been reported in patients with ET or PMF. Patients with exon 12 mutations can develop thrombotic events and can also evolve into post-PV myelofibrosis (MF) and acute leukemia.

Clinical manifestations of polycythemia vera (PV)

The principal clinical manifestations of PV can be attributed to the excessive production of cells of myeloid lineage affected by the malignant clone. Symptomatic patients can present with a myriad of generalized symptoms, such as weakness, dizziness, pruritus, headaches, visual disturbances, excessive sweating, abdominal discomfort, weight loss, and thrombotic or hemorrhagic episodes. Thrombosis is a frequent presenting event with two-thirds of these episodes occurring either at presentation or before diagnosis.[76] The principal findings on physical examination of a patient with PV include ruddy cyanosis, conjunctival plethora, hepatomegaly, splenomegaly, and hypertension. Untreated patients are at a particularly high risk for thrombotic complications. Arterial thrombotic events account for two-thirds of these episodes, with transient ischemic attacks, ischemic strokes, and myocardial infarctions being the most frequent complications.[77,78] The cumulative rate of thrombosis ranges from 2.5% to 5% per patient per year. It is usual for these patients to develop thrombosis in unusual sites, such as splanchnic veins including hepatic, splenic, or mesenteric vessels, or in a cerebral sinus. Budd-Chiari syndrome is one of the most serious thrombotic complications of PV, and results from hepatic venous or inferior vena cava thrombosis and can culminate in the development of liver cirrhosis.[79] Patients can present with portal or hepatic vein thrombosis and have normal values of hemoglobin and hematocrit.[80] They often have leukocytosis, increased platelet count, and splenomegaly. Screening for JAK2[V617F] mutation should be performed in these patients.[81] In patients with splanchnic vein thrombosis who are JAK2[V617F] negative, a bone marrow biopsy should be performed to assess for a JAK2[V617F]-negative MPN.[82] In these patients, gastrointestinal bleeding or increased plasma volume caused by splenomegaly may be responsible for normal hematocrit.

PV can often present with symptoms of peripheral vascular disease, such as intense redness or cyanosis of the digits, classic erythromelalgia, digital ischemia with normal pulses, or thrombophlebitis. Erythromelalgia is described as a sensation of burning pain and increased temperature in the digits. PV is the most common cause of erythromelalgia, and is one of the few disorders in which digital ischemia exists in the presence of palpable pulses.[83] Foot pain at rest is another distressing symptom of PV. The pain is most severe at night and is dull in nature. These symptoms have been shown to be a result of platelet aggregation and activation in vivo, which preferentially occurs in arterioles.[84] Phlebotomy alone does not relieve erythromelalgia. These symptoms can be abolished by reducing the platelet counts to normal levels. Symptoms also improve with antiplatelet therapy.[85]

Neurologic abnormalities can occur in up to 60% to 80% of untreated or poorly controlled patients with PV and include transient ischemic attacks, cerebral ischemia, cerebral hemorrhage, fluctuating dementia, and confusion.[86] In addition, symptoms of dizziness, visual disturbances, tinnitus, paresthesias, and headaches are commonly reported. These symptoms are attributed to increased blood viscosity and reduced cerebral blood flow caused by erythrocytosis.[87]

Patients with PV have greater than expected incidence of pulmonary hypertension.[88] Possible mechanisms include extramedullary hematopoiesis in lung parenchyma, direct obstruction of pulmonary vessels by circulating megakaryocytes, smooth muscle hyperplasia induced by release of platelet-derived growth factor from activated platelets, and recurrent thrombotic events.

Up to 30% to 40% of patients with PV experience some type of hemorrhagic event, ranging from inconsequential epistaxis or gingival bleeding to life-threatening gastrointestinal hemorrhages.[89]

Patients with PV undergoing a surgical procedure are at high risk of developing postoperative complications. Complications can be caused by thrombosis or hemorrhage.[90] A retrospective study by an Italian group evaluated 311 surgical interventions in 105 patients with PV and 150 with ET: 24 arterial or venous thrombosis (7.7%), 23 major hemorrhages (7.3%), and 5 surgery-related deaths (1.6%) were observed within 3 months of the procedure. Patients with PV with uncontrolled erythrocytosis before surgery have the highest rate of complications after surgery. These complications can be greatly reduced by achieving normalization of blood counts before surgery. The risk seems to be even lower in patients who achieved long-term blood count control before surgery.

Generalized pruritus occurs in 40% of patients. Water contact such as during a shower or bath can induce attacks of intolerable pruritus.[91] The degree of pruritus has no correlation with severity of disease and 20% of patients continue to experience severe pruritus despite adequate control of their blood counts.

There have been reports of patients with PV suffering nonhematologic complications of iron deficiency. However, there is no convincing evidence that undue fatigue caused by iron deficiency occurs in patients with normal or increased hematocrit levels.[92] These patients do not experience esophageal changes or dysphagia that is known to be associated with chronic iron deficiency.

The risk of development of post-PV MF increases with prolonged duration of disease and should be considered the natural evolution of disease.[77] For patients with disease duration greater than 10 years, the hazard ratio was reported to be 15.24 (95% confidence interval 4.22–55.06, $P<.0001$). The median interval between diagnosis of PV and development of post-PV MF is 13 years.[93] Post-PV MF is characterized by increasing splenomegaly, leukoerythroblastic characteristics on peripheral blood smear review (tear drop morphology of red cells, nucleated red cells), development of extensive bone marrow fibrosis, and normal or decreased red cell mass. The patients can complain of fatigue, dizziness, and weight loss. Splenomegaly can lead to abdominal pain and early satiety. Patients with post-PV MF are virtually all JAK2[V617F] positive and have high JAK2[V617F] allele burden.

The median survival for patients with post-PV MF is 5.7 years and these patients are at high risk of developing acute leukemia.[94] Eighteen percent of patients with post-PV MF undergo leukemic transformation after 3 years. Patients with hemoglobin of less than 10 g/dL, platelet count less than 100×10^9/L, and white blood cell counts more than 30×10^9/L have a poorer prognosis than patients who have fewer of these prognostic factors.

Differential diagnosis
The first step in establishing the cause of erythrocytosis is to confirm that it is absolute erythrocytosis. A hematocrit level greater than 60% on several occasions in men or greater than 55% in women is associated with an increased red cell mass in virtually every case. Documentation of an absolute increase in red cell mass by direct measurement is rarely required and this test is now available in few institutions.

Initially, it is important to differentiate PV from other causes of secondary erythrocytosis (see **Box 1**). Characteristically, the patient with PV presents with erythrocytosis, leukocytosis, thrombocytosis, splenomegaly, and positivity for JAK2[V617F]. The bone marrow biopsy shows hypercellularity with trilineage hyperplasia. In patients with only some of the characteristics listed earlier, it is important to determine the arterial oxygen saturation using an arterial blood gas and the carboxyhemoglobin level to rule out smokers polycythemia. The $P_{50}O_2$ should be established in patients with other family members with erythrocytosis to exclude congenital disorders with high-oxygen-affinity hemoglobins leading to tissue hypoxia and erythrocytosis. A Pao_2 greater than 67 mm Hg or an O_2 saturation greater than 95% on an arterial blood gas helps to rule out hypoxic conditions that lead to erythrocytosis. Other essential tests are serum EPO levels, the ability of bone marrow cells to form erythroid colonies in the absence of exogenous EPO, and JAK2[V617F] determination. Increase of EPO levels with erythrocytosis indicates a hypoxic cause of secondary erythrocytosis, whereas extremely low levels of EPO (<4 mIU/mL) are virtually diagnostic of PV.

Clinical criteria for diagnosis of PV have been defined by the World Health Organization (WHO) and include molecular testing for JAK2 mutations and histopathologic parameters (**Box 2**).[95] Individual patients may not meet the diagnostic criteria for PV as defined by WHO, but may clearly have a PV-like MPN.

Patients with isolated erythrocytosis who are negative for JAK2[V617F] mutation and JAK2 exon 12 mutation can present a diagnostic dilemma. The familial congenital form of polycythemia caused by truncation of the EPOR, characterized by increased sensitivity of erythroid progenitor cells to EPO, can be easily distinguished from PV. These patients frequently present in childhood, have a strong family history, and

---

Box 2
The 2008 WHO diagnostic criteria for PV

Diagnosis requires meeting both major criteria and 1 minor criterion or the first major criterion and 2 minor criteria

Major criteria

1. Hemoglobin >18.5 g/dL in men, 16.5 g/dL in women, or other evidence of increased red cell volume[a]

2. Presence of JAK2[V617F] or other functionally similar mutation such as JAK2 exon 12

Minor criteria

1. Bone marrow biopsy showing hypercellularity for age with trilineage growth with prominent erythroid, granulocytic, and megakaryocytic proliferation

2. Serum EPO level less than the reference range for normal

3. Endogenous erythroid colonies formation in vitro

[a] Hemoglobin or hematocrit greater than the 99th percentile of method-specific reference range for age, sex, altitude of residence, or hemoglobin greater than 17 g/dL in men and 15 g/dL in women if associated with a documented and sustained increase of at least 2 g/dL from an individual's baseline value that cannot be attributed to correction of iron deficiency, or increased red cell mass greater than 25% more than the mean normal predicted value.

Data from Tefferi A, Thiele J, Orazi A, et al. Proposals and rationale for revision of the World Health Organization diagnostic criteria for polycythemia vera, essential thrombocythemia, and primary myelofibrosis: From an ad hoc international expert panel. Blood 2007;110:1092–7.

---

this disorder is characterized by isolated erythrocytosis. In contrast with PV, the marrow progenitor cells are hypersensitive to EPO, but no colonies form in the absence of EPO.[96] Other patients with isolated erythrocytosis who are negative for JAK2[V617F] mutation and JAK2 exon 12 mutations and do not fulfill criteria for other acquired causes of erythrocytosis should be evaluated for mutations in the hypoxia-responsive element of the human EPO gene, HIF-1a, HIF-2a, VHL, PHD1,2,3, STAT5, LNK, and TET2.[50] Some of these tests can be performed by commercial laboratories, but most require contacting an academic reference laboratory.

PV must also be distinguished from other MPNs, such as chronic myeloid leukemia (CML), ET, and PMF because it has important prognostic distinctions and different therapeutic options. With the distinctive cytogenetic and molecular abnormality (BCR-ABL) associated with CML, these 2 disorders should be easy to differentiate.

Therapy

Cumulative duration of survival for patients with PV treated with modern strategies is reported to be 15 to 17 years.[93,97] The mortality of patients with PV is increased by 1.84 compared with sex-matched and age-matched controls. The goal of therapy is to normalize blood counts to minimize the risk of thrombotic events.[98] In addition, therapy is stratified based on the perceived baseline risk for thrombosis, with low-risk patients treated with phlebotomy plus an antiplatelet agent.[99] High-risk patients are additionally treated with some form of myelosuppressive therapy.[100] The current therapeutic goal is to reduce hematocrit to 45% in men and 42% in women, although the relationship between keeping the hematocrit at less than this target and clinical outcomes is still a matter of debate.

Low-risk patients with PV are defined as patients less than 60 years of age, without any prior history of thrombosis, with platelet count less than 1.5×10^6.[101] These low-risk patients should be treated with low-dose aspirin (81 mg daily) and phlebotomy to maintain hematocrit targets as described earlier. Aspirin should be avoided in patients with history of hemorrhagic episodes, acquired Von Willebrand syndrome, and extreme thrombocytosis. Patients who develop thrombosis or hemorrhage, painful splenomegaly, refractory pruritus, or other systemic symptoms should be offered additional therapy. Pegylated interferon or interferon α is often used as first-line therapy if available and tolerated. More than 80% of patients on interferon achieve hematologic response with normalization of their blood counts, and up to 20% of patients treated with pegylated interferon achieve molecular remission as well.[102] Patients also benefit from reduction in splenomegaly and pruritus. If interferon is not available or not tolerated, anagrelide can be used to control platelet count.[103] If patients continue to have thrombotic events or worsening splenomegaly, hydroxyurea therapy should be considered. If the disease is not controlled with adequate doses of hydroxyurea (2–3 g daily), busulfan can be considered as the next line of treatment.

High-risk patients are defined as patients more than 60 years of age or patients with previous history of thrombotic or hemorrhagic events. These patients should be placed on low-dose aspirin, phlebotomy, and myelosuppressive therapy. Presently, hydroxyurea is considered first-line therapy.[93] If patients are intolerant or resistant to hydroxyurea, interferon can be considered as the next line of treatment. Randomized clinical trials comparing hydroxyurea versus pegylated interferon as first-line treatment of patients with high-risk PV are ongoing.

A great deal of interest has been generated lately by the development of oral JAK inhibitors in the treatment of MPN. In November of 2011, the US Food and Drug Administration approved ruxolitinib (a JAK1 and JAK2 inhibitor) for use in patients with MF. Several JAK inhibitors have also been evaluated for the treatment of PV and ET. Phlebotomy independence and spleen reduction were observed as well as alleviation of pruritus and other systemic symptoms. However, no reduction in JAK2^{V617F} allele burden was noted. At present time, the role of JAK inhibitors in PV seems to be limited, but they may be useful in specific circumstances, such as intractable pruritus or massive splenomegaly in patients who are resistant to, or intolerant of, standard agents.[104]

SUMMARY

Polycythemia is defined as hematocrit of more than 48% in women and 52% in men.

- Relative polycythemia is an increase in hematocrit without an increase in red cell mass. It is usually caused by an acute state of hemoconcentration.
- Accurate history and careful physical examination are essential to determine the cause of erythrocytosis. Many causes of secondary erythrocytosis can be elucidated from history (drug use, pulmonary disease, living at high altitude, smoking, family history). Splenomegaly is commonly found in patients with PV.
- Low serum EPO level strongly suggests the diagnosis of PV. High EPO level indicates secondary polycythemia and rules out PV.
- If PV is a likely diagnosis, molecular testing for JAK2 mutations should be performed.
- PV is a chronic clonal progressive MPN with high risk of thrombotic and hemorrhagic complications.
- The goal of therapy for PV is to reduce the risk of thrombotic complications. Patients with low-risk disease are treated with low-risk aspirin and phlebotomy for a goal hematocrit of 42% in women and 45% in men. Patients with high-risk disease are treated with myelosuppressive therapy in addition to aspirin and phlebotomy.
- Patients with PV are at high risk of developing post-PV MF and acute leukemia.

REFERENCES

1. Messinezy M, Westwood NB, El-Hemaidi I, et al. Serum erythropoietin values in erythrocytoses and in primary thrombocythaemia. Br J Haematol 2002;117: 47–53.
2. Adamson JW. The erythropoietin-hematocrit relationship in normal and polycythemic man: implications of marrow regulation. Blood 1968;32:597–609.
3. Zanjani ED, Ascensao JL. Erythropoietin. Transfusion 1989;29:46–57.
4. Ebert BL, Bunn HF. Regulation of the erythropoietin gene. Blood 1999;94: 1864–77.
5. Khwaja A. The role of Janus kinases in haemopoiesis and haematological malignancy. Br J Haematol 2006;134:366–84.
6. Witthuhn BA, Quelle FW, Silvennoinen O, et al. JAK2 associates with the erythropoietin receptor and is tyrosine phosphorylated and activated following stimulation with erythropoietin. Cell 1993;74:227–36.
7. Krantz SB. Erythropoietin. Blood 1991;77:419–34.
8. Donnelly S. Why is erythropoietin made in the kidney? The kidney functions as a critmeter. Am J Kidney Dis 2001;38:415–25.
9. Semenza GL, Wang GL. A nuclear factor induced by hypoxia via de novo protein synthesis binds to the human erythropoietin gene enhancer at a site required for transcriptional activation. Mol Cell Biol 1992;12:5447–54.
10. Semenza GL. Involvement of oxygen-sensing pathways in physiologic and pathologic erythropoiesis. Blood 2009;114:2015–9.
11. Semenza GL, Jiang BH, Leung SW, et al. Hypoxia response elements in the aldolase A, enolase 1, and lactate dehydrogenase A gene promoters contain essential binding sites for hypoxia-inducible factor 1. J Biol Chem 1996;271: 32529–37.
12. Carmeliet P, Dor Y, Herbert JM, et al. Role of HIF-1alpha in hypoxia-mediated apoptosis, cell proliferation and tumour angiogenesis. Nature 1998;394:485–90.
13. Kaelin WG Jr. The von Hippel-Lindau protein, HIF hydroxylation, and oxygen sensing. Biochem Biophys Res Commun 2005;338:627–38.
14. Maxwell PH, Wiesener MS, Chang GW, et al. The tumour suppressor protein VHL targets hypoxia-inducible factors for oxygen-dependent proteolysis. Nature 1999;399:271–5.
15. Ivan M, Kondo K, Yang H, et al. HIFalpha targeted for VHL-mediated destruction by proline hydroxylation: implications for O_2 sensing. Science 2001;292:464–8.
16. McDonough MA, Li V, Flashman E, et al. Cellular oxygen sensing: crystal structure of hypoxia-inducible factor prolyl hydroxylase (PHD2). Proc Natl Acad Sci U S A 2006;103:9814–9.
17. Formenti F, Beer PA, Croft QP, et al. Cardiopulmonary function in two human disorders of the hypoxia-inducible factor (HIF) pathway: von Hippel-Lindau disease and HIF-2alpha gain-of-function mutation. FASEB J 2011;25:2001–11.
18. Weinreb NJ, Shih CF. Spurious polycythemia. Semin Hematol 1975;12:397–407.
19. Biswas M, Prakash PK, Cossburn M, et al. Life-threatening thrombotic complications of relative polycythaemia. J Intern Med 2003;253:481–3.
20. Huang LJ, Shen YM, Bulut GB. Advances in understanding the pathogenesis of primary familial and congenital polycythaemia. Br J Haematol 2010;148:844–52.
21. Prchal JT, Sokol L. "Benign erythrocytosis" and other familial and congenital polycythemias. Eur J Haematol 1996;57:263–8.
22. Sokol L, Prchal J, Prchal JT. Primary familial and congenital polycythaemia. Lancet 1993;342:115–6.

23. Kent BD, Mitchell PD, McNicholas WT. Hypoxemia in patients with COPD: cause, effects, and disease progression. Int J Chron Obstruct Pulmon Dis 2011;6:199–208.
24. Boyer L, Chaar V, Pelle G, et al. Effects of polycythemia on systemic endothelial function in chronic hypoxic lung disease. J Appl Physiol 2011;110:1196–203.
25. Thorne SA. Management of polycythaemia in adults with cyanotic congenital heart disease. Heart 1998;79:315–6.
26. Trojnarska O, Plaskota K. Therapeutic methods used in patients with Eisenmenger syndrome. Cardiol J 2009;16:500–6.
27. DeFilippis AP, Law K, Curtin S, et al. Blood is thicker than water: the management of hyperviscosity in adults with cyanotic heart disease. Cardiol Rev 2007;15:31–4.
28. Spence MS, Balaratnam MS, Gatzoulis MA. Clinical update: cyanotic adult congenital heart disease. Lancet 2007;370:1530–2.
29. Carlson JT, Hedner J, Fagerberg B, et al. Secondary polycythaemia associated with nocturnal apnoea–a relationship not mediated by erythropoietin? J Intern Med 1992;231:381–7.
30. Moore-Gillon JC, Treacher DF, Gaminara EJ, et al. Intermittent hypoxia in patients with unexplained polycythaemia. Br Med J (Clin Res Ed) 1986;293:588–90.
31. Weitzenblum E, Kessler R, Chaouat A. Alveolar hypoventilation in the obese: the obesity-hypoventilation syndrome. Rev Pneumol Clin 2002;58:83–90 [in French].
32. Penaloza D, Arias-Stella J. The heart and pulmonary circulation at high altitudes: healthy highlanders and chronic mountain sickness. Circulation 2007;115:1132–46.
33. Leon-Velarde F, Gamboa A, Chuquiza JA, et al. Hematological parameters in high altitude residents living at 4,355, 4,660, and 5,500 meters above sea level. High Alt Med Biol 2000;1:97–104.
34. Lorenzo VF, Yang Y, Simonson TS, et al. Genetic adaptation to extreme hypoxia: study of high-altitude pulmonary edema in a three-generation Han Chinese family. Blood Cells Mol Dis 2009;43:221–5.
35. Aitchison R, Russell N. Smoking–a major cause of polycythaemia. J R Soc Med 1988;81:89–91.
36. Schwarcz TH, Hogan LA, Endean ED, et al. Thromboembolic complications of polycythemia: polycythemia vera versus smokers' polycythemia. J Vasc Surg 1993;17:518–22 [discussion: 522–3].
37. Tadmor T, Mishchenko E, Polliack A, et al. Hookah (narghile) smoking: a new emerging cause of secondary polycythemia. Am J Hematol 2011;86:719–20.
38. Kessler M, Hestin D, Mayeux D, et al. Factors predisposing to post-renal transplant erythrocytosis. A prospective matched-pair control study. Clin Nephrol 1996;45:83–9.
39. Vlahakos DV, Marathias KP, Agroyannis B, et al. Posttransplant erythrocytosis. Kidney Int 2003;63:1187–94.
40. Marinella MA. Hematologic abnormalities following renal transplantation. Int Urol Nephrol 2010;42:151–64.
41. Danovitch GM, Jamgotchian NJ, Eggena PH, et al. Angiotensin-converting enzyme inhibition in the treatment of renal transplant erythrocytosis. Clinical experience and observation of mechanism. Transplantation 1995;60:132–7.
42. Wiesener MS, Seyfarth M, Warnecke C, et al. Paraneoplastic erythrocytosis associated with an inactivating point mutation of the von Hippel-Lindau gene in a renal cell carcinoma. Blood 2002;99:3562–5.
43. Matsuyama M, Yamazaki O, Horii K, et al. Erythrocytosis caused by an erythropoietin-producing hepatocellular carcinoma. J Surg Oncol 2000;75:197–202.
44. Kuhne M, Sidler D, Hofer S, et al. Challenging manifestations of malignancies. Case 1. Polycythemia and high serum erythropoietin level as a result of hemangioblastoma. J Clin Oncol 2004;22:3639–40.

45. Zoppoli G, Bianchi F, Bruzzone A, et al. Polycythemia as rare secondary direct manifestation of acromegaly: management and single-centre epidemiological data. Pituitary 2011. [Epub ahead of print].

46. Dickerman RD, Pertusi R, Miller J, et al. Androgen-induced erythrocytosis: is it erythropoietin? Am J Hematol 1999;61:154–5.

47. Hajjar RR, Kaiser FE, Morley JE. Outcomes of long-term testosterone replacement in older hypogonadal males: a retrospective analysis. J Clin Endocrinol Metab 1997;82:3793–6.

48. Wajcman H, Galacteros F. Hemoglobins with high oxygen affinity leading to erythrocytosis. New variants and new concepts. Hemoglobin 2005;29:91–106.

49. Galacteros F, Rosa R, Prehu MO, et al. Diphosphoglyceromutase deficiency: new cases associated with erythrocytosis. Nouv Rev Fr Hematol 1984;26:69–74 [in French].

50. McMullin MF. HIF pathway mutations and erythrocytosis. Expert Rev Hematol 2010;3:93–101.

51. Sergeyeva A, Gordeuk VR, Tokarev YN, et al. Congenital polycythemia in Chuvashia. Blood 1997;89:2148–54.

52. Ang SO, Chen H, Gordeuk VR, et al. Endemic polycythemia in Russia: mutation in the VHL gene. Blood Cells Mol Dis 2002;28:57–62.

53. Gordeuk VR, Sergueeva AI, Miasnikova GY, et al. Congenital disorder of oxygen sensing: association of the homozygous Chuvash polycythemia VHL mutation with thrombosis and vascular abnormalities but not tumors. Blood 2004;103: 3924–32.

54. Percy MJ, McMullin MF, Jowitt SN, et al. Chuvash-type congenital polycythemia in 4 families of Asian and western European ancestry. Blood 2003;102:1097–9.

55. Albiero E, Ruggeri M, Fortuna S, et al. Isolated erythrocytosis: study of 67 patients and identification of three novel germ-line mutations in the prolyl hydroxylase domain protein 2 (PHD2) gene. Haematologica 2012;97:123–7.

56. Kutti J, Ridell B. Epidemiology of the myeloproliferative disorders: essential thrombocythaemia, polycythaemia vera and idiopathic myelofibrosis. Pathol Biol (Paris) 2001;49:164–6.

57. Johansson P, Kutti J, Andreasson B, et al. Trends in the incidence of chronic Philadelphia chromosome negative (Ph−) myeloproliferative disorders in the city of Goteborg, Sweden, during 1983-99. J Intern Med 2004;256:161–5.

58. Chaiter Y, Brenner B, Aghai E, et al. High incidence of myeloproliferative disorders in Ashkenazi Jews in northern Israel. Leuk Lymphoma 1992;7:251–5.

59. Kurita S. Epidemiological studies of polycythemia vera in Japan (author's translation). Nihon Ketsueki Gakkai Zasshi 1974;37:793–5 [in Japanese].

60. Lawrence JH, Goetsch AT. Familial occurrence of polycythemia and leukemia. Calif Med 1950;73:361–4.

61. Landgren O, Goldin LR, Kristinsson SY, et al. Increased risks of polycythemia vera, essential thrombocythemia, and myelofibrosis among 24,577 first-degree relatives of 11,039 patients with myeloproliferative neoplasms in Sweden. Blood 2008;112:2199–204.

62. Marsh GM, Enterline PE, McCraw D. Mortality patterns among petroleum refinery and chemical plant workers. Am J Ind Med 1991;19:29–42.

63. Seaman V, Jumaan A, Yanni E, et al. Use of molecular testing to identify a cluster of patients with polycythemia vera in eastern Pennsylvania. Cancer Epidemiol Biomarkers Prev 2009;18:534–40.

64. Danish EH, Rasch CA, Harris JW. Polycythemia vera in childhood: case report and review of the literature. Am J Hematol 1980;9:421–8.

65. Adamson JW, Fialkow PJ, Murphy S, et al. Polycythemia vera: stem-cell and probable clonal origin of the disease. N Engl J Med 1976;295:913–6.

66. Gilliland DG, Blanchard KL, Levy J, et al. Clonality in myeloproliferative disorders: analysis by means of the polymerase chain reaction. Proc Natl Acad Sci U S A 1991;88:6848–52.

67. Zanjani ED, Lutton JD, Hoffman R, et al. Erythroid colony formation by polycythemia vera bone marrow in vitro. Dependence on erythropoietin. J Clin Invest 1977;59:841–8.

68. Ash RC, Detrick RA, Zanjani ED. In vitro studies of human pluripotential hematopoietic progenitors in polycythemia vera. Direct evidence of stem cell involvement. J Clin Invest 1982;69:1112–8.

69. James C, Ugo V, Le Couedic JP, et al. A unique clonal JAK2 mutation leading to constitutive signalling causes polycythaemia vera. Nature 2005;434:1144–8.

70. Levine RL, Wadleigh M, Cools J, et al. Activating mutation in the tyrosine kinase JAK2 in polycythemia vera, essential thrombocythemia, and myeloid metaplasia with myelofibrosis. Cancer Cell 2005;7:387–97.

71. Kralovics R, Passamonti F, Buser AS, et al. A gain-of-function mutation of JAK2 in myeloproliferative disorders. N Engl J Med 2005;352:1779–90.

72. Baxter EJ, Scott LM, Campbell PJ, et al. Acquired mutation of the tyrosine kinase JAK2 in human myeloproliferative disorders. Lancet 2005;365:1054–61.

73. Tefferi A, Lasho TL, Gilliland G. JAK2 mutations in myeloproliferative disorders. N Engl J Med 2005;353:1416–7 [author reply: 7].

74. Jones AV, Kreil S, Zoi K, et al. Widespread occurrence of the JAK2 V617F mutation in chronic myeloproliferative disorders. Blood 2005;106:2162–8.

75. Scott LM, Tong W, Levine RL, et al. JAK2 exon 12 mutations in polycythemia vera and idiopathic erythrocytosis. N Engl J Med 2007;356:459–68.

76. Pearson TC, Wetherley-Mein G. Vascular occlusive episodes and venous haematocrit in primary proliferative polycythaemia. Lancet 1978;2:1219–22.

77. Marchioli R, Finazzi G, Landolfi R, et al. Vascular and neoplastic risk in a large cohort of patients with polycythemia vera. J Clin Oncol 2005;23:2224–32.

78. Harrison CN. Platelets and thrombosis in myeloproliferative diseases. Hematology Am Soc Hematol Educ Program 2005;409–15.

79. Menon KV, Shah V, Kamath PS. The Budd-Chiari syndrome. N Engl J Med 2004; 350:578–85.

80. Lamy T, Devillers A, Bernard M, et al. Inapparent polycythemia vera: an unrecognized diagnosis. Am J Med 1997;102:14–20.

81. Darwish Murad S, Plessier A, Hernandez-Guerra M, et al. Etiology, management, and outcome of the Budd-Chiari syndrome. Ann Intern Med 2009;151: 167–75.

82. Goulding C, Uttenthal B, Foroni L, et al. The JAK2(V617F) tyrosine kinase mutation identifies clinically latent myeloproliferative disorders in patients presenting with hepatic or portal vein thrombosis. Int J Lab Hematol 2008;30:415–9.

83. Michiels JJ, van Genderen PJ, Lindemans J, et al. Erythromelalgic, thrombotic and hemorrhagic manifestations in 50 cases of thrombocythemia. Leuk Lymphoma 1996;22(Suppl 1):47–56.

84. Michiels JJ, Abels J, Steketee J, et al. Erythromelalgia caused by platelet-mediated arteriolar inflammation and thrombosis in thrombocythemia. Ann Intern Med 1985;102:466–71.

85. van Genderen PJ, Michiels JJ, van Strik R, et al. Platelet consumption in thrombocythemia complicated by erythromelalgia: reversal by aspirin. Thromb Haemost 1995;73:210–4.

86. Michiels JJ, van Genderen PJ, Jansen PH, et al. Atypical transient ischemic attacks in thrombocythemia of various myeloproliferative disorders. Leuk Lymphoma 1996;22(Suppl 1):65–70.
87. Kwaan HC, Wang J. Hyperviscosity in polycythemia vera and other red cell abnormalities. Semin Thromb Hemost 2003;29:451–8.
88. Dingli D, Utz JP, Krowka MJ, et al. Unexplained pulmonary hypertension in chronic myeloproliferative disorders. Chest 2001;120:801–8.
89. Schafer AI. Bleeding and thrombosis in the myeloproliferative disorders. Blood 1984;64:1–12.
90. Ruggeri M, Rodeghiero F, Tosetto A, et al. Postsurgery outcomes in patients with polycythemia vera and essential thrombocythemia: a retrospective survey. Blood 2008;111:666–71.
91. Steinman HK, Kobza-Black A, Lotti TM, et al. Polycythaemia rubra vera and water-induced pruritus: blood histamine levels and cutaneous fibrinolytic activity before and after water challenge. Br J Dermatol 1987;116:329–33.
92. Rector WG Jr, Fortuin NJ, Conley CL. Non-hematologic effects of chronic iron deficiency. A study of patients with polycythemia vera treated solely with venesections. Medicine (Baltimore) 1982;61:382–9.
93. Kiladjian JJ, Chevret S, Dosquet C, et al. Treatment of polycythemia vera with hydroxyurea and pipobroman: final results of a randomized trial initiated in 1980. J Clin Oncol 2011;29:3907–13.
94. Passamonti F, Rumi E, Caramella M, et al. A dynamic prognostic model to predict survival in post-polycythemia vera myelofibrosis. Blood 2008;111: 3383–7.
95. Tefferi A, Thiele J, Orazi A, et al. Proposals and rationale for revision of the World Health Organization diagnostic criteria for polycythemia vera, essential thrombocythemia, and primary myelofibrosis: recommendations from an ad hoc international expert panel. Blood 2007;110:1092–7.
96. Sokol L, Luhovy M, Guan Y, et al. Primary familial polycythemia: a frameshift mutation in the erythropoietin receptor gene and increased sensitivity of erythroid progenitors to erythropoietin. Blood 1995;86:15–22.
97. Polycythemia vera: the natural history of 1213 patients followed for 20 years. Gruppo Italiano Studio Policitemia. Ann Intern Med 1995;123:656–64.
98. McMullin MF, Bareford D, Campbell P, et al. Guidelines for the diagnosis, investigation and management of polycythaemia/erythrocytosis. Br J Haematol 2005; 130:174–95.
99. Landolfi R, Marchioli R, Kutti J, et al. Efficacy and safety of low-dose aspirin in polycythemia vera. N Engl J Med 2004;350:114–24.
100. Vannucchi AM, Guglielmelli P. Advances in understanding and management of polycythemia vera. Curr Opin Oncol 2010;22:636–41.
101. Barbui T, Barosi G, Birgegard G, et al. Philadelphia-negative classical myeloproliferative neoplasms: critical concepts and management recommendations from European LeukemiaNet. J Clin Oncol 2011;29:761–70.
102. Kiladjian JJ, Cassinat B, Chevret S, et al. Pegylated interferon-alfa-2a induces complete hematologic and molecular responses with low toxicity in polycythemia vera. Blood 2008;112:3065–72.
103. Petitt RM, Silverstein MN, Petrone ME. Anagrelide for control of thrombocythemia in polycythemia and other myeloproliferative disorders. Semin Hematol 1997;34:51–4.
104. Tefferi A. JAK inhibitors for myeloproliferative neoplasms: clarifying facts from myths. Blood 2012. [Epub ahead of print].

Why Does My Patient Have Thrombocytosis?

Nanna H. Sulai, MD[a], Ayalew Tefferi, MD[b],*

KEYWORDS

- Thrombocytosis • Platelets • Gene mutation
- Molecular therapy

Thrombocytosis is defined as having excess platelets in the blood. The normal platelet count in adults ranges between 150,000 and 450,000/μL (mean ± 2 standard deviations), regardless of sex and ethnicity.[1,2] Based on the normal distribution, this implies that a platelet count exceeding 450,000/μL exists in about 2.5% of the population.

An increased platelet count usually has an acquired cause. It is rarely congenital. Congenital thrombocytosis results from gain-of-function mutations in either thrombopoietin (TPO) or its receptor (MpL).[3–5] The altered regulation is usually transmitted in an autosomal dominant fashion and often involves the 5′-untranslated region of the TPO mRNA (a donor splice site), resulting in increased translational efficiency.[5] Increases in serum TPO concentrations are noted in those patients with a TPO gene mutation.[4]

Acquired thrombocytosis may be either a primary or secondary process. Essential thrombocytosis (ET) is also known as primary thrombocytosis, essential thrombocythemia, and autonomous thrombocytosis. It is a disease of the bone marrow associated with myeloproliferative neoplasms that lead to an increase in platelets. This process may be growth factor independent or growth factor hypersensitive.[6] Acquired thrombocytosis may be reactive and secondary to an unrelated condition such as infection, chronic inflammation, hemolysis, iron deficiency anemia, or splenectomy, and is referred to as reactive thrombocytosis (RT).

REACTIVE THROMBOCYTOSIS (RT)
Prevalence and Relevance

RT refers to an increase in platelet count associated with conditions other than chronic myeloproliferative or myelodysplastic disorders. It is observed in a variety of conditions that may cause an acute, transient, or sustained increase in platelet counts (**Table 1**). It is generally accompanied by the signs and symptoms of the underlying disease and normalizes, or is expected to normalize, after resolution of this condition.[10] In routine clinical practice, RT accounts for more than 85% of cases

[a] Department of Internal Medicine, Mayo Clinic, 200 First Street SW, Rochester, MN 55905, USA
[b] Division of Hematology, Department of Internal Medicine, Mayo Clinic, 200 First Street SW, Rochester, MN 55905, USA
* Corresponding author.
E-mail address: tefferi.ayalew@mayo.edu

Hematol Oncol Clin N Am 26 (2012) 285–301
doi:10.1016/j.hoc.2012.01.003
0889-8588/12/$ – see front matter © 2012 Elsevier Inc. All rights reserved.

Table 1
Causes of thrombocytosis (platelet count of 500 × 10⁹/L or more) in unselected cohorts of consecutive patients (values are approximate percentages)

Condition	Adults (n = 777)[7]	Platelet Count of 1 Million/μL or More (n = 280)[8]	Children (n = 663)[9]
Infection	22	31	31
Rebound thrombocytosis	19	3	15
Tissue damage (eg, surgery)	18	14	15
Chronic inflammation	13	9	4
Malignancy	6	14	2
Renal disorders	5	NS	4
Hemolytic anemia	4	NS	19
After splenectomy	2	19	1
Blood loss	NS	6	NS
Primary thrombocythemia	3	14	0

Abbreviation: NS, not specified.

of thrombocytosis,[11] even in patients with extreme thrombocytosis (platelet count >1000 × 10^3/μL).[8,12]

It is important to distinguish between RT and ET because of their different clinical manifestations and treatment strategies. There is a well-established association of ET with vasomotor symptoms and thrombotic or bleeding complications.[13,14] In general, thromboembolic complications are rare in RT compared with ET, unless clinically provoked by underlying conditions such as malignancy or atherosclerosis.[10] More often, high-risk patients with ET require cytoreductive therapy to prevent catastrophic thrombohemorrhagic complications, whereas the prothrombotic potential of RT may be too low to even justify the use of platelet directed therapy,[8,15,16] even in the context of surgical procedures.[17] Because of the low likelihood of vascular complications, there is no evidence to support the use of cytoreductive agents in patients with RT.

Pathogenesis

A list of the causes of RT is shown in **Table 1**. Several cytokines and lymphokines are increased in the blood of patients with RT, especially those associated with infection, inflammation, malignancy, and tissue damage. These cytokines include interleukin (IL)-6, thrombopoietin, IL-1, IL-4, interferon γ, and tumor necrosis factor-α.[18,19] Of all the cytokines implicated, the most compelling evidence for their pathogenic role is noted with IL-6 and interferon γ. The administration of a transcription factor that mimics interferon γ led to the correction of thrombocytopenia in a genetic model.[20] IL-6 stimulates TPO production in the liver.[21–23] Thrombocytosis and induction of other acute phase reactants are noted with the administration of human recombinant IL-6 in patients with metastatic cancer.[24]

RT is a predictable finding after splenectomy, with an incidence approaching 50% in large series.[25] Thrombocytosis is commonly seen immediately after splenectomy and normalizes in most cases within several months, and rarely only after many years. Hyposplenism-associated RT may reflect platelet redistribution in the peripheral blood as well as altered metabolism of thrombopoietic cytokines.[26–28] Persistent thrombocytosis has been described in congenital and functional asplenia (celiac sprue, amyloidosis). Whatever the cause, in the absence of a chronic myeloproliferative disorder (MPD), hyposplenic-associated thrombocytosis is rarely associated with an increased risk of thrombosis.[27]

Reactive Thrombocytosis Versus Essential Thrombocytosis (ET)

ET is a clonal proliferation process with subsequent increase in platelet counts. A thorough history and physical examination are the most important elements in differentiating RT from ET. Determining the duration of thrombocytosis is a key diagnostic step of the initial workup. If no obvious explanation is provided, longstanding and persistent thrombocytosis strongly suggests ET. A history of vasomotor symptoms, thrombohemorrhagic complications, and physical examination findings such as splenomegaly and acral erythema also strongly suggest ET. An increased platelet count in the presence of conditions associated with RT, as outlined in **Table 1**, may favor the diagnosis of RT. However, if thrombocytosis is noted in the absence of associated clinical conditions such as vasculitis and infection, then ET may be more likely.

Complete blood count with differential counts, red blood cell indices, and peripheral blood smear examination, as well as iron studies, provide additional information for differentiating ET from RT (**Fig. 1**). Laboratory findings that suggest RT include microcytosis, which may indicate iron deficiency anemia. Although a normal ferritin level may reduce the likelihood of iron deficiency anemia associated with RT, a low level does not necessarily eliminate the possibility of ET. Increased acute phase reactants such as C-reactive protein, erythrocyte sedimentation rate,[29] plasma fibrinogen,[30] and

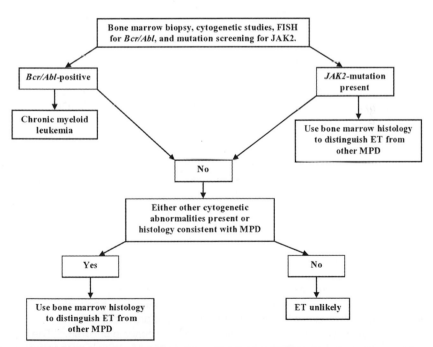

Fig. 1. A diagnostic algorithm for thrombocythemia that is clinically not consistent with reactive thrombocytosis. MPD, myeloproliferative disorder. (*Modified from* Tefferi A, Gilliland DG. The JAK2^{V617F} tyrosine kinase mutation in myeloproliferative disorders: status report and immediate implications for disease classification and diagnosis. Mayo Clin Proc 2005;80:954; with permission.)

IL-6[31] levels have been shown to be increased in RT. The presence of Howell-Jolly bodies on the peripheral blood smear suggests hyposplenism, supporting a diagnosis of RT, whereas a leukoerythroblastic smear suggests primary myelofibrosis (PMF) (also known as myelofibrosis with myeloid metaplasia).

It is difficult to discriminate between ET and RT based on the degree of thrombocytosis, regardless of how high the platelet counts might be.[8,32] There is no diagnostic usefulness of platelet indices (mean volume, size distribution width) in discriminating between ET and RT because of the considerable overlap in the measured values. Although abnormalities of platelet function as measured by prolonged bleeding time,[33] decreased adenosine triphosphate secretion,[34] and altered thromboxane generation are seen in ET,[35] these laboratory assays are not routinely used because they require substantial expertise to perform and interpret.

The presence of cytogenetic abnormalities, such as the Janus kinase 2 (JAK2^{V617F}) mutation, is strongly associated with MPDs.[36] This abnormality has not been detected in healthy controls or in patients with secondary erythrocytosis or RT,[37,38] thus making mutation screening an important part of the diagnostic workup (see **Fig. 1**).[39] Although clonal cytogenetic abnormalities can be detected and are diagnostic of ET, not all causes of ET have detectable cytogenetic abnormalities (<5% of patients with ET).

Consequently, bone marrow histology evaluation is still a critical part of the evaluation process. Although the bone marrow histology is normal in RT, it displays a wide variety of abnormalities in ET depending on the cause of the underlying chronic myeloproliferative disease (CMD). These abnormalities include aberrations in cellular morphology, increased numbers of megakaryocytes, presence of megakaryocyte clusters, and reticulin fibrosis.[40]

ESSENTIAL THROMBOCYTOSIS (ET) AND MYELOPROLIFERATIVE STATES

ET is a clonal expansion of a multipotential stem cell observed in the presence of a chronic MPD or myelodysplastic syndrome (MDS).[41] Clonal or autonomous thrombocytosis is part of ET and is seen in 50% of patients with polycythemia vera (PV).[42] It is also seen in about 35% of patients with chronic myeloid leukemia (CML).[43]

These disorders (MPD and MDS) may be classified as those that exhibit trilineage morphologic dysplasia (in MDS) and those that do not (in MPD). The classification of chronic myeloid disorders is shown in **Box 1**.[44] Although thrombocytosis in MDS has been associated with the presence of ringed sideroblasts and may be linked with certain cytogenetic abnormalities including trisomy 8,[45] 5q− syndrome,[31,46] and abnormalities of chromosome 3,[47] the underlying pathogenic connection between these defects and thrombocytosis is unclear. Except for a few atypical myelodysplasia states and CML, the molecular pathogenesis of the MPDs is also unclear.[48]

ET
Epidemiology

ET is a diagnosis of exclusion once other causes of thrombocytosis such as reactive conditions, MDS, and other myeloproliferative states have been eliminated (see **Table 1**). Among the classic MPDs, ET has the highest prevalence (about 24/100,000) and carries the best prognosis.[49] ET does not routinely occur in children.[50] The median age at diagnosis is 40 to 60 years.[51] There is a suggestion of a female preponderance.[52]

Distinction from Other Causes of ET

Because of MDS,[53] PMF, and CML[54,55] can all mimic ET in their presentation, it is important to clinically distinguish these separate entities when a working diagnosis

---

Box 1
A semimolecular classification of chronic myeloid disorders

1. MPS

2. MPDs

  a. Classic MPDs

    i. Molecularly defined

      1. CML (*Bcr/Abl$^+$*)

    ii. Clinicopathologically assigned (Bcr/Abl$^-$ and frequently associated with JAK2^{V617F} mutation)

      1. Essential thrombocythemia

      2. PV

      3. Myelofibrosis with myeloid metaplasia

  b. Atypical MPDs

    i. Molecularly defined

      1. *PDGFRA*-rearranged eosinophilic/mast cell disorders (eg, *FIP1L1-PDGFRA*)

      2. *PDGFRB*-rearranged eosinophilic disorders (eg, *TEL/ETV6-PDGFRB*)

      3. Systemic mastocytosis associated with *c-kit* mutation (eg, *c-kit^{D816V}*)

      4. 8p11 Myeloproliferative syndrome (eg, *ZNF198/FIM/RAMP-FGFR1*)

    ii. Clinicopathologically assigned

      1. Chronic neutrophilic leukemia

      2. Chronic eosinophilic leukemia, molecularly not defined

      3. Hypereosinophilic syndrome

      4. Chronic basophilic leukemia

      5. Chronic myelomonocytic leukemia

      6. Juvenile myelomonocytic leukemia (associated with recurrent mutations of RAS signaling pathway molecules including *PTPN11* and *NF1*)

      7. Systemic mastocytosis, molecularly not defined

      8. Unclassified MPD

Data From Tefferi A, Gilliland G. Classification of myeloproliferative disorders: from Dameshek toward a semi-molecular system. Best Pract Res Clin Haematol 2006;19(3):365–85.

---

of ET is considered. Workup should include exclusion of CML by conventional cytogenetics and fluorescence in situ hybridization (FISH) testing for BCR/ABL.[56] Bone marrow histology should be examined for features that suggest MDS and PMF, such as the presence of trilineage dysplasia and increased marrow cellularity with atypical megakaryocyte hyperplasia and myelofibrosis, respectively.

Pathophysiology

Before the discovery of the JAK2^{V617F} mutation, scant information existed regarding the molecular pathogenesis of ET. This new discovery has advanced knowledge of the pathophysiology of the condition, as well as the development of new therapeutic tools.[57] The JAK2^{V617F} mutation, which rarely exists in a homozygous state, is estimated to occur at a frequency of 23% to 60% in ET and 95% in PV.[58] JAK2^{V617F} is part of the cytoplasmic protein tyrosine kinases. This mutation is an acquired G to T nucleotide shift at position 1849 in exon 12, which leads to a valine to phenylalanine substitution at codon 617 (JAK2^{V617F}).[58,59] This mutation is located in the pseudokinase domain (JH2) of the JAK2 protein and interferes with autoinhibitory function. Consequently, mutated JAK2 exists in a constitutively phosphorylated state.

JAK2^{V617F} mutation has been associated with induction of erythropoietin hypersensitivity, a hallmark of PV and other classic MPDs.[58] In vivo, a retrovirus containing JAK2^{V617F}, when transduced into murine bone marrow, induced erythrocytosis in the transplanted mice.[60,61] These findings suggest some pathogenic relevance for this particular mutation in MPDs.

Clinical Features of ET

The diagnosis of ET is usually incidental.[62] Many patients with ET are asymptomatic at diagnosis and have a prolonged, stable, or uneventful clinical course. The signs and symptoms may be non–life threatening, such as the presence of vasomotor features (headaches, erythromelalgia, and lightheadedness), splenomegaly, or hypertension, or life threatening, such as thrombohemorrhagic complications.

Erythromelalgia

Erythromelalgia is a classic vasomotor symptom of essential thrombocythemia. It has been described even in patients with only marginal increase in platelet counts. It is defined as a burning sensation associated with a red discoloration of the hands or feet. This condition can be precipitated by heat or exercise.[63] The ensuing digital ischemic changes may be caused by arteriolar inflammation secondary to abnormal platelet-endothelium interaction.[64] Histopathologic studies in erythromelalgia have shown platelet-rich arteriolar microthrombi with endothelial inflammation and intimal proliferation. The prompt response of erythromelalgia to aspirin (40–325 mg/d) is consistent with a diagnosis of a vasomotor symptom as opposed to a thrombotic complication.[64]

Thrombosis

Age greater than 60 years, thrombotic history, leukocytosis greater than $11 \times 10^3/\mu L$, and presence of the JAK2^{V617F} mutation are considered important factors in assessing the risk of thrombosis.[65,66] In general, thrombotic events are more frequent than bleeding episodes, with more arterial events than venous events. **Tables 2** and **3** list the incidence of thrombotic and hemorrhagic events in ET, respectively.[68] It is common to have both microcirculatory and large vessel involvement.[11] Abdominal large vessel occlusions and cerebral sinus thrombosis are potentially catastrophic events that occasionally occur in patients with ET.[69,70]

The pathogenesis of thrombosis in ET is complex. It centers around the combination of endothelial dysfunction, abnormal platelet shapes and function, and the presence of circulating platelet-leukocyte aggregates.[66] Potential risk factors include leukocytosis[66] and defects in arachidonic acid metabolism. These theories are strengthened by the beneficial clinical response associated with myelosuppressive therapy[71] and low-dose aspirin, respectively.[72]

Bleeding

Bleeding, including epistaxis, gingival bleeding, and mild gastrointestinal or genitourinary hemorrhage, occurs less frequently in ET than thrombosis.[62] Although thrombocytosis by itself may not be a risk factor for bleeding, the concurrent use of aspirin therapy may reveal the bleeding tendency in patients.[73] The pathogenesis of bleeding in ET is thought to arise from altered Von Willebrand factor (VWF) function, which is

Table 2
Thrombotic and hemorrhagic events in ET reported at diagnosis

	n	Platelet × 10⁹/L (Median/Mean)	Asymptomatic (%)	Major Thrombosis (%)	Major Arterial Thrombosis[a] (%)	Major Venous Thrombosis[a] (%)	MVD (%)	Total Bleeds (%) (Major)
ET								
Bellucci et al,[105] 1986	94	1200	67	22	81	19	43	37 (3.2)
Fenaux et al,[51] 1990	147	1150	36	18	83	17	34	18 (4)
Cortelazzo et al,[52] 1990	100	1135	34	11	91	9	30	9 (3)
Colombi et al,[106] 1991	103	1200	73	23.3	87.5	12.5	33	3.6 (1.9)
Basses et al,[83] 1999	148	898	57	25	NA	NA	29	6.1 (NA)
Jensen et al,[67] 2000	96	1102	52	14	85	15	23	9 (5.2)

Abbreviations: IAVT, intra-abdominal venous thrombosis; MVD, microvascular disturbances; NA, not available.

[a] Percentage of total major thrombotic events.

Data from Elliott MA, Tefferi A. Thrombosis and haemorrhage in polycythaemia vera and essential thrombocythaemia. Br J Haematol 2005;128:275–90.

Table 3
Thrombotic and hemorrhagic events in ET reported at follow-up

	n	Major Thrombosis (%)	Major Arterial Thrombosis (%)[a]	Major Venous Thrombosis (%)[a]	MVD (%)	Total Bleeds (%) (Major)	Percentage of Deaths From Hemorrhage (%)	Percentage of Deaths From Thrombosis (%)
ET								
Bellucci et al,[105] 1986	94	17	62.5	37.5	17	14 (3.2)	0	0
Fenaux et al,[51] 1990	147	13.6	86	14	4.1	NA (0.7)	0	25
Cortelazzo et al,[52] 1990	100	20	71	29	NA	NA (1)	0	100 (1 patient, IAVT)
Colombi et al,[106] 1991	103	10.6	91	9	33	8.7 (5.8)	0	27.3
Besses et al,[83] 1999	148	22.3	94	6	27.7	11.5 (4.1)	0	13.3
Jensen et al,[67] 2000	96	16.6	69	31	16.7	13.6 (7.3)	3.3	16.7

Abbreviations: IAVT, intra-abdominal venous thrombosis; MVD, microvascular disturbances; NA, not available.
[a] Percentage of total major thrombotic events.
Data from Elliott MA, Tefferi A. Thrombosis and haemorrhage in polycythaemia vera and essential thrombocythaemia. Br J Haematol 2005;128:275–90.

platelet dependent. In the presence of extreme thrombocytosis (platelet count >1 million/μL), the ADAMTS13 cleaving protease is activated, which leads to increased proteolysis of high-molecular-weight VWF.[74] Other potential causes of excessive bleeding in ET include platelet dysfunction. Platelet abnormalities such as storage pool deficiency, decreased adrenergic receptor expression, impaired response to epinephrine, and decreased membrane glycoprotein receptor expression have been described.[67,68]

Pregnancy complications

ET is the most common MPD among women of childbearing age and is associated with an increased risk of fetal and maternal complications. The most common complication is first trimester abortion caused by placental infarctions associated with platelet dysfunction.[75,76] Treatment recommendations depend on the risk stratification (**Table 4**). Aspirin is usually sufficient, but therapy with interferon α or low-molecular-weight heparin are indicated in high-risk individuals such as those with a prior history of thrombosis.[77]

Disease transformation

In the absence of leukemogenic therapy, conversion of ET to acute myeloid leukemia (AML) rarely occurs.[78] The 15-year cumulative risk of evolution into either AML or PMF is 2% and 4% respectively.[13,78,79] An increase in myelofibrosis transformation is seen as the disease progresses and with the use of anagrelide.[78]

Diagnosis

In establishing a diagnosis of ET, other causes of thrombocytosis must first be considered. This process includes eliminating the possibility of reactive thrombocytosis and CML with relevant laboratory work such as cytogenetic studies and FISH for the BCR/ABL gene rearrangement. In addition, mutation screening for JAK2[V617F] aids in distinguishing ET from RT, but not necessarily other MPDs (see **Fig. 1**). The second step in determining whether thrombocytosis is caused by ET involves histopathologic analysis of the bone marrow, which helps eliminate the possibility of other myeloid disorders.

Prognosis

ET is an indolent disorder. There are few valid prospective data regarding long-term survival in ET. Most data are gathered from retrospective studies.[80] Compared with the general population, a 2-fold decrease in survival is seen in patients with ET, starting from the first decade after diagnosis. Most deaths are associated with thrombotic events.[58]

Table 4
Risk stratification in essential thrombocythemia

Low risk	Age less than 60 y and No history of thrombosis, and Platelet count less than 1.5 million/μL, and Absence of cardiovascular risk factors (smoking, hypertension, hyperlipidemia, diabetes)
Indeterminate risk	Neither low risk nor high risk
High risk	Age 60 y or older, or a positive history of thrombosis

Treatment

Before considering treatment, affected individuals must be stratified based on their risk category (see **Table 4**).[52,81] A step-by-step approach is involved in management based on the defined goals of therapy, existing evidence that supports such an action, and the risk of the patient. Treatment involves the use of antiplatelet aggregating agents and cytoreductive therapy. In the low-risk individual, treatment with aspirin (40–325 mg daily) to reduce vasomotor symptoms may be sufficient once the possibility of clinically significant acquired Von Willebrand syndrome has been excluded in patients with extreme thrombocytosis.[68,82] Cytoreductive therapy is generally not indicated in low-risk individuals given the low risk of thrombosis,[51,52,69,83] but may be considered in the treatment of refractory symptoms.

The goal of therapy with the use of cytoreductive agents is to prevent thrombohemorrhagic events. As a result, we recommend cytoreductive therapy in high-risk patients (see **Table 4**).[84,85] Cytoreduction is also considered in patients with extreme thrombocytosis (platelet count >1.5 million/μL) in the setting of a bleeding diathesis or aspirin-resistant microvascular symptoms. The desired platelet count in this instance is the level that provides symptomatic relief or corrects the bleeding diathesis.

Although various cytoreductive agents have been used to treat thrombocytosis, hydroxyurea is currently the treatment of choice. Compared with anagrelide, both alone and in combination with aspirin, there was a significantly decreased number of thrombotic and bleeding events in the hydroxyurea treatment arm (36 vs 55 events in the anagrelide group). A dose of 500 to 1000 mg daily should result in decreased platelet numbers. The therapeutic goal in terms of platelet count, based on anecdotal evidence of optimal thrombosis control, is less than 400,000/μL.[86] Although there is concern about the leukemogenic effect of hydroxyurea, the presumed association has not been shown by large retrospective or prospective controlled trials. In addition, no association with leukemic transformation has been documented in other disease states treated with hydroxyurea.[84,87] However, leg ulcers are a complication associated with hydroxyurea.

In patients who are intolerant of hydroxyurea, anagrelide or interferon α has been used as a second-line cytoreductive agent. Anagrelide works by altering megakaryocyte maturation. It is associated with side effects such as headaches, palpitations, diarrhea, and fluid retention, which are intolerable to many patients. These symptoms are dose dependent and generally abate after 4 to 8 weeks of therapy. Interferon is commonly used at a dose of 3 million units 3 times a week and has an inhibitory effect on megakaryopoiesis. It is particularly safe to use in pregnancy and has been shown to induce a stable state of remission in about 80% to 90% of patients.[62] Although the addition of antiplatelet therapy has not yet been shown prospectively to reduce the incidence of thrombosis in ET, we recommend its use in combination with cytoreductive therapy in all high-risk patients (**Table 5**).[88]

JAK2[V617F] inhibitors have been shown to be tolerable, with benefits in alleviating symptoms such as fatigue. Although there are data showing control of myeloproliferation in patients with ET, information about effects on thrombosis and disease transformation into more aggressive states, such as leukemia, is currently lacking.[89] Additional studies on these potential therapeutic modalities need to be undertaken.

Plateletpheresis has been reserved for patients with extreme thrombocytosis with a platelet count greater than 1 million/μL and those with acute thrombotic or hemorrhagic complications. Because the benefits of plateletpheresis are not permanent, this should be followed with cytoreductive therapy. Patients most likely to benefit include those with severe organ dysfunction.[90]

Table 5 Treatment algorithm in ET			
Risk Category	Age <60 y	Age ≥60 y	Women of Childbearing Age
Low risk	Low-dose aspirin[a]	Not applicable	Low-dose aspirin[a]
Indeterminate risk[b]	Low-dose aspirin[a]	Not applicable	Low-dose aspirin[a]
High risk	Hydroxyurea and low-dose aspirin	Hydroxyurea and Low-dose aspirin	Interferon α and low-dose aspirin

[a] In the absence of a contraindication including evidence for acquired Von Willebrand syndrome (ie, a ristocetin cofactor activity of <50%).
[b] The decision to use cytoreductive agents in indeterminate-risk patients should be made on an individual basis (see text for elaboration).

POLYCYTHEMIA VERA (PV)

PV is a disease often diagnosed by laboratory assessment that is ordered because of symptoms or signs such as headaches, visual changes, erythromelalgia, spleno-megaly, and postbath pruritus. Diagnostic criteria include an increased hemoglobin level (>18.5 g/dL for men or 16.5 g/dL for women) and a $JAK2^{V617F}$ gene mutation.[91] Thrombocytosis is commonly a feature of PV.[92] Although the presence of a $JAK2^{V617F}$ or mutation involving MpL reduces the possibility that thrombocytosis is caused by a reactive process, it does not distinguish among the different types of myeloprolifer-ative neoplasms. The presence of a $JAK2^{V617F}$ mutation and increased red cell mass is consistent with PV 95% of the time.[58,93]

The clinical course of PV, much like that of ET, is characterized primarily by throm-bohemorrhagic complications, myelofibrosis, or leukemic transformation.[58] The pres-ence of a $JAK2^{V617F}$ mutation status[78,94] and high allelic burden of greater than 75%[95,96] are associated with a high risk of thrombosis. Mortality is increased compared with the general population and is age dependent, with a 2-fold increase in patients more than 50 years old (1.6-fold vs 3.3-fold in patients >50 years old).[58,97]

Similar to the recommendations for ET, the treatment of PV depends on the classi-fied risk status. Low-dose aspirin and repeated phlebotomies are sufficient for low-risk patients. In contrast, cytoreductive agents are necessary for patients considered high risk, such as those with a history of thrombotic events, or patients with massive splenomegaly and extreme leukocytosis or thrombocytosis. Treatment with hydroxy-urea or interferon α is frequently used.[91]

CHRONIC MYELOGENOUS LEUKEMIA (CML)

CML is one of the myeloproliferative neoplasms and is characterized by the unregu-lated proliferation of mature and maturing granulocytes. The clinical picture of CML consists of leukocytosis, splenomegaly, and thrombocytosis.[10] An increased platelet count is seen in as many as 35% of patients with CML.[43] Diagnostic confirmation is accomplished with FISH or polymerase chain reaction analysis for the Philadelphia chromosome, BCR-ABL gene rearrangement, or the mRNA gene product. A low leukocyte alkaline phosphatase (LAP) score differentiates CML from PV, in which the LAP score is increased.[98] The use of tyrosine kinase inhibitors is now the mainstay of therapy, with cytogenetic remission observed in about 80% of patients.[91]

PRIMARY MYELOFIBROSIS

Primary myelofibrosis (PMF) is one of the least common myeloproliferative neoplasms, with an estimated incidence of 1.5 per 100,000 per year in Olmsted County, Minnesota.[85] It clinically presents with splenomegaly, hepatomegaly, and extramedullary hematopoiesis. Thrombocytosis occurs in about 13% to 50% of patients at diagnosis, with thrombocytopenia becoming apparent as the disease progresses.[43,99] Peripheral blood smear and histologic bone marrow findings such as the presence of tear drop–shaped cells and fibrosis, respectively, are key in distinguishing this disease entity from other causes of primary thrombocytosis. Unlike PV and ET, which have a good prognosis, patients with PMF have a median survival of less than 5 years.[100] Poor prognostic factors include the presence of circulating blasts (>3%) and platelet count less than 100,000/μL.

JAK2^{V617F} mutations have been described in primary myelofibrosis and are estimated to occur in 43% to 57% of patients with PMF,[101] with apparent homozygosity in 13% of patients.[102] Although it is uncertain whether the clinical course differs based on the JAK2^{V617F} mutation status,[39,103] in transplant patients, achievement of JAK2^{V617F} negativity is linked to a decreased relapse rate.[101] Mutations involving MpL have been documented and are thought to be partially responsible for thrombocytosis observed in PMF.[104]

Treatment of PMF is targeted toward symptoms instead of the underlying molecular disorder.[103] For instance, splenectomy is indicated in patients with severe pain and red cell transfusions, with iron chelation therapy for those with symptomatic anemia. Drugs such as danazol and thalidomide have been used with good results to correct cytopenias and to halt splenomegaly.[100,103] Studies evaluating the therapeutic role of JAK2^{V617F} kinase inhibitors in patients with PMF are currently underway.[91]

SUMMARY

Thrombocytosis is a common clinical problem frequently encountered during routine evaluation. The diagnostic workup entails a step-by-step approach, which allows for an accurate assessment of the underlying cause. A through clinical history and physical examination may help differentiate thrombocytosis secondary to a reactive process versus an underlying clonal proliferation process. Once ET is evident, relevant laboratory evaluation for an ongoing MPD is paramount. With the recent advances in JAK2^{V617F} mutation analysis, more appropriate diagnostic conclusions may be achieved.

With regard to treatment, various modalities targeted toward correction of the underlying cause in the case of reactive thrombocytosis and, in the case of ET, the use of agents such as aspirin, hydroxyurea, anagrelide, and interferon (based on identified risk profiles) have all been proved to be beneficial. With further scientific investigation underway, molecular therapies targeted at identified JAK2^{V617F} mutations may soon be cornerstones of therapy in ET.

REFERENCES

1. Del Corso L, Romanelli AM, Pentimone F, et al. New hematological indices in healthy elderly. J Investig Med 1999;47:156a.
2. Lozano M, Narvaez J, Faundez A, et al. Platelet count and mean platelet volume in the Spanish population. Med Clin (Barc) 1998;110:774–7 [in Spanish].
3. Wiestner A, Padosch SA, Ghilardi N, et al. Hereditary thrombocythaemia is a genetically heterogeneous disorder: exclusion of TPO and MPL in two families with hereditary thrombocythaemia. Br J Haematol 2000;110:104–9.

4. Ghilardi N, Wiestner A, Kikuchi M, et al. Hereditary thrombocythaemia in a Japanese family is caused by a novel point mutation in the thrombopoietin gene. Br J Haematol 1999;107:310–6.

5. Wiestner A, Schlemper RJ, van der Maas AP, et al. An activating splice donor mutation in the thrombopoietin gene causes hereditary thrombocythaemia. Nat Genet 1998;18:49–52.

6. Skoda RC. Thrombocytosis. Hematology Am Soc Hematol Educ Program 2009;159–67.

7. Santhosh-Kumar CR, Yohannan MD, Higgy KE, et al. Thrombocytosis in adults: analysis of 777 patients. J Intern Med 1991;229:493–5.

8. Buss DH, Cashell AW, O'Connor ML, et al. Occurrence, etiology, and clinical significance of extreme thrombocytosis: a study of 280 cases. Am J Med 1994; 96:247–53.

9. Yohannan MD, Higgy KE, al-Mashhadani SA, et al. Thrombocytosis. Etiologic analysis of 663 patients. Clin Pediatr (Phila) 1994;33:340–3.

10. Vannucchi AM, Barbui T. Thrombocytosis and thrombosis. Hematology Am Soc Hematol Educ Program 2007;363–70.

11. Griesshammer M, Bangerter M, Sauer T, et al. Aetiology and clinical significance of thrombocytosis: analysis of 732 patients with an elevated platelet count. J Intern Med 1999;245:295–300.

12. Chuncharunee S, Archararit N, Ungkanont A, et al. Etiology and incidence of thrombotic and hemorrhagic disorders in Thai patients with extreme thrombocytosis. J Med Assoc Thai 2000;83(Suppl 1):S95–100.

13. Harrison CN. Essential thrombocythaemia: challenges and evidence-based management. Br J Haematol 2005;130:153–65.

14. Tefferi A. Polycythemia vera: a comprehensive review and clinical recommendations. Mayo Clin Proc 2003;78:174–94.

15. Coon WW, Penner J, Clagett P, et al. Deep venous thrombosis and postsplenectomy thrombocytosis. Arch Surg 1978;113:429–31.

16. Coon WW, Willis PW. Deep venous thrombosis and pulmonary embolism: prediction, prevention and treatment. Am J Cardiol 1959;4:611–21.

17. Meekes I, van der Staak F, van Oostrom C. Results of splenectomy performed on a group of 91 children. Eur J Pediatr Surg 1995;5:19–22.

18. Ishiguro A, Ishikita T, Shimbo T, et al. Elevation of serum thrombopoietin precedes thrombocytosis in Kawasaki disease. Thromb Haemost 1998;79:1096–100.

19. Wolber EM, Jelkmann W. Interleukin-6 increases thrombopoietin production in human hepatoma cells HepG2 and Hep3B. J Interferon Cytokine Res 2000;20: 499–506.

20. Huang Z, Richmond TD, Muntean AG, et al. STAT1 promotes megakaryopoiesis downstream of GATA-1 in mice. J Clin Invest 2007;117:3890–9.

21. Blay JY, Rossi JF, Wijdenes J, et al. Role of interleukin-6 in the paraneoplastic inflammatory syndrome associated with renal-cell carcinoma. Int J Cancer 1997;72:424–30.

22. Barton BE. The biological effects of interleukin 6. Med Res Rev 1996;16:87–109.

23. Takagi M, Egawa T, Motomura T, et al. Interleukin-6 secreting phaeochromocytoma associated with clinical markers of inflammation. Clin Endocrinol (Oxf) 1997;46:507–9.

24. Stouthard JM, Goey H, de Vries EG, et al. Recombinant human interleukin 6 in metastatic renal cell cancer: a phase II trial. Br J Cancer 1996;73:789–93.

25. Traetow WD, Fabri PJ, Carey LC. Changing indications for splenectomy. 30 years' experience. Arch Surg 1980;115:447–51.

26. Chuncharunee S, Archararit N, Hathirat P, et al. Levels of serum interleukin-6 and tumor necrosis factor in postsplenectomized thalassemic patients. J Med Assoc Thai 1997;80(Suppl 1):S86–91.

27. Gordon DH, Schaffner D, Bennett JM, et al. Postsplenectomy thrombocytosis: its association with mesenteric, portal, and/or renal vein thrombosis in patients with myeloproliferative disorders. Arch Surg 1978;113:713–5.

28. Boxer MA, Braun J, Ellman L. Thromboembolic risk of postsplenectomy thrombocytosis. Arch Surg 1978;113:808–9.

29. Espanol I, Hernandez A, Cortes M, et al. Patients with thrombocytosis have normal or slightly elevated thrombopoietin levels. Haematologica 1999;84:312–6.

30. Messinezy M, Westwood N, Sawyer B, et al. Primary thrombocythaemia: a composite approach to diagnosis. Clin Lab Haematol 1994;16:139–48.

31. Tefferi A, Ho TC, Ahmann GJ, et al. Plasma interleukin-6 and C-reactive protein levels in reactive versus clonal thrombocytosis. Am J Med 1994;97:374–8.

32. Schilling RF. Platelet millionaires. Lancet 1980;2:372–3.

33. Murphy S, Davis JL, Walsh PN, et al. Template bleeding time and clinical hemorrhage in myeloproliferative disease. Arch Intern Med 1978;138:1251–3.

34. Lofvenberg E, Nilsson TK. Qualitative platelet defects in chronic myeloproliferative disorders: evidence for reduced ATP secretion. Eur J Haematol 1989;43:435–40.

35. Zahavi J, Zahavi M, Firsteter E, et al. An abnormal pattern of multiple platelet function abnormalities and increased thromboxane generation in patients with primary thrombocytosis and thrombotic complications. Eur J Haematol 1991;47:326–32.

36. Steensma DP, Tefferi A. Cytogenetic and molecular genetic aspects of essential thrombocythemia. Acta Haematol 2002;108:55–65.

37. Kralovics R, Passamonti F, Buser AS, et al. A gain-of-function mutation of JAK2 in myeloproliferative disorders. N Engl J Med 2005;352:1779–90.

38. Jones AV, Kreil S, Zoi K, et al. Widespread occurrence of the JAK2 V617F mutation in chronic myeloproliferative disorders. Blood 2005;106:2162–8.

39. Tefferi A, Lasho TL, Schwager SM, et al. The JAK2(V617F) tyrosine kinase mutation in myelofibrosis with myeloid metaplasia: lineage specificity and clinical correlates. Br J Haematol 2005;131:320–8.

40. Buss DH, O'Connor ML, Woodruff RD, et al. Bone marrow and peripheral blood findings in patients with extreme thrombocytosis. A report of 63 cases. Arch Pathol Lab Med 1991;115:475–80.

41. Vardiman JW, Harris NL, Brunning RD. The World Health Organization (WHO) classification of the myeloid neoplasms. Blood 2002;100:2292–302.

42. Thiele P, Muller M. On the clinical aspects, pathological anatomy and case reports of aortic arch syndromes. Dtsch Gesundheitsw 1966;21:145–53 [in German].

43. Thiele J, Kvasnicka HM, Diehl V, et al. Clinicopathological diagnosis and differential criteria of thrombocythemias in various myeloproliferative disorders by histopathology, histochemistry and immunostaining from bone marrow biopsies. Leuk Lymphoma 1999;33:207–18.

44. Tefferi A, Vardiman JW. Classification and diagnosis of myeloproliferative neoplasms: the 2008 World Health Organization criteria and point-of-care diagnostic algorithms. Leukemia 2008;22:14–22.

45. Patel K, Kelsey P. Primary acquired sideroblastic anemia, thrombocytosis, and trisomy 8. Ann Hematol 1997;74:199–201.

46. Brusamolino E, Orlandi E, Morra E, et al. Hematologic and clinical features of patients with chromosome 5 monosomy or deletion (5q). Med Pediatr Oncol 1988;16:88–94.

47. Jenkins RB, Tefferi A, Solberg LA Jr, et al. Acute leukemia with abnormal thrombopoiesis and inversions of chromosome 3. Cancer Genet Cytogenet 1989;39: 167–79.
48. Nowell PC. The minute chromosome (Phl) in chronic granulocytic leukemia. Blut 1962;8:65–6.
49. Ma X, Vanasse G, Cartmel B, et al. Prevalence of polycythemia vera and essential thrombocythemia. Am J Hematol 2008;83:359–62.
50. Hasle H. Incidence of essential thrombocythaemia in children. Br J Haematol 2000;110:751.
51. Fenaux P, Simon M, Caulier MT, et al. Clinical course of essential thrombocythemia in 147 cases. Cancer 1990;66:549–56.
52. Cortelazzo S, Viero P, Finazzi G, et al. Incidence and risk factors for thrombotic complications in a historical cohort of 100 patients with essential thrombocythemia. J Clin Oncol 1990;8:556–62.
53. Gupta R, Abdalla SH, Bain BJ. Thrombocytosis with sideroblastic erythropoiesis: a mixed myeloproliferative myelodysplastic syndrome. Leuk Lymphoma 1999;34:615–9.
54. Stoll DB, Peterson P, Exten R, et al. Clinical presentation and natural history of patients with essential thrombocythemia and the Philadelphia chromosome. Am J Hematol 1988;27:77–83.
55. Michiels JJ, Berneman Z, Schroyens W, et al. Philadelphia (Ph) chromosome-positive thrombocythemia without features of chronic myeloid leukemia in peripheral blood: natural history and diagnostic differentiation from Ph-negative essential thrombocythemia. Ann Hematol 2004;83:504–12.
56. Tefferi A, Dewald GW, Litzow ML, et al. Chronic myeloid leukemia: current application of cytogenetics and molecular testing for diagnosis and treatment. Mayo Clin Proc 2005;80:390–402.
57. Wernig G, Mercher T, Okabe R, et al. Expression of Jak2V617F causes a polycythemia vera-like disease with associated myelofibrosis in a murine bone marrow transplant model. Blood 2006;107:4274–81.
58. Vannucchi AM, Guglielmelli P, Tefferi A. Advances in understanding and management of myeloproliferative neoplasms. CA Cancer J Clin 2009;59:171–91.
59. Lindauer K, Loerting T, Liedl KR, et al. Prediction of the structure of human Janus kinase 2 (JAK2) comprising the two carboxy-terminal domains reveals a mechanism for autoregulation. Protein Eng 2001;14:27–37.
60. James C, Ugo V, Le Couedic JP, et al. A unique clonal JAK2 mutation leading to constitutive signalling causes polycythaemia vera. Nature 2005;434:1144–8.
61. Levine RL, Wadleigh M, Cools J, et al. Activating mutation in the tyrosine kinase JAK2 in polycythemia vera, essential thrombocythemia, and myeloid metaplasia with myelofibrosis. Cancer Cell 2005;7:387–97.
62. Frenkel EP, Mammen EF. Sticky platelet syndrome and thrombocythemia. Hematol Oncol Clin North Am 2003;17:63–83.
63. van Genderen PJ, Michiels JJ, van Strik R, et al. Platelet consumption in thrombocythemia complicated by erythromelalgia: reversal by aspirin. Thromb Haemost 1995;73:210–4.
64. Michiels JJ, van Genderen PJ, Lindemans J, et al. Erythromelalgic, thrombotic and hemorrhagic manifestations in 50 cases of thrombocythemia. Leuk Lymphoma 1996;22(Suppl 1):47–56.
65. Carobbio A, Thiele J, Passamonti F, et al. Risk factors for arterial and venous thrombosis in WHO-defined essential thrombocythemia: an international study of 891 patients. Blood 2011;117:5857–9.

66. Vianello F, Battisti A, Cella G, et al. Defining the thrombotic risk in patients with myeloproliferative neoplasms. ScientificWorldJournal 2011;11:1131–7.
67. Jensen MK, de Nully Brown P, Lund BV, et al. Increased platelet activation and abnormal membrane glycoprotein content and redistribution in myeloproliferative disorders. Br J Haematol 2000;110(1):116–24.
68. Elliott MA, Tefferi A. Thrombosis and haemorrhage in polycythaemia vera and essential thrombocythaemia. Br J Haematol 2005;128:275–90.
69. Bazzan M, Tamponi G, Schinco P, et al. Thrombosis-free survival and life expectancy in 187 consecutive patients with essential thrombocythemia. Ann Hematol 1999;78:539–43.
70. Anger BR, Seifried E, Scheppach J, et al. Budd-Chiari syndrome and thrombosis of other abdominal vessels in the chronic myeloproliferative diseases. Klin Wochenschr 1989;67:818–25.
71. Cortelazzo S, Finazzi G, Ruggeri M, et al. Hydroxyurea for patients with essential thrombocythemia and a high risk of thrombosis. N Engl J Med 1995;332:1132–6.
72. Schafer AI. Deficiency of platelet lipoxygenase activity in myeloproliferative disorders. N Engl J Med 1982;306:381–6.
73. Finazzi G, Carobbio A, Thiele J, et al. Incidence and risk factors for bleeding in 1104 patients with essential thrombocythemia or prefibrotic myelofibrosis diagnosed according to the 2008 WHO criteria. Leukemia 2011. [Epub ahead of print].
74. Tsai HM. Physiologic cleavage of von Willebrand factor by a plasma protease is dependent on its conformation and requires calcium ion. Blood 1996;87: 4235–44.
75. Beressi AH, Tefferi A, Silverstein MN, et al. Outcome analysis of 34 pregnancies in women with essential thrombocythemia. Arch Intern Med 1995;155:1217–22.
76. Falconer J, Pineo G, Blahey W, et al. Essential thrombocythemia associated with recurrent abortions and fetal growth retardation. Am J Hematol 1987;25:345–7.
77. Valera MC, Parant O, Vayssiere C, et al. Essential thrombocythemia and pregnancy. Eur J Obstet Gynecol Reprod Biol 2011;158(2):141–7.
78. Antonioli E, Guglielmelli P, Poli G, et al. Influence of JAK2V617F allele burden on phenotype in essential thrombocythemia. Haematologica 2008;93:41–8.
79. Passamonti F, Rumi E, Pungolino E, et al. Life expectancy and prognostic factors for survival in patients with polycythemia vera and essential thrombocythemia. Am J Med 2004;117:755–61.
80. Beer PA, Green AR. Pathogenesis and management of essential thrombocythemia. Hematology Am Soc Hematol Educ Program 2009;621–8.
81. Watson KV, Key N. Vascular complications of essential thrombocythaemia: a link to cardiovascular risk factors. Br J Haematol 1993;83:198–203.
82. McCarthy L, Eichelberger L, Skipworth E, et al. Erythromelalgia due to essential thrombocythemia. Transfusion 2002;42:1245.
83. Besses C, Cervantes F, Pereira A, et al. Major vascular complications in essential thrombocythemia: a study of the predictive factors in a series of 148 patients. Leukemia 1999;13:150–4.
84. Lanzkron S, Strouse JJ, Wilson R, et al. Systematic review: hydroxyurea for the treatment of adults with sickle cell disease. Ann Intern Med 2008;148:939–55.
85. Mesa RA, Silverstein MN, Jacobsen SJ, et al. Population-based incidence and survival figures in essential thrombocythemia and agnogenic myeloid metaplasia: an Olmsted County Study, 1976-1995. Am J Hematol 1999;61:10–5.
86. Regev A, Stark P, Blickstein D, et al. Thrombotic complications in essential thrombocythemia with relatively low platelet counts. Am J Hematol 1997;56: 168–72.

87. Beer PA, Erber WN, Campbell PJ, et al. How I treat essential thrombocythemia. Blood 2011;117:1472–82.
88. Jensen MK, de Nully Brown P, Nielsen OJ, et al. Incidence, clinical features and outcome of essential thrombocythaemia in a well defined geographical area. Eur J Haematol 2000;65:132–9.
89. Harrison C. Rethinking disease definitions and therapeutic strategies in essential thrombocythemia and polycythemia vera. Hematology Am Soc Hematol Educ Program 2010;2010:129–34.
90. Schafer AI. Bleeding and thrombosis in the myeloproliferative disorders. Blood 1984;64:1–12.
91. Hellmann A. Myeloproliferative syndromes: diagnosis and therapeutic options. Pol Arch Med Wewn 2008;118:756–60.
92. Schafer AI. Thrombocytosis. N Engl J Med 2004;350:1211–9.
93. Campbell PJ, Green AR. The myeloproliferative disorders. N Engl J Med 2006; 355:2452–66.
94. Antonioli E, Guglielmelli P, Pancrazzi A, et al. Clinical implications of the JAK2 V617F mutation in essential thrombocythemia. Leukemia 2005;19:1847–9.
95. Vannucchi AM, Antonioli E, Guglielmelli P, et al. Clinical profile of homozygous JAK2 617V>F mutation in patients with polycythemia vera or essential thrombocythemia. Blood 2007;110:840–6.
96. Vannucchi AM, Antonioli E, Guglielmelli P, et al. Prospective identification of high-risk polycythemia vera patients based on JAK2(V617F) allele burden. Leukemia 2007;21:1952–9.
97. Cervantes F, Passamonti F, Barosi G. Life expectancy and prognostic factors in the classic BCR/ABL-negative myeloproliferative disorders. Leukemia 2008;22: 905–14.
98. Faderl S, Talpaz M, Estrov Z, et al. The biology of chronic myeloid leukemia. N Engl J Med 1999;341:164–72.
99. Visani G, Finelli C, Castelli U, et al. Myelofibrosis with myeloid metaplasia: clinical and haematological parameters predicting survival in a series of 133 patients. Br J Haematol 1990;75:4–9.
100. Barosi G, Hoffman R. Idiopathic myelofibrosis. Semin Hematol 2005;42:248–58.
101. Baxter EJ, Scott LM, Campbell PJ, et al. Acquired mutation of the tyrosine kinase JAK2 in human myeloproliferative disorders. Lancet 2005;365:1054–61.
102. Mesa RA, Powell H, Lasho T, et al. A longitudinal study of the JAK2(V617F) mutation in myelofibrosis with myeloid metaplasia: analysis at two time points. Haematologica 2006;91:415–6.
103. Hoffman R, Rondelli D. Biology and treatment of primary myelofibrosis. Hematology Am Soc Hematol Educ Program 2007;346–54.
104. Pikman Y, Lee BH, Mercher T, et al. MPLW515L is a novel somatic activating mutation in myelofibrosis with myeloid metaplasia. PLoS Med 2006;3:e270.
105. Bellucci S, Janvier M, Tobelem G, et al. Essential thrombocythemias. Clinical evolutionary and biological data. Cancer 1986;58:2440–7.
106. Colombi M, Radaelli F, Zocchi L, et al. Thrombotic and hemorrhagic complications in essential thrombocythemia. A retrospective study of 103 patients. Cancer 1991;67:2926–30.

Why Does My Patient Have Leukocytosis?

Jan Cerny, MD, PhD[a,b], Alan G. Rosmarin, MD[a,b,*]

KEYWORDS

- Leukocytosis • Neutrophilia • Lymphocytosis
- Diagnostic evaluation • Leukemia
- Myeloproliferative neoplasm

Leukocytosis is an increase of the white blood cell (WBC, or leukocyte) count; for adults, this is usually more than 11,000/μL. The term leukocyte refers collectively to granulocytes (neutrophils, eosinophils, and basophils), monocytes, and lymphocytes. Any of these individual lineages, or combinations of them, may account for increased WBC.

Leukocytosis is one of the most commonly encountered laboratory abnormalities in clinical medicine, and is a frequent reason for both outpatient and inpatient consultation by a hematologist. Leukocytosis may be an acute or chronic process. It is most often caused by an appropriate physiologic response of normal bone marrow to an infectious or inflammatory stimulus. Less frequently, leukocytosis is caused by a primary bone marrow disorder, such as leukemia, lymphoma, or a myeloproliferative neoplasm. Defining the cause of leukocytosis demands a thorough clinical history, physical examination, and review of the peripheral blood smear, and may require additional laboratory testing, radiologic imaging, bone marrow examination, and molecular or cytogenetic analyses.

WHITE BLOOD CELL (WBC) DEVELOPMENT

Three-quarters of all nucleated cells in the bone marrow are committed to the production of leukocytes. Each day, approximately 1.6 billion leukocytes are produced per kilogram of body weight, and more than half are neutrophils.[1]

The peripheral WBC count is an indirect measure of the body's total mass of leukocytes, because only 2% to 3% of total leukocytes circulate in the bloodstream; 90% of

---

There are no commercial relationships or entanglements to disclose.

[a] University of Massachusetts Medical School, University Hospital, H8-533, 55 Lake Avenue North, Worcester, MA 01655, USA

[b] University of Massachusetts Memorial Medical Center, 55 Lake Avenue North, Worcester, MA 01655, USA

* Corresponding author. University of Massachusetts Medical School, University Hospital, H8-533, 55 Lake Avenue North, Worcester, MA 01655.

E-mail address: Alan.Rosmarin@umassmed.edu

Hematol Oncol Clin N Am 26 (2012) 303–319

doi:10.1016/j.hoc.2012.01.001

WBCs are present in bone marrow stores and 7% to 8% are stored in other tissues.[1] The WBC count, as measured in a peripheral blood complete blood count (CBC), is influenced by changes in: (1) the size of the bone marrow storage pool; (2) the rate of WBC release from storage pools; (3) the balance of actively circulating WBC versus reversibly adherent (marginated) cells; and (4) rates of migration to, and consumption of, leukocytes in peripheral tissues.

DEVELOPMENT, MATURATION, AND SURVIVAL OF GRANULOCYTES

Despite their distinctive appearances, functions, and patterns of gene/protein expression, all cellular elements of peripheral blood, that is, red blood cells (RBCs), platelets, and WBCs, ultimately arise from hematopoietic stem cells (HSCs). This rare population of bone marrow cells (<0.2%) has the ability to both self-renew and give rise to more differentiated committed progenitor cells, which are committed to specific cellular lineages, including precursors to granulocytes, monocytes, lymphocytes, RBCs, and megakaryocytes. HSCs and progenitor cells are mononuclear cells morphologically indistinguishable from lymphocytes, but they can be identified in the bone marrow by their expression of antigens such as CD34.[1]

Differentiating granulocytes pass through 6 successive, morphologically distinct stages of maturation. The earliest recognizable form is the myeloblast, followed in turn by promyelocytes and myelocytes; together, these cells constitute the proliferative pool of myeloid cells. The later stages of neutrophil maturation, that is, metamyelocytes, bands and, ultimately, polymorphonuclear neutrophils (polys), are postmitotic.[1] Maturation of granulocytes is marked by nuclear condensation and eventual segmentation (hence the term polymorphonuclear), and acquisition of cytoplasmic granules, which contain pools of degradative enzymes and other products required for effective bacterial killing.

The bone marrow reserve of maturing neutrophils represents approximately a 1-week supply. This storage pool allows a rapid response to demand for WBCs and can triple the level of circulating leukocytes within hours. Neutrophils that leave the marrow can circulate, marginate, or enter peripheral tissues. Margination is the process whereby neutrophils reversibly adhere to the blood vessel wall using specialized adhesion molecules. When stimulated by infection, inflammation, drugs, or metabolic toxins, these cells can demarginate to enter the pool of freely circulating leukocytes. Granulocytes remain in circulation or in peripheral tissues for only a few hours before cell death. The estimated total life span of maturing granulocytes is 11 to 16 days, most of which involves bone marrow maturation and storage.[1]

Based on the staining qualities of their cytoplasmic granules, 3 major granulocytic subgroups are recognized. Most granulocytes are neutrophils (50%–70% of circulating leukocytes), whereas eosinophils and basophils typically constitute only 1% to 2% each. The specialized contents of their distinctive granules support their important roles in bacterial killing (neutrophils), parasitic infections (eosinophils), and viral infections or allergic immune reactions (basophils).

DEVELOPMENT OF MONOCYTES

Monocytes develop from a granulocyte-monocyte precursor that also gives rise to the granulocyte lineage. Under the influence of specialized cytokines, monocytes transform into macrophages that reside in peripheral tissues. Monocytes are the largest mature cells in circulation, and play major roles in phagocytosis and regulation of the immune response.[1]

LYMPHOCYTE DEVELOPMENT

There are 2 major categories of lymphocytes, B cells and T cells, and lesser lympho-cyte populations, including natural killer (NK) cells. B lymphocytes are responsible for generating the enormous range of highly specific antibodies (immunoglobulins) that are required for effective immune function. B cells arise in the bone marrow, rearrange their immunoglobulin genes in lymph nodes after antigen exposure, and take up resi-dence in lymph nodes. A subset of B lymphocytes further matures into plasma cells, which primarily reside in bone marrow and generate large quantities of immunoglob-ulins in response to infectious or inflammatory challenges.

T lymphocytes originate in the bone marrow, mature in the thymus, and take up residence in lymph nodes, bone marrow, and peripheral tissues. Cytotoxic T cells can directly attack abnormal or infected cells (ie, bearing viral antigens on their cell surface), and modulate the activity of B cells and other aspects of the immune system. T-helper cells secrete cytokines that augment specific immune responses. By con-trast, T-suppressor or regulatory cells secrete cytokines that can dampen the intensity of immune response after the infectious agent is cleared. NK cells, a subpopulation of lymphocytes, lack most of the recognizable surface markers of mature T or B cells. NK cells can nonspecifically target cancer cells or microorganisms. The term large gran-ular lymphocytes (LGLs) usually refers to NK cells, because up to 75% of LGLs func-tion as NK cells.[1]

EVALUATION OF LEUKOCYTOSIS

The clinical evaluation of leukocytosis is influenced by (1) the nature of the cells involved, (2) the duration of the leukocytosis, and (3) the presence of associated clin-ical findings. The differential count from a CBC and review of the peripheral blood smear will define whether the increased leukocytes are predominantly granulocytes or lymphocytes, detect abnormalities of WBC morphology, and identify abnormalities of other lineages (eg, anemia, polycythemia, or platelet abnormalities).

The duration of leukocytosis, that is, hours to days versus weeks, months, or years, influences the likely underlying cause. A short duration of leukocytosis suggests an acute event, such an infection or acute leukemia. By contrast, long-standing leukocy-tosis may represent chronic inflammatory states or hematologic malignancies, such as chronic leukemias or lymphomas. Similarly, the presence of associated clinical findings may point to an underlying systemic illness or reflect consequences of a primary hematologic disorder.

CLASSIFICATION OF LEUKOCYTOSIS

The following terms refer to the level and nature of leukocytosis, but do not have strict definitions and may be applied loosely by clinicians. Left shift refers to an increased percentage of immature granulocyte forms in the peripheral blood, which may exhibit toxic granulations (prominent primary granules) and Döhle bodies (prom-inent secondary granules) in response to severe infections. The presence of myelo-cytes or even less mature granulocyte forms in peripheral blood should raise the question of an underlying hematologic malignancy or severe trauma.

Leukemoid reactions represent exaggerated leukocytosis (typically 50,000–100,000/μL) and may include in the peripheral blood all recognizable stages of neutro-phil maturation, that is, from myeloblasts to mature granulocytes. Leukemoid reactions typically last hours to days and may be caused by either benign or malignant conditions. A leukoerythroblastic reaction caused by myelophthisis is similar (but the total WBC does not need to be high) and also includes nucleated RBCs. Leukoery-throblastosis indicates severe disruption of the marrow by overwhelming infection, myelofibrosis, or bone marrow invasion by cancer, and may be associated with extra-medullary hematopoiesis. A leukoerythroblastic reaction in infants can occur with severe hemolytic anemia (eg, erythroblastosis fetalis) or the rare bone disorder, osteo-petrosis, in which failure of osteoclasts to resorb bone causes loss of hematopoietic marrow space and resultant extramedullary hematopoiesis.

Hyperleukocytosis refers to a WBC count greater than 100,000/μL, and is seen almost exclusively in leukemias and myeloproliferative disorders. Leukostasis, or sludging of WBC in small vessels of the brain, lungs, and kidneys, is an oncologic emergency that may cause life-threatening cerebral infarcts, cerebral hemorrhage, or pulmonary insufficiency caused by impaired blood flow. Leukostasis is more common in acute myelogenous leukemia than in acute lymphoblastic leukemia, because myeloblasts are larger and more adhesive than lymphoblasts; it is rarely seen in chronic leukemias, even with extremely high WBC counts.[2,3]

DISTINGUISHING A PRIMARY HEMATOLOGIC DISORDER FROM A REACTIVE (SECONDARY) LEUKOCYTOSIS

When evaluating leukocytosis, attempts should be made to distinguish a primary hematologic disorder (such as leukemias and myeloproliferative neoplasms) from a secondary effect, that is, the response of normal bone marrow to an infectious or inflam-matory challenge. A careful history and physical examination, review of the peripheral blood smear, and laboratory studies are important for making this distinction. Ultimately bone marrow examination, including morphology, chromosome analysis, molecular testing, and imaging studies may be required to conclusively distinguish between these categories of leukocytosis.

True Leukocytosis Versus Pseudoleukocytosis

Leukocytosis may result from (1) increased production, (2) mobilization of storage pools, (3) reduced adhesion to vascular endothelium, (4) decreased migration to periph-eral tissues, (5) increased cell survival, or (6) combinations of these processes. Pseudo-neutrophilia may result from granulocyte demargination due to exercise, epinephrine, or anesthesia. Because the normal spleen retains a large number of leukocytes, asplenia is associated with an increased WBC count. Corticosteroids, which demarginate granu-locytes, decrease neutrophil release from the marrow, and reduce neutrophil egress from the circulation, frequently cause leukocytosis.

CAUSES OF SECONDARY LEUKOCYTOSIS
Infections

Bacterial infections typically cause mild to moderate leukocytosis (11,000–30,000/μL), with a preponderance of mature neutrophils and bands (**Box 1**). The granulocytosis is usually of short duration, and may be associated with a left shift and toxic granulations or Döhle bodies. WBC counts may transiently decline early in the course of over-whelming sepsis, only to increase later. Some patients with *Clostridium difficile* infec-tion or tuberculosis may manifest a leukemoid reaction with a WBC count greater than 50,000/μL. Conversely, typhoid fever, brucellosis, tularemia, rickettsial diseases, ehr-lichiosis, leishmaniasis, and some cases of *Staphylococcus aureus* infection may be associated with leukopenia. Viral infections do not typically cause neutrophilia, but leukocytosis may be observed in the early phases of viral infection.

Box 1
Causes of neutrophilia

1. Secondary to other disease entities
   a. Infection
      i. Acute via release from marginated and storage pools
      ii. Chronic via increased myelopoiesis (eg, tuberculosis, fungal infection, chronic abscess, other chronic infections)
   b. Chronic inflammation
      i. Rheumatic disease: juvenile rheumatoid arthritis, rheumatoid arthritis, Still disease, and others
      ii. Inflammatory bowel disease
      iii. Granulomatous disease
      iv. Chronic hepatitis
   c. Cigarette smoking
   d. Stress
   e. Drug induced
      i. Corticosteroids
      ii. β-Agonists
      iii. Lithium
      iv. Recombinant cytokine administration
      v. Administration of inhibitors of adhesion molecules
   f. Nonhematologic malignancy
      i. Cytokine-secreting tumors (lung, tongue, kidney, urothelial tumors)
      ii. Marrow metastasis (myelophthisis)
   g. Marrow stimulation
      i. Hemolytic anemia, immune thrombocytopenia
      ii. Recovery from marrow suppression
      iii. Recombinant cytokine administration
   h. Postsplenectomy
2. Primary hematologic etiology
   a. Congenital neutrophilia
      i. Hereditary neutrophilia
      ii. Chronic idiopathic neutrophilia
      iii. Down syndrome
      iv. Leukocyte adhesion deficiency (LAD): LAD I and LAD II
   b. Acquired hematologic neoplasms
      i. Acute myelogenous leukemia
      ii. Myeloproliferative neoplasms
         1. Chronic myelogenous leukemia
         2. Polycythemia vera
         3. Essential thrombocytosis
         4. Idiopathic fibrosis

Infectious lymphocytosis (generally 20,000–50,000/μL small, mature-appearing lymphocytes) is mainly a disease of children. It may be related to coxsackievirus A or B6, echovirus, and adenovirus 12, and is rarely associated with splenomegaly or lymphadenopathy. Infection with Epstein-Barr virus (EBV) can cause atypical lymphocytosis (large and reactive lymphocytes with abundant basophilic cytoplasm) and lymphadenopathy. Human T-lymphotropic virus type 1 (HTLV-1) may produce a transient lymphocytosis (usually <20,000/μL) with fever, rash, and lymphadenopathy. In contrast to most other bacterial infections, pertussis (whooping cough) is frequently accompanied by lymphocytosis.

Noninfectious Causes of Leukocytosis

Leukocytosis can be caused by a variety of malignancies, chronic inflammatory conditions, medications, splenectomy, and in association with hemolytic anemia. Postsplenectomy leukocytosis may last weeks to months and has no clinical importance, but may lead to evaluation for other sources of abnormality. Patients with hemolytic anemia may experience a nonspecific increase in leukocyte production and release, in parallel with the increase in RBC production. Chronic smokers may exhibit a mildly increased WBC count that can persist for years.

Chronic inflammatory conditions, including rheumatoid arthritis, juvenile rheumatoid arthritis, and Still disease; inflammatory bowel disorders, such as Crohn disease and ulcerative colitis; vasculitides; granulomatous infections; and chronic hepatitis are often associated with leukocytosis. These processes are associated with increased expression of cytokines that stimulates neutrophil and monocyte production, but can deplete mature neutrophil pools over time. Leukocytosis associated with these inflammatory conditions is typically more modest than in acute infection or inflammation.

Neutrophilia may occur as a result of physical and emotional stress.[4,5] This transient increase in circulating neutrophils occurs within minutes of exercise, surgery, or other forms of stress, and typically reverses within hours of elimination of the trigger. Stress leukocytosis is presumed to be caused by catecholamine-induced demargination of neutrophils, and some cases can be prevented by pretreatment with β-adrenergic antagonists. Exercise-induced neutrophilia, however, is not blocked by propranolol, and may be due to redistribution of neutrophils from the lungs. An increased WBC count may be seen in the setting of acute myocardial infarction, but whether this is a risk factor for cardiac ischemia or a result of inflammation is unclear.[6]

Drug Effect

Medications commonly associated with leukocytosis include corticosteroids, lithium, and β-agonists.[7–9] Steroid administration typically leads to decreased egress from the circulation and increased demargination. Lithium causes neutrophilia by increasing the production of endogenous colony-stimulating factors (CSFs). The cytokines, granulocyte CSF (G-CSF) and granulocyte-macrophage CSF (GM-CSF), are routinely used to mobilize hematopoietic stem and progenitor cells for autologous and allogeneic hematopoietic stem cell transplantation,[10,11] and can cause pronounced neutrophilia if not appropriately managed. Mobilization is achieved within hours of administration of certain chemokines (interleukin-8),[12] small-molecule antagonists of the CXCR4 receptor (eg, AMD3100),[13] or a small-molecule antagonist of VLA-4 (BIO4860).[13,14]

Almost any kind of malignancy may cause leukocytosis, as tumors nonspecifically stimulate the production of leukocytes in bone marrow. Some tumors (eg, lung, tongue, kidney, bladder) can secrete G-CSF as an ectopic hematopoietic growth factor. Other tumors (eg, lung, stomach, breast) can cause a leukoerythroblastic reaction when they spread to bone marrow.[15] Patients with Hodgkin lymphoma typically have mild to moderate neutrophilia, but neutrophilia can be associated with many nonhematologic malignancies.

Recovery of cell counts after marrow suppression, as in the case of chemotherapy, may cause rebound leukocytosis that can last for days to weeks. Similarly, hemolytic anemia and idiopathic thrombocytopenic purpura can result in generalized stimulation of the bone marrow and result in a so-called spillover leukocytosis.

Lymphocytosis

Lymphocytes normally represent 20% to 45% of circulating WBCs. Lymphocytosis conventionally refers to a lymphocyte count greater than 4000/μL, and is the second most common cause of leukocytosis (**Box 2**). The lymphocyte count increases in certain acute and chronic infections. Marked lymphocytosis is observed in individuals infected with pertussis ($\geq$40,000/μL), and lymphocyte counts greater than 100,000/μL indicate a poor prognosis. Chronic brucellosis[16] and syphilis infections[17] may occasionally cause an atypical lymphocytosis.

Viral infections may cause relative or absolute lymphocytosis, with or without neutropenia. Infectious mononucleosis is a self-limited infection caused by EBV infection of B lymphocytes. During the second week of illness, proliferating activated cytotoxic/suppressor T lymphocytes are seen in the peripheral blood as they attack and kill the infected B cells. Such large atypical lymphocytes are not unique to infectious mononucleosis, but can be seen in other viral infections. Infectious mononucleosis, which is

---

Box 2
Causes of lymphocytosis

1. Infection
   a. Viral infection
      i. Epstein-Barr virus
      ii. Cytomegalovirus
      iii. Hepatitis
   b. Bacterial infection
      i. Pertussis
      ii. Bartonella
      iii. Tuberculosis
      iv. Syphilis
      v. Rickettsia
      vi. Babesia
2. Hypersensitivity reactions
   a. Serum sickness
   b. Drug hypersensitivity
3. Primary hematologic disease
   a. Chronic lymphocytic leukemia
   b. Monoclonal B-cell lymphocytosis
   c. Non-Hodgkin lymphoma

most common in adolescents and young adults, typically presents with fever, sore throat, cervical lymphadenopathy, and splenomegaly. Cytomegalovirus (CMV) occasionally causes lymphocytosis with similar symptoms. Toxoplasmosis may cause similar atypical lymphocytosis with fever and lymphadenopathy. Other viral causes of lymphocytosis include infectious lymphocytosis and HTLV-1–related transient lymphocytosis.[18]

Relative, rather than absolute, leukocytosis occurs in infancy, and in association with some viral infections, connective tissue diseases, thyrotoxicosis, and Addison disease. Splenomegaly may cause relative lymphocytosis as a result of splenic sequestration of granulocytes.[19]

Monocytosis (>950/μL; **Box 3**) is commonly caused by bacterial infections, such as tuberculosis, subacute endocarditis, and brucellosis. Other infections include viral infections (eg, infectious mononucleosis), protozoal and rickettsial infections (eg, kala azar, malaria, Rocky Mountain spotted fever), and syphilis. Monocytosis can be seen during the recovery from neutropenia or an acute infection, autoimmune disease, and vasculitis (systemic lupus erythematosus, rheumatoid arthritis, ulcerative colitis, and inflammatory bowel disease). Sarcoidosis and lipid storage disease can be also heralded by monocytosis.[20]

Eosinophilia is defined as an absolute eosinophil count greater than 500/μL. The most common causes of eosinophilia are drug hypersensitivity and allergic conditions,

---

Box 3
Causes of monocytosis

1. Infection
    a. Granulomatous disease (tuberculosis, fungal disease)
    b. Endocarditis
    c. Syphilis
2. Autoimmune diseases
    a. Lupus, rheumatoid arthritis
    b. Giant cell arteritis
    c. Vasculitis
3. Inflammatory bowel disease
4. Sarcoid
5. Malignancy
    a. Primary hematologic malignancy
        i. Chronic myelomonocytic leukemia
        ii. Acute myelomonocytic leukemia
        iii. Lymphoma
    b. Solid tumors
6. Neutropenia
    a. Associated with chronic neutropenia
    b. Recovery from marrow suppression
7. Postsplenectomy

including asthma, hay fever, angioneurotic edema, urticaria, atopic dermatitis and eczema, eosinophilic esophagitis and enteritis, and others.

Eosinophils play an important role in the immune response to parasites. The most common parasitic infections in the United States that are associated with marked eosinophilia are parasites that cause visceral larva migrans by tissue invasion, such as *Toxocara canis* and *Toxocara cati*. Recovery from scarlet fever and some viral infections can also be associated with eosinophilia. Chlamydial infection causes an absolute increase in eosinophils, but generally does not result in leukocytosis. Eosinophilia is associated with dermatologic disorders, such as dermatitis herpetiformis, pemphigus, and erythema multiforme. Eosinophilia, together with basophilia, is seen in some cases of chronic myelogenous leukemia, and increasing counts may herald the onset of the blast phase of this disorder. Other intrinsic hematologic disorders that cause eosinophilia are discussed in the following paragraphs.

Basophilia, defined as a basophil count greater than 100/μL, is seen in association with some allergic conditions and parasitic infections, but rarely leads to leukocytosis. Basophilia is most commonly seen in association with chronic myelogenous leukemia.

Nonmalignant Hematologic Disorders Associated with Leukocytosis

Familial neutrophilia, an autosomal dominant disorder of prominent leukocytosis (>20,000/μL), splenomegaly, and widened diploë of the skull, is caused by a mutation in the G-CSF receptor gene (CSF3R) (see **Box 1**).[21] Neutrophils in this disorder are functionally normal and the leukocytosis has no clinical consequences.

Chronic idiopathic neutrophilia (CIN) is marked by leukocytosis of 11,000/μL to 40,000/μL with a normal bone marrow. Smoking and obesity are significantly associated with CIN and may be causative, but CIN is unlikely to develop into a clinically recognizable myeloproliferative neoplasm, other than chronic myelogenous leukemia (CML).[22] A study with 20-year follow-up of patients with CIN indicated that no medical sequelae arise from the increased WBC count.[22]

Pelger-Huët anomaly (PHA) is characterized by mature neutrophils with bilobed nuclei, rather than the characteristic multilobed nuclear morphology. Because of their resemblance to old-fashioned eyeglasses, such granulocytes are described as pince-nez cells. PHA is caused by a mutation in the lamin B receptor gene.[23] Neutrophil function in PHA is normal, but automated cell counters may indicate a left-shifted WBC because they mistakenly classify the cells as immature granulocytes.

Acquired conditions that may be associated with bilobed granulocytes, so-called pseudo-PHA, include patients with myelodysplasia.[24] Treatment with colchicine, sulfonamides, ibuprofen, and valproate can cause reversible pseudo-PHA.[25] Because deficiencies of vitamin B_{12} or folate increase neutrophil nuclear lobation, these disorders may mask the diagnosis of PHA, but the aberrant neutrophil nuclear morphology returns with correction of the vitamin deficiency.

Transient myeloproliferative disorder (TMD) is seen in up to 10% of patients with Down syndrome (trisomy 21). TMD is characterized by peripheral blood leukocytosis in early infancy, and may include circulating myeloblasts in association with an accumulation of megakaryoblasts in the blood, liver, and marrow. TMD typically persists for several weeks and resolves spontaneously in most patients, but up to 30% of affected patients later develop acute megakaryoblastic leukemia.[26] TMD may also be seen in patients with trisomy 21 mosaicism who are phenotypically normal.

Patients with leukocyte adhesion deficiency (LAD) have persistent leukocytosis, defects in neutrophil activation, recurrent infections, and delayed separation of the umbilical stump. LAD is a congenital abnormality of leukocyte adhesion molecules. LAD I is attributable to the absence or marked reduction in the common β chain of β2 integrins, resulting in loss of expression of leukocyte function-associated antigen 1 (LFA-1), the C3bi receptor, and GP150;95. Babies born with this disorder have persistent neutrophilia in the absence of clinical signs of infection, and increased susceptibility to infection. The diagnosis is confirmed by the absence of CD11b/CD18 on the patient's leukocytes by flow cytometry. In LAD II, neutrophils lack sialyl Lewis X, the ligand for L-selectin expressed on endothelial cells. Neutrophils appear morphologically normal, but are defective in chemotaxis, adherence, and phagocytosis.[27]

Familial cold urticaria is a rare autosomal dominant inflammatory disorder characterized by leukocytosis, episodic fevers, urticaria, rash, conjunctivitis, and muscle and skin tenderness with cold exposure. The rash consists of infiltrating neutrophils. The syndrome seems to be related to decreased levels of C1-esterase inhibitor and is associated with mutations in the CIAS1 gene on chromosome 1q.[28]

HEMATOLOGIC MALIGNANCIES

Leukocytosis is often the initial finding that leads to the diagnosis of a primary hematologic disorder, such as leukemia or a myeloproliferative neoplasm. Careful evaluation of the peripheral blood smear may suggest the underlying disorder and will help to generate the differential diagnosis. However, bone marrow evaluation for histology, flow cytometry, chromosome analysis, and molecular diagnostics are usually required to confirm the diagnosis of a primary hematologic disorder. Even when a pathognomonic finding is available from peripheral blood (eg, detection of the BCR-ABL rearrangement in CML), bone marrow evaluation provides crucial additional information (eg, the degree of marrow fibrosis).

Acute Myelogenous Leukemia

Acute leukemia arises from malignant transformation of an early hematopoietic progenitor cell (see **Box 1**). Instead of proliferating and differentiating normally, the affected cell gives rise to a clone of cells that fail to differentiate normally, and may proliferate in an uncontrolled fashion or fail to undergo programmed cell death, or apoptosis.

Because normal cellular elements in bone marrow may be decreased or absent, acute myelogenous leukemia (AML) often presents clinically as bone marrow failure. Symptoms include fever, infection, anemia, and bleeding or bruising, with corresponding signs on physical examination. Leukemic blasts may not be apparent in peripheral blood (so-called aleukemic leukemia) or may be abundant, ranging up to hyperleukocytosis. Abnormalities of WBCs are typically accompanied by variable degrees of anemia and thrombocytopenia. It is important to quickly recognize acute leukemias, as they may be associated with rapid life-threatening complications including bleeding, disseminated intravascular coagulopathy, leukostasis, brain infarction, and severe infections.

Morphology is an important clue to the nature of acute leukemia, but many cases cannot be definitively classified based on morphology alone. Myeloblasts are large cells with a high nuclear/cytoplasmic ratio; the nuclei may contain several distinct nucleoli, and a thin rim of cytoplasm may contain faint granularity. Bundles of cytoplasmic granules forming Auer rods are a pathognomonic finding in AML.

The diagnosis of AML requires confirmation by histochemical stains or immunophenotyping, and cytogenetic or fluorescent in situ hybridization (FISH) chromosome analysis of bone marrow specimens. More than half of all adults with AML exhibit characteristic nonrandom chromosomal abnormalities, and these anomalies are useful for categorizing patients with good, intermediate, or poor prognosis.[29]

The diagnosis of acute leukemia typically requires bone marrow aspiration and biopsy, usually from the posterior iliac crest. The bone marrow is usually hypercellular and contains at least 20% myeloblasts. Bone marrow should also be examined for fibrosis and dysplasia. However, the normal marrow architecture may be largely effaced, which makes it difficult to identify underlying hematologic disorders such as myelodysplasia or a myeloproliferative neoplasm.

Patients with AML require prompt diagnosis and therapy. WBC counts in excess of 100,000/μL constitute a medical emergency because of the risk of leukostasis (described earlier). Such patients may require therapeutic pheresis or emergent chemotherapy to reduce levels of circulating leukemic blasts and prevent life-threatening vascular complications. Patients with AML may require immediate transfusion of RBCs or platelets. In patients who are judged able to withstand the intensity of leukemia induction therapy, treatment with anthracyclines and cytarabine is usually administered. The resultant profound and prolonged cytopenias may result in infectious complications and threats to all bodily systems.

It is essential to promptly recognize and treat a distinct subset of AML known as acute promyelocytic leukemia (APL). APL is caused by rearrangement of the *retinoic acid receptor* α (*RARA*) gene to one of several partners. APL is unique among AML subsets because of its distinctive clinical presentation, therapy, and natural history. Prompt recognition and treatment of APL can avoid death from disseminated intravascular coagulation (DIC) or infection.[30,31] APL treatment uses all-*trans* retinoic acid (ATRA) in combination with cytotoxic chemotherapy or arsenicals, and has an excellent prognosis for cure if early death from DIC and infection can be avoided.

Acute Lymphoblastic Leukemia

Acute lymphoblastic leukemia (ALL) is the most common childhood leukemia, but it is also seen in adults (although less commonly than AML) (see **Box 2**). Presentation in children may include lethargy, pallor, listlessness, fever, hepatosplenomegaly, and bruising. In adults, the clinical presentation is similar to AML. Most cases of ALL are of B-cell origin. Leukemic blasts in ALL exhibit a high nuclear/cytoplasmic ratio, fine chromatin, inconspicuous nucleoli, bluish cytoplasm, and no cytoplasmic granules. The diagnosis can be confirmed by histochemistry, immunophenotyping, karyotyping, and molecular diagnostics. Intensive induction therapy is usually followed by consolidation therapy and prolonged maintenance therapy.

Chronic Leukemias

Patients with chronic leukemias typically present with less severe symptoms than those with acute leukemias. Chronic leukemia is usually diagnosed by incidental leukocytosis found on routine CBC. Chronic leukemias can be broadly divided into chronic lymphocytic leukemia and CML, depending on the cell of origin. The two categories of chronic leukemia have different underlying molecular defects, clinical manifestations, natural histories, and therapies.

CML (see **Box 1**) is a myeloproliferative neoplasm marked by clonal expansion of bone marrow myeloid precursor cells and increased numbers of circulating mature and immature myeloid cells. At presentation, CML must be distinguished from a leukemoid reaction but, in contrast to a leukemoid reaction, CML is characterized by the presence of abnormalities of other blood cell lines (panmyelosis). Therefore, the peripheral blood smear in CML (but not the leukemoid reaction) may display concomitant basophilia, eosinophilia, anemia, and thrombocytosis.

Most patients with CML are diagnosed incidentally on routine CBC, and many patients are asymptomatic for a long period. However, symptoms of CML include fatigue, bleeding, weight loss, and abdominal discomfort or early satiety caused by splenomegaly; lymphadenopathy is uncommon.

The hallmark of CML is the Philadelphia chromosome (reciprocal translocation of chromosomes 9 and 22), which generates the *BCR-ABL* gene rearrangement that can be identified in peripheral blood by FISH or reverse transcriptase–polymerase chain reaction (RT-PCR). Previously a low leukocyte alkaline phosphatase (LAP) score was used as a diagnostic marker for CML, but this has been supplanted by direct molecular tests for *BCR-ABL* or the 9;22 chromosomal rearrangement.

The chronic phase of CML evolves into the accelerated phase, characterized by fever, sweats, weight loss, bone pain, bruising, and hepatosplenomegaly, and later, a blastic phase that resembles AML. The median time for transformation to blast phase is between 2 and 5 years. However, treatment of CML has been revolutionized by the development of targeted therapy with tyrosine kinase inhibitors (TKIs), which antagonize abnormal signal transduction signaling of the aberrant BCR-ABL protein. Treatment with TKIs is not curative, but survival of treated patients is significantly greater than for patients treated in the pre-TKI era.[32] Treatment with TKIs decreases the blastic transformation rates, perhaps because TKIs eliminate cells that are susceptible to blastic transformation. The blastic phase of CML remains very difficult to treat, even with TKIs and allogeneic stem cell transplantation.[33,34]

Chronic lymphocytic leukemia (CLL; see **Box 2**) results in accumulation of relatively mature-appearing lymphocytes in bone marrow, peripheral blood, lymph nodes, spleen, and other organs. Molecular defects in the normal processes of apoptosis cause accumulation of these malignant lymphocytes. Immunity is decreased because the malignant lymphocytes exhibit impaired immune function.

The lymphocytes in CLL generally appear mature, with condensed nuclei and a thin rim of bluish cytoplasm. These lymphocytes are fragile, and result in so-called smudge cells in the peripheral smear. CLL may be often accompanied by anemia and/or thrombocytopenia caused by impaired bone marrow production, splenic sequestration, or immune destruction. The diagnosis of CLL is established definitively by flow cytometry, which demonstrates a clonal population of lymphocytes that coexpress markers of both B cells (eg, CD19) and T cells (eg, CD5). Evaluation of the bone marrow can define the degree and pattern of bone marrow involvement and the status of other cellular lineages. In the absence of constitutional symptoms (fever, sweats, weight loss), critical cytopenias, troublesome adenopathy, or organ dysfunction, CLL may be managed by careful observation.

The group of BCR-ABL–negative myeloproliferative neoplasms (MPNs) includes chronic myelomonocytic leukemia (CMML), polycythemia vera (PV), myelofibrosis (MF), and essential thrombocythemia (ET). Because all of these entities may present with leukocytosis, distinguishing between them can be difficult, and may require special laboratory studies and bone marrow examinations.[35]

Although superficially resembling CML in its clinical and morphologic presentation, CMML is considered a separate entity because of its particular clinical, therapeutic, and prognostic aspects. CMML is manifest as a myeloproliferative neoplasm that involves the monocytic series and dysplasia of the erythroid-megakaryocytic series. Patients with CMML are older (65–70 years) than most patients with CML. Cytogenetics are usually normal or trisomy 8, and patients with CMML have *RAS* mutations in 40% to 60% of cases, whereas *JAK2* mutation is rare (4%).[36]

PV, MF, and ET are associated with activating mutations in the *JAK2* gene (PV: 65%–97%; ET: 23%–57%; MF: 35%–57%).[37] PV usually is characterized by deregulated and excessive production of RBCs, but increased WBC and platelet counts may also be evident. Symptoms resulting from hypervolemia and hyper viscosity, such as headache, dizziness, visual disturbances, and paresthesias, are sometimes present. Less frequently, patients with PV present with myocardial infarction, stroke, venous thrombosis, and congestive heart failure. Overall survival is generally long (10–20 years).[38]

MF is a bone marrow disorder in which fibroblasts replace normal elements of the marrow. Patients with myelofibrosis are usually 50 years or older and have a median survival of less than 10 years. As bone marrow fibrosis develops, patients can develop leukocytosis, although decreased WBC, RBC, and platelet counts are more common. Patients are asymptomatic early in the course of the disease and are usually diagnosed incidentally based on changes in blood cell counts. Symptomatic patients have fatigue, shortness of breath, weight loss, bleeding, or abdominal discomfort related to splenomegaly. Acute leukemia can develop over time and, when it occurs, usually progresses rapidly.

Leukocytosis is also found in patients with ET. Although increased platelet counts occur in all myeloproliferative disorders, ET is distinguished by the singular prominence of platelets. This diagnosis is one of exclusion, in which t(9;22) and bone marrow fibrosis are absent. It is also important to exclude secondary thrombocytosis caused by nonmarrow disorders (eg, iron deficiency or bleeding). Most patients with ET are asymptomatic and require little, if any, therapy, but some patients develop thrombosis or hemorrhage secondary to increased numbers of dysfunctional platelets.

Several primary hematologic disorders may affect eosinophils. Hypereosinophilic syndrome (HES), in which eosinophil counts of more than 1500/μL persist for at least 6 months, is associated with infiltration of essential organs, such as the heart and the nervous syndrome. Some patients with HES have rearrangements of the *PDGFRA* and *FIP1L* genes that create an activated tyrosine kinase.[39] Patients may respond to steroids, cytotoxic agents, imatinib (especially in patients with *PDGFRA-FIP1L* rearrangements), or mepolizumab (anti–interleukin-5 monoclonal antibody).[40] Untreated, HES inevitably leads to progressive disability and death. Eosinophilic leukemia exhibits accumulation of incompletely differentiated eosinophils.

DIAGNOSTIC WORKUP OF LEUKOCYTOSIS

Leukocytosis is most commonly the result of acute or chronic infection, inflammation, nonhematologic malignancy, or medications. In such clinical settings, leukocytosis represents an appropriate physiologic response of the hematopoietic system to stress. These diagnoses can generally be identified by careful clinical history and physical examination, examination of the peripheral blood smear, and other laboratory and imaging studies. In such settings, direct evaluation of the bone marrow is rarely warranted, unless it is to document infection involving the bone marrow itself.

However, leukocytosis in the absence of such signs and symptoms, coincident anemia or thrombocytopenia, or evidence of a leukoerythroblastic reaction should prompt consideration of bone marrow examination. These findings may point toward an intrinsic hematologic disorder, such as an MPN, leukemia, or lymphoma, or may suggest metastatic cancer or fibrosis involving the bone marrow.

Medical History

A careful history is essential for accurate diagnosis of the cause of leukocytosis. Symptoms such as fever, cough, gastrointestinal symptoms, rash, or swelling may suggest an underlying infection. Infections may present acutely, but longer-term complaints such as fever, rash, or joint pain may broaden the differential diagnosis to include chronic infections, inflammation, or autoimmune diseases. Weight loss, fatigue, and night sweats should prompt consideration of an underlying hematologic or nonhematologic malignancy. Medications such as corticosteroids or epinephrine cause a transitory increase in neutrophil count, and a rebound from recent treatment with chemotherapy, especially if therapeutic cytokines have been used, may account for leukocytosis. History of cigarette smoking and exercise should be defined. In children, sickle cell disease should be considered, and in infants the transient leukemoid reaction seen in Down syndrome or LAD syndromes should be considered.

Physical Examination

A careful examination for infection, including cellulitis, otitis, pharyngitis, pneumonia, urinary tract infection, or abscesses should be sought. The heart and extremities should be carefully examined for stigmata of infective endocarditis. Lymphadenopathy or hepatosplenomegaly points toward a possible viral cause, but may also reflect an underlying malignancy. Tender or swollen joints may indicate juvenile rheumatoid arthritis, septic arthritis, or systemic lupus erythematosus. Stigmata of Down syndrome may explain leukocytosis.

Laboratory Tests

CBC

A confirmatory CBC with differential count should be obtained, and previous CBCs can document the duration of leukocytosis. The nature of the increased cells, that is, granulocytes versus lymphocytes, will often set the direction of further evaluation. It is critical to personally examine the peripheral blood smear. The blood smear in bacterial infection may demonstrate a left shift of granulocytes, accompanied by Döhle bodies, toxic granulations, or vacuolization. Immature granulocyte forms, such as myeloblasts, promyelocytes, and myelocytes, should prompt consideration of acute or chronic leukemias. Pelger-Huët cells or other evidence of granulocyte dysplasia may suggest underlying myelodysplasia, and an increased lymphocyte count accompanied by smudge cells suggests CLL.

Abnormalities of other cellular lineages may provide important clues about the underlying diagnosis. Schistocytes may point toward disseminated intravascular coagulopathy, and a leukoerythroblastic appearance with anemia or thrombocytopenia may suggest a marrow infiltrative disorder, such as cancer, infection, or fibrosis. Anemia with spherocytosis and thrombocytopenia may suggest extravascular hemolysis, as is seen in lymphoma. RBC inclusions may point toward malaria or other intracellular parasites, whereas target cells or sickle cells may indicate an underlying hemoglobinopathy. Recovering or stressed marrow may exhibit an increased monocyte count. Increased numbers of eosinophils and/or basophils may suggest CML.

Other laboratory studies

No single panel of laboratory studies is useful in evaluating all patients with leukocytosis. Thus, laboratory studies should be selected to clarify and perhaps broaden the differential diagnosis.

Liver function tests may point to a possible viral or bacterial infection. Appropriate cultures of blood, urine, stool, or throat may define the underlying disorder. Other useful studies may include Mono spot, heterophil antibodies, EBV, or CMV titers to evaluate infectious mononucleosis.

Uric acid and lactate dehydrogenase are often increased in leukemias and lymphomas. Serologic studies, such as antinuclear antibody, may point toward a rheumatologic origin. LAP was used previously to distinguish infection (increased LAP score) from CML (decreased LAP score), but this has largely been supplanted by more precise testing. RT-PCR performed on peripheral blood for *BCR-ABL* and *JAK2* mutation may document CML or other MPNs, and FISH or cytogenetics can demonstrate the t(9;22) found in CML.

Radiologic examination, such as chest radiographs, may indicate pneumonia, tuberculosis, or other infections. Ultrasonography, computed tomography (CT), positron-emission tomography combined with CT, and other imaging modalities may demonstrate abscesses, tumor masses, or even bone marrow infiltration.

SUMMARY

Leukocytosis is one of the most common laboratory findings in medicine, and represents one of the most frequent sources of requests for hematologic consultation. Because the differential diagnosis potentially encompasses the entirety of medical disorders, the consulting hematologist must make a thoughtful evaluation. The evaluation requires an attentive history, careful physical examination, meticulous review of the CBC and peripheral blood smear, and judicious application of laboratory and radiologic testing. The resultant findings may prompt bone marrow aspiration and biopsy to document cellular morphology and immunophenotype, culture for infectious agents, chromosome analysis, and molecular studies. The results of this evaluation should indicate the appropriate treatment for the underlying disorder.

REFERENCES

1. Turgeon ML. Clinical hematology: theory and procedures. 4th edition. Philadelphia: Lippincott Williams & Wilkins; 2004.
2. Novotny JR, Müller-Beißenhirtz H, Herget-Rosenthal S, et al. Grading of symptoms in hyperleukocytic leukaemia: a clinical model for the role of different blast types and promyelocytes in the development of leukostasis syndrome. Eur J Haematol 2005;74:501–10.
3. Novotny JR, Nückel H, Dührsen U. Correlation between expression of CD56/NCAM and severe leukostasis in hyperleukocytic acute myelomonocytic leukaemia. Eur J Haematol 2006;76:299–308.
4. Steel JM, Steel CM, Johnstone FD. Leukocytosis induced by exercise. Br Med J (Clin Res Ed) 1987;295:1135–6.
5. Darko DF, Rose J, Gillin JC, et al. Neutrophilia and lymphopenia in major mood disorders. Psychiatry Res 1988;25:243–51.
6. Green SM, Vowels J, Waterman B, et al. Leukocytosis: a new look at an old marker for acute myocardial infarction. Acad Emerg Med 1996;3:1034–41.
7. Dale DC, Fauci AS, Guerry DI, et al. Comparison of agents producing a neutrophilic leukocytosis in man. Hydrocortisone, prednisone, endotoxin, and etiocholanolone. J Clin Invest 1975;56:808–13.
8. Lapierre G, Stewart RB. Lithium carbonate and leukocytosis. Am J Hosp Pharm 1980;37:1525–8.
9. Dimitrov S, Lange T, Born J. Selective mobilization of cytotoxic leukocytes by epinephrine. J Immunol 2010;184:503–11.
10. Sato N, Sawada K, Takahashi TA, et al. A time course study for optimal harvest of peripheral blood progenitor cells by granulocyte colony-stimulating factor in healthy volunteers. Exp Hematol 1994;22:973–8.
11. Matsunaga T, Sakamaki S, Kohgo Y, et al. Recombinant human granulocyte colony-stimulating factor can mobilize sufficient amounts of peripheral blood stem cells in healthy volunteers for allogeneic transplantation. Bone Marrow Transplant 1993;11:103–8.

12. Laterveer L, Lindley IJ, Hamilton MS, et al. Interleukin-8 induces rapid mobilization of hematopoietic stem cells with radioprotective capacity and long-term myelolymphoid repopulating ability. Blood 1995;85:2269–75.
13. Bensinger W, DiPersio JF, McCarty JM. Improving stem cell mobilization strategies: future directions. Bone Marrow Transplant 2009;43:181–95.
14. Papayannopoulou T. Current mechanistic scenarios in hematopoietic stem/progenitor cell mobilization. Blood 2004;103:1580–5.
15. Granger JM, Kontoyiannis DP. Etiology and outcome of extreme leukocytosis in 758 nonhematologic cancer patients: a retrospective, single-institution study. Cancer 2009;115:3919–23.
16. Sharda DC, Lubani M. A study of brucellosis in childhood. Clin Pediatr (Phila) 1986;25:492–5.
17. Wood TA, Frenkel EP. The atypical lymphocyte. Am J Med 1967;42:923–36.
18. Tsaparas YF, Brigden ML, Mathias R, et al. Proportion positive for Epstein-Barr virus, cytomegalovirus, human herpesvirus 6, Toxoplasma, and human immunodeficiency virus types 1 and 2 in heterophile-negative patients with an absolute lymphocytosis or an instrument-generated atypical lymphocyte flag. Arch Pathol Lab Med 2000;124:1324–30.
19. Abramson N, Melton B. Leukocytosis: basics of clinical assessment. Am Fam Physician 2000;62:2053–60.
20. Hillman RS, Ault KA, Rinder HM, et al. Hematology in clinical practice: a guide to diagnosis and management. 4th edition. New York: McGraw-Hill; 2005.
21. Plo I, Zhang Y, Le Couedic JP, et al. An activating mutation in the CSF3R gene induces a hereditary chronic neutrophilia. J Exp Med 2009;206:1701–7.
22. Weir AB, Lewis JB Jr, Arteta-Bulos R. Chronic idiopathic neutrophilia: experience and recommendations. South Med J 2011;104:499–504.
23. Shultz LD, Lyons BL, Burzenski LM, et al. Mutations at the mouse ichthyosis locus are within the lamin B receptor gene: a single gene model for human Pelger-Huët anomaly. Hum Mol Genet 2003;12:61–9.
24. Shetty VT, Mundle SD, Raza A. Pseudo Pelger-Huët anomaly in myelodysplastic syndrome: hyposegmented or apoptotic neutrophil? Blood 2001;98:1273–5.
25. Wang E, Boswell E, Siddiqi I, et al. Pseudo-Pelger-Huët anomaly induced by medications. Am J Clin Pathol 2011;135:291–303.
26. Mundschau G, Gurbuxani S, Gamis AS, et al. Mutagenesis of GATA1 is an initiating event in Down syndrome leukemogenesis. Blood 2003;101:4298–300.
27. Alizadeh P, Rahbarimanesh AA, Bahram MG, et al. Leukocyte adhesion deficiency type 1 presenting as leukemoid reaction. Indian J Pediatr 2007;74:1121–3.
28. Hoffman HM, Wright FA, Broide DH, et al. Identification of a locus on chromosome 1q44 for familial cold urticaria. Am J Hum Genet 2000;66:1693–8.
29. Grimwade D, Hills RK, Moorman AV, et al. Refinement of cytogenetic classification in acute myeloid leukemia: determination of prognostic significance of rare recurring chromosomal abnormalities among 5876 younger adult patients treated in the United Kingdom Medical Research Council trials. Blood 2010;116: 354–65.
30. Sanz MA, Grimwade D, Tallman MS, et al. Management of acute promyelocytic leukemia: recommendations from an expert panel on behalf of the European LeukemiaNet. Blood 2009;113:1875–91.
31. Sanz MA, Lo-Coco F. Modern approaches to treating acute promyelocytic leukemia. J Clin Oncol 2011;29:495–503.
32. Druker BJ, Guilhot F, O'Brien SG, et al. Five-year follow-up of patients receiving imatinib for chronic myeloid leukemia. N Engl J Med 2006;355:2408–17.

33. Kantarjian H, Shah NP, Hochhaus A, et al. Dasatinib versus imatinib in newly diagnosed chronic-phase chronic myeloid leukemia. N Engl J Med 2010;362: 2260–70.
34. Saglio G, Kim DW, Issaragrisil S, et al. Nilotinib versus imatinib for newly diagnosed chronic myeloid leukemia. N Engl J Med 2010;362:2251–9.
35. Gilbert HS. The spectrum of myeloproliferative disorders. Med Clin North Am 1973;57:355–93.
36. Wang SA, Galili N, Cerny J, et al. Chronic myelomonocytic leukemia evolving from preexisting myelodysplasia shares many features with de novo disease. Am J Clin Pathol 2006;126:789–97.
37. Tefferi A, Gilliland DG. JAK2 in myeloproliferative disorders is not just another kinase. Cell Cycle 2005;4:4053–6.
38. Vakil E, Tefferi A. BCR-ABL1-negative myeloproliferative neoplasms: a review of molecular biology, diagnosis, and treatment. Clin Lymphoma Myeloma Leuk 2011;11(Suppl 1):S37–45.
39. Cools J, DeAngelo DJ, Gotlib J, et al. A tyrosine kinase created by fusion of the PDGFRA and FIP1L1 genes as a therapeutic target of imatinib in idiopathic hypereosinophilic syndrome. N Engl J Med 2003;348:1201–14.
40. Rothenberg ME, Klion AD, Roufosse FE. Treatment of patients with the hypereosinophilic syndrome with mepolizumab. N Engl J Med 2008;358:2530.

Why Is My Patient Bleeding Or Bruising?

Natalia Rydz, MD[a], Paula D. James, MD[b,*]

KEYWORDS

- Mucocutaneous bleeding • Bleeding scores • Bruising
- Epistaxis • Menorrhagia • Von Willebrand disease (VWD)
- Hemophilia • Platelet function disorder (PFD)

The initial assessment of a patient presenting with bleeding complaints includes a thorough history to determine several points regarding the bleeding symptoms: the pattern (primary vs secondary hemostasis), the severity, and the onset (congenital vs acquired). Bleeding assessment tools (BATs) may be useful In determining whether bleeding symptoms are outside the normal range. The laboratory investigations are directed by the clinical pattern of bleeding and family history; however, because Von Willebrand disease (VWD) comprises the most common and best characterized of the primary hemostatic disorders, VWD is often the first diagnosis within the broad differential to be considered. Clinical management of bleeding disorders is highly individualized and focuses on the particular symptoms experienced by the patient. Potential therapies include replacement of the factor that is deficient or defective (eg, Von WIllebrand factor [VWF]/factor VIII [FVIII] concentrates in VWD, and platelet transfusion in platelet function disorder [PFD]) or indirect treatments, such as antifibrinolytics [tranexamic acid], desmopressin 1-deamino-8-D-arginine vasopressin [DDAVP], and hormone-based therapy (oral contraceptive pill [OCP] for menorrhagia).

The evaluation of a patient presenting with bleeding symptoms is complicated by several challenges. In contrast to severe bleeding disorders, such as severe hemophilia A (HA) and B (HB), or type 3 VWD, milder mucocutaneous bleeding symptoms are frequently reported by a normal population, and show a great deal of overlap with bleeding disorders, such as type 1 VWD.[1–5] Bleeding histories are subjective, and significant symptoms may be interpreted as part of the spectrum of normal bleeding. The differential diagnosis is broad, ranging from defects in primary hemostasis (VWD, or PFDs), coagulation deficiencies, or dysfunction (mild HA/HB or dysfibrinogenemia) to connective tissue disorders (Ehlers-Danlos syndrome [EDS]). Many of the available laboratory investigations are not well standardized and can be difficult

a Department of Pathology and Molecular Medicine, Queen's University, Room 2025, Etherington Hall, Kingston, ON, Canada K7L 3N6
b Department of Medicine, Queen's University, Room 2025, Etherington Hall, Kingston, ON, Canada K7L 3N6
* Corresponding author.
E-mail address: jamesp@queensu.ca

Hematol Oncol Clin N Am 26 (2012) 321–344
doi:10.1016/j.hoc.2012.01.002
0889-8588/12/$ – see front matter © 2012 Elsevier Inc. All rights reserved.

hemonc.theclinics.com

to interpret.[6,7] Finally, despite significant clinical evidence of abnormal bleeding, many patients are not categorizable into any specific diagnostic category despite extensive testing.[8] Awareness of these issues is of paramount importance and is discussed in the following sections.

PATIENT HISTORY
Bleeding History

The bleeding history includes a detailed assessment of the reported symptoms and is summarized in **Table 1**. The following details should be determined:

- The consultant should investigate the nature of the bleeding, which includes inciting factors, frequency, duration, and severity, as well as complications, which include need and type of medical intervention for each bleeding symptom. Locations of bleeding include oral mucosal, cutaneous, gastrointestinal, genitourinary, intracranial, intramuscular, or intra-articular tissues.
- A thorough inquiry into past events is important. This inquiry includes the identification of past hemostatic challenges, associated bleeding complications, and level of intervention required. Hemostatic challenges include invasive surgical procedures, dental extractions, injuries, and wounds. In pediatrics, relevant hemostatic challenges include umbilical stump bleeding or bleeding at the time of circumcision.
- With easy or spontaneous bruising, the consultant should identify the location, size, and associated subcutaneous hematomas.
- When investigating menorrhagia, there are many relevant historical facts. The hematology consultant should determine the onset of menorrhagia (whether it was since menarche), duration of menses, number of pads/tampons needed

Table 1 Summary of clinical history	
Symptom	**Details**
Bruising	Location, associated trauma, associated hematomas
Epistaxis	Frequency, duration, interventions required
Bleeding from minor wounds	Duration
Dental extractions	Duration of bleeding, intervention required
Menorrhagia	Duration of menses, amount of blood loss (pads/tampons used), size of clots seen
Postpartum hemorrhage	Amount and duration of blood loss, intervention required
Bleeding with surgery or injury	Amount and duration of blood loss, intervention required
Muscle hematomas, hemarthrosis	Associated trauma, history of recurrence
History of gastrointestinal/genitourinary/ central nervous system bleeds	Associated anatomic lesions and treatment required
Iron deficiency	Requiring oral/intravenous iron and red cell transfusion
Family history	Of bleeding symptoms or bleeding disorder, consanguinity
Medical history	Medications and comorbidities

throughout the day, history of iron deficiency, and previous treatments such as OCPs, progesterone impregnated intrauterine devices (IUDs), uterine ablation, or hysterectomy. Three findings predict abnormal blood loss: clots larger than approximately 2.5 cm, low serum ferritin, and the need to change a pad or tampon more than hourly.[9] Bleeding symptoms surrounding childbirth, including postpartum hemorrhage, should be explored. Reproductive complications, such as recurrent miscarriages, are also pertinent.

- What measures have been used to treat or alleviate the bleeding symptoms?
- Has the patient ever had anemia requiring treatment with iron supplementation or transfusion?

In addition, the clinician should determine whether the bleeding history supports a primary versus an acquired disorder by the presence of:

- A family history of increased bleeding symptoms or a bleeding disorder
- Consanguinity
- Comorbidities such as renal disease, liver disease, autoimmune disease, lymphoproliferative disease, myeloproliferative neoplasm, plasma cell dyscrasia, cardiac valve disease, hypothyroidism
- Medications with particular attention paid to the use of aspirin (ASA), nonsteroidal antiinflammatory drugs (NSAIDs), clopidogrel, and anticoagulants (both generic and trade names should be used when asking patients about these medications). It is also important to inquire about alternative and complementary medications. For example, the commonly used herbal medications garlic, ginkgo, and ginseng may have an effect on platelet function and increase in bleeding symptoms.[10]

The number and quality of symptoms reported by a patient may be influenced not only by education, family background, and personality but also by the type of data ascertainment because bleeding histories are subject to physicians' interpretation. These factors contribute to the overlap between mild mucocutaneous bleeding symptoms reported by patients with mild to moderate bleeding disorders and those reported by normal individuals; healthy controls may report bleeding symptoms as frequently as individuals with known bleeding disorders.[1–5] A review of the information that compared individuals with VWD with normal populations is presented in **Table 2** to highlight this issue. Similarly, a positive family history is also frequently reported among healthy individuals. For example, in 1 cohort study, in 44% of healthy children undergoing tonsillectomy, parents and guardians reported a family history of bleeding.[11] The points in the history, which are most supportive of a bleeding disorder, include bleeding after hemostatic challenges, intramuscular or intra-articular bleeds, a positive family history of an established bleeding disorder, and positive responses to multiple questions pertaining to bleeding.[4,12] Conversely, a negative family history does not exclude a bleeding disorder. For example, 30% to 40% of patients with hemophilia have de novo mutations and lack a family history.

Bleeding Assessment Tools (BAT)

Much of the recent effort to improve the accuracy of bleeding assessments has focused on quantitative scoring systems, also known as BATs. A group of Italian investigators have pioneered this work and developed a bleeding questionnaire that has been validated for the diagnosis of VWD in a primarily adult population.[3] Since this initial work, several different scoring systems,[13–15] each an adaptation of its

Table 2
Incidence (%) of bleeding symptoms in patients with VWD and in healthy individuals

Symptoms	Normal Individuals (n = 500,[1] n = 341,[4,a] n = 215)[3]	All Types VWD (n = 264)[1]	Type 1 VWD (n = 671,[5] n = 84)[3]	Type 2 VWD (n = 497)[5]	Type 3 VWD (n = 348,[2] n = 66)[5]
Epistaxis	5–11	63	54–61	63	66–77
Menorrhagia	17–44	60	32–67	32	56–69
Postdental extraction bleeding	5–11	52	31–72	39	53–77
Hematomas	12	49	13	14	33
Bleeding from minor wounds	0.2–5	36	36–46	40	50
Gum bleeding	7–37	35	31	35	56
Postsurgical bleeding	1–6	28	20–38	23	41
Postpartum bleeding	3–23	23	17–61	18	15–26
Gastrointestinal bleeding	1	14	5	8	19.2
Joint bleeding	6	8	3	4	37–45
Hematuria	1-8	7	2	5	1–12
Cerebral bleeding	NR	NR	1	2	9

Abbreviation: NR, not reported.
[a] 341 controls were sent a questionnaire. Exact number of respondents is not reported.

predecessor, have been created and validated for VWD. This tool has also been adapted to the pediatric population and validated for both VWD and PDF.[16,17] All versions are based on the principle of summing the severity of bleeding symptoms. **Table 3** shows an example of the MCMDM-1 (Molecular and Clinical Markers for the Diagnosis and Management of VWD type 1) bleeding score.

The main utility of the current BATs occurs at the time of new patient assessments: a positive bleeding score helps identify individuals in need of additional testing, whereas negative bleeding scores can be used to avoid unnecessary investigations. A bleeding history with a significant BAT score is a good predictor of future bleeding, whereas the absence of abnormal investigations or mildly abnormal investigations such as a mildly decreased VWF level (0.30–0.50 u/mL) are not.[13] These scoring systems can determine if there is a greater bleeding risk than in the normal population and thereby may justify the diagnosis of a bleeding disorder.

The currently available BATs have some limitations: when scoring severe bleeding disorders, the BATs become saturated because they take into account the worst episode of bleeding within each category but do not account for other important features such as the frequency of bleeding. In an attempt to standardize the BAT and bleeding score, the International Society on Thrombosis and Haemostasis (ISTH)/Scientific and Standardization Committee (SSC) Joint VWF and Perinatal/Pediatric Hemostasis Subcommittees Working Group have established a revised BAT (http://www.isth.org/default/assets/File/Bleeding_Type1_VWD.pdf).[15]   Studies   to establish the validity and reliability of this new tool are under way.

PHYSICAL EXAMINATION

The examination should be guided by the patient's history and may include the following:

- A dermatologic assessment for the distribution and characteristics of petechiae and ecchymoses; the observation of skin abnormalities or abnormal scars may indicate a collagen defect
- Signs of anemia
- Joint examination in the case of a positive history of hemarthrosis
- Joint hypermobility assessment using the Beighton scale.[18] This involves 5 simple maneuvers that can be performed at the bedside (**Table 4**); a score of 5/9 or greater defines joint hyperflexibility and may indicate a connective tissue disorder
- Assessment for cardiac murmurs, lymphadenopathy, splenomegaly, hepatomegaly, thyroid goiter, evidence of cirrhosis, and so forth.

CLINICAL MANIFESTATIONS
General Considerations

The classic symptoms/characteristics of the bleeding disorder categories are summarized in **Table 5**. Clinical symptoms may be modified by coexisting illnesses or medications such as OCP, which can decrease bleeding in women with menorrhagia. Symptoms may become apparent only after hemostatic provocation (such as menses, surgery, or trauma).

Defects of Primary Hemostasis: Platelet Function Defects (PFD) and Von Willebrand Disease (VWD)

The characteristic bleeding symptoms in PFD and VWD involve the skin and mucous membranes. They include petechiae, ecchymoses, epistaxis, menorrhagia, excessive bleeding after minor wounds, dental extractions, surgery or childbirth, and bleeding from the oral cavity or gastrointestinal tract. Musculoskeletal bleeding such as hemarthrosis and intramuscular hematomas is rare and usually occurs only in severe forms of VWD, and in association with significantly decreased FVIII, which may occur in certain subtypes of VWD and HA.[2,5] Severe bleeding (central nervous system or gastrointestinal tract) can occur in individuals with type 3 VWD and in some with type 2 VWD, but is rare in individuals with type 1 VWD.[19] Bleeding with hemostatic challenges is immediate.

Defects of Secondary Hemostasis: Deficiencies or Defects in Coagulation Factors

Coagulation disorders manifest deep tissue bleeding such as large palpable ecchymoses, deep soft tissue hematomas, and intramuscular hematomas. Hemarthrosis tends to occur only in severe deficiencies, such as HA with an FVIII less than 1 IU/dL (normal range 50–150 IU/dL). Mild deficiencies often present after hemostatic challenges with delayed postsurgical bleeding complications.

Abnormalities of Connective Tissue/Collagen. Ehlers Danlos Syndrome (EDS)

Connective tissue disease manifests with symptoms that reflect vascular fragility. Easy or spontaneous bruising is often the presenting complaint and recurs in the same areas, causing a characteristic discoloration of the skin from hemosiderin

Table 3
MCMDM-1VWD bleeding score key

Symptom		Score					
	-1	0	1	2	3	4
Epistaxis	—	No or trivial (<5)	>5 or more than 10 min	Consultation only	Packing or cauterization or antifibrinolytic	Blood transfusion or replacement therapy or desmopressin
Cutaneous	—	No or trivial (<1 cm)	>1 cm and no trauma	Consultation only		
Bleeding from minor wounds	—	No or trivial (<5)	>5 or more than 5 min	Consultation only	Surgical hemostasis	Blood transfusion or replacement therapy or desmopressin
Oral cavity	—	No	Referred at least 1	Consultation only	Surgical hemostasis or antifibrinolytic	Blood transfusion or replacement therapy or desmopressin
Gastrointestinal bleeding	—	No	Associated with ulcer, portal hypertension, hemorrhoids, angiodysplasia	Spontaneous	Surgical hemostasis, blood transfusion, replacement therapy, desmopressin, antifibrinolytic	
Tooth extraction	No bleeding in at least 2 extractions	None or no bleeding in 1 extraction	Referred in <25% of all procedures	Referred in >25% of all procedures, no intervention	Resuturing or packing	Blood transfusion or replacement therapy or desmopressin

Surgery	No bleeding in at least 2 surgeries	None or no bleeding in 1 surgery	Referred in <25% of all surgeries	Referred in >25% of all procedures, no intervention	Surgical hemostasis or antifibrinolytic	Blood transfusion or replacement therapy or desmopressin
Menorrhagia	—	No	Consultation only	Antifibrinolytics, OCP use	Dilatation and curettage, iron therapy	Blood transfusion or replacement therapy or desmopressin or hysterectomy
Postpartum hemorrhage	No bleeding in at least 2 deliveries	No deliveries or no bleeding in 1 delivery	Consultation only	Dilatation and curettage, iron therapy, antifibrinolytics	Blood transfusion or replacement therapy or desmopressin	Hysterectomy
Muscle hematomas	—	Never	After trauma no therapy	Spontaneous, no therapy	Spontaneous or traumatic, requiring desmopressin or replacement therapy	Spontaneous or traumatic, requiring surgical intervention or blood transfusion
Hemarthrosis	—	Never	After trauma no therapy	Spontaneous, no therapy	Spontaneous or traumatic, requiring desmopressin or replacement therapy	Spontaneous or traumatic, requiring Surgical intervention or blood transfusion
Central nervous system bleeding	—	Never	—	—	Subdural, any intervention	Intracerebral, any intervention

Reproduced from Tosetto A, Rodeghiero F, Castaman G, et al. A quantitative analysis of bleeding symptoms in type 1 Von Willebrand disease: results from a multi-center European study (MCMDM-1 VWD). J Thromb Haemost 2006;4:768; with permission.

Table 4
Beighton scale: a score ≥5 indicated joint hypermobility and raises the possibility of an underlying connective tissue disorder. A score of ≥5/9 is significant for joint hypermobility

Maneuver	Points
Passive dorsiflexion of the little (fifth) finger >90°	1 point for each hand
Passive apposition of the thumbs to the flexor aspects of the forearm	1 point for each hand
Hyperextension of the elbows beyond 10°	1 point for each elbow
Hyperextension of the knees beyond 10°	1 point for each knee
Forward flexion of the trunk with knees fully extended so that the palms of the hands rest flat on the floor	1 point

Adapted from Beighton P, Solomon L, Soskolne CL. Articular mobility in an African population. Ann Rheum Dis 1973;32:413–8; with permission.

deposition.[20,21] A wide range of bleeding symptoms, from severe bruising, subcutaneous hematomas, oral mucosal bleeding, menorrhagia, to internal bleeding as a result of arterial rupture, may also occur. Bleeding complications with invasive procedures are immediate. Other clinical manifestations include skin hyperextensibility, delayed wound healing with atrophic scarring, joint hypermobility, and generalized connective tissue fragility.[22]

Acquired Bleeding Disorders

Acquired bleeding disorders can affect any of the components of hemostasis: platelets, coagulation factors, and even the vessel wall. Therefore the pattern of bleeding depends on the underlying pathologic process. However, an important distinction from the hereditary causes is that the patient has a negative past personal history and family history for bleeding symptoms.

LABORATORY TESTING

The laboratory evaluation of a patient with bleeding symptoms involves several screening tests that direct subsequent investigations. These tests include a complete blood count (CBC) with a peripheral blood smear (PBS), activated partial thromboplastin time (aPTT), prothrombin time (PT), thrombin time (TT), and fibrinogen concentration. Tests that may be included with the initial investigations to identify common, easily diagnosable causes of acquired bleeding disorders include renal, liver, and thyroid function tests. Iron stores should be assessed with a ferritin. Other screening tests such as bleeding time or platelet function analyzer (PFA-100) may be available in some laboratories. Any abnormalities in the screening tests should be pursued with further investigations. Second-line testing will include specific tests that are necessary to diagnose VWD (VWF antigen level [VWF:Ag], VWF ristocetin cofactor [VWF:Rco], FVIII) or PFD, because these two diagnoses make up the most commonly diagnosed bleeding disorders. If no abnormality has been discovered at this point, testing of factor assays, fibrinolysis, and thrombin generation completes the available diagnostic workup, albeit with a low diagnostic yield. An approach is summarized in **Box 1**.

Despite a significant history of bleeding symptoms, and extensive laboratory testing, a large portion of patients will have no identifiable cause. This finding was shown in a large prospective study[8] of 280 patients with mucocutaneous bleeding: 17.9%, 23.2%, and 3.9% were found to have VWD, PFD, or mild clotting factor

Table 5
Clinical manifestations of bleeding disorder categories

Symptom	PFD/VWD	Clotting Factor Deficiencies	Connective Tissue Disorders
Location of bleeding symptoms	Mucocutaneous bleeding: oral cavity, nasal, gastrointestinal, and genitourinary	Deep tissue bleeding: joints and muscles	Mucocutaneous bleeding, but can have a variable clinical picture
Ecchymoses	Common, superficial, can be associated with small subcutaneous hematomas	Large subcutaneous and soft tissue hematomas, out of proportion to inciting trauma	Common, often spontaneous, recurring in the same location, and associated with hemosiderin deposition. May also have subcutaneous hematomas
Petechiae	Common	Uncommon	Common
Bleeding after minor cuts	Common	Uncommon	Common with abnormal healing and scar formation
Deep tissue bleeding (joint and muscle bleeds)	Uncommon	Common and spontaneous in severe factor deficiencies. Provoked by injury in moderate to mild deficiencies	Uncommon
Bleeding with invasive procedures	Immediate	Delayed	Immediate
Manifestations other than bleeding	Generally none. Rare subtypes of PFD can be associated with hearing loss, mental retardation, albinism (see **Table 8**)	Generally none. Afibrinogenemia/dysfibrinogenemia is associated with increased risk of thrombosis. FXIII may be marked by poor wound healing. Both are associated with recurrent miscarriages	Skin hyperextensibility Delayed wound healing Atrophic scarring Joint hypermobility Generalized connective tissue fragility

deficiencies, respectively; 11.5% had combined defects. However, 59.6% of patients had bleeding of unknown cause (BUC), with a prolonged bleeding time in 18.6%, despite significant clinical evidence of a bleeding diathesis and extensive laboratory testing. All of the reported diseases, including the category of BUC, were undistinguishable as far as severity of bleeding symptoms.

Screening Tests

Any abnormal result warrants further investigation. (**Table 6** shows the approach to abnormal coagulation tests.)

Box 1
Suggested approach to investigations

First Line

    Includes screening tests and causes/consequences of bleeding disorders:

- CBC, PBS, aPTT, PT, TT, fibrinogen
- Ferritin, renal, and liver function tests, TSH
- Consider PFA-100, or BT

Second Line

    In the presence of normal screening tests, this line of investigations identifies the 2 most common causes of mild to moderate bleeding disorders:

- VWF:Ag, VWF:RCo, FVIII
- Platelet function testing (LTA and EM)

Third Line

    Performance of the following tests should be based on abnormal screening tests or in the presence of severe bleeding symptoms with unremarkable testing thus far:

- Mixing studies
- Factor assays (eg, II, V, VII, XI, XIII)
- Inhibitor assays (Bethesda assay with Nijmegen modification)
- Urea clot stability or euglobulin clot lysis time
- α_2-Antiplasmin level and PAI-1 activity
- Reptilase time

1. Only those with a high clinical index of suspicion should be investigated

2. If the history clearly indicates a particular disorder, the appropriate investigations should be performed at first-line testing

Abbreviations: BT, bleeding time; EM, electron microscopy; LTA, light transmission aggregometry; PAI-1, plasminogen activator inhibitor 1; TSH, thyroid-stimulating hormone.

- CBC and PBS assess the platelet count and allow for the morphologic assessment of all the cell lines, with special attention to the platelets.
- aPTT and PT measure the intrinsic and extrinsic coagulation pathways, respectively, and may be prolonged in factor deficiencies, factor inhibitors, liver disease, and vitamin K deficiency.
- TT measures the conversion of fibrinogen to fibrin after the addition of thrombin, and is increased in hereditary or acquired deficiencies or dysfunctions of fibrinogen.
- Fibrinogen concentration is a functional assay based on the time for fibrin clot formation.
- Bleeding time is the only in vivo hemostasis test and screens for functional platelet disorders.[23] Although it is consistently prolonged in patients with severe diseases (ie, Glanzmann thrombasthenia and type 3 VWD), it lacks sensitivity in individuals with mild bleeding disorders.[24–26] In addition, bleeding time is poorly reproducible and invasive. As a result, its utility has been called into question and many laboratories no longer perform bleeding times. However, the bleeding time may be useful in centers where second-line and third-line testing are not available.

Table 6
The differential diagnosis of abnormal screening coagulation tests and further investigations

PT	aPTT	TT	Fibrinogen	Interpretation
N	N	N	N	Normal profile, which can be seen with mild factor deficiencies, mild VWD, PFD, FXIII deficiency, PAI-1 deficiency, α_2-antiplasmin deficiency and connective tissue disorders
↑	N	N	N	FVII deficiency, warfarin therapy, early liver failure, early DIC
N	↑	N	N	Deficiencies of FVIII, IX, XI, XII VWD if FVIII is significantly decreased
↑	↑	N	N	Deficiencies of FII, FV, FX Supratherapeutic warfarin
↑	↑	↑	↓	Dysfibrinogenemia or afibrinogenemia Late DIC or liver failure
↑	↑	↑	N	Large amounts of heparin (reptilase time is normal)
N	N	↑	↓	Mild cases of dysfibrinogenemia or hypofibrinogenemia
N	↑	↑	N	Heparin (reptilase time is normal)

Abbreviations: DIC, disseminated intravascular coagulation; N, within normal range.

- PFA-100 measures platelet function under conditions of high shear. It is a simple, rapid noninvasive test that does not require specialized training.[23] Similar to the bleeding time, PFA-100 is abnormal in patients with severe PFD but lacks sensitivity in persons with mild bleeding, calling into question its use as a screening tool.[23–26]

Second Line of Testing

Any abnormalities in the screening tests direct further investigations. If the screening tests are normal, testing for VWD and PFD should be performed.

- VWD testing includes:
  - VWF:Ag, a measure of the quantity of VWF protein in the plasma
  - VWF:RCo, a measure of the ability of VWF to agglutinate platelets
  - FVIII:C, an FVIII assay because VWF functions as the carrier protein for FVIII in the plasma.

Intrapatient variation in VWF studies is influenced by several environmental factors, which include physiologic stressors and hormones. In addition, several analytical issues (for example, the high degree of assay variability) and preanalytical issues with sample handling can complicate the diagnostic workup of VWD.[6] As a result, at least 2 sets of tests using appropriately handled samples are needed to confirm or refute the diagnosis of VWD, and testing should be avoided in stressed, ill, or pregnant patients.

- Platelet function testing includes:
  - LTA methods to assess platelet function
  - EM to assess for dense granule deficiency.

These tests are time-consuming, time-sensitive, poorly standardized, and subject to significant preanalytical and analytical variables. Efforts to standardize LTA methods are ongoing.[27,28] An abnormal result should be confirmed with repeat testing on another sample. North American consensus guidelines[28] provide recommendations on how to further investigate abnormalities that suggest specific diagnoses.

Third Line of Testing

These investigations include either the follow-up of abnormalities identified with screening investigations or further evaluations of the patient when the investigations mentioned earlier have not yet yielded a diagnosis. In the latter case, the likelihood of obtaining a diagnosis, when VWD and PFD have been excluded, is low.[8]

- Mixing study, involving a 1:1 mix of control plasma to patient plasma, differentiates the presence of a factor deficiency versus an inhibitor, in the face of a prolonged aPTT or PT. This test has no clinical usefulness if the baseline aPTT or PT is normal.
- Factor assays specifically for FIX (VIII has already been assessed in the VWD investigations) should be considered because deficiencies in VIII and IX make up the 2 most common hemophilias[29] and the coagulation screen may not be prolonged in mild deficiencies. Other deficiencies, such as XI, II, V, VII, and X, are rare, but should be considered in certain populations, such as FXI deficiency in the Ashkenazi Jewish population[30] and consanguineous families.
- Urea clot stability or euglobulin clot lysis time tests the ability of urea or monochloroacetic acid to solubilize the clot, reflecting a deficiency of FXIII that cross-links fibrin and stabilizes clots.
- α_2-Antiplasmin level and PAI-I activity are measures of fibrinolytic activity, and abnormalities in either are rare causes of bleeding.
- Reptilase time is similar to TT in that it measures the conversion of fibrinogen to fibrin, but instead of thrombin, reptilase, a thrombinlike snake enzyme, is added, which is resistant to inhibition by drugs such as heparin; the usefulness of this test is in ruling out heparin contamination. For example, if TT is prolonged and reptilase time is normal, the presence of heparin should be suspected.

DIAGNOSTIC ALGORITHM AND DIFFERENTIAL DIAGNOSIS

A brief discussion of the differential diagnosis follows.

Von Willebrand Disease (VWD)

VWF is an adhesive multimeric plasma glycoprotein that performs 2 functions in hemostasis: it mediates platelet adhesion to injured subendothelium via glycoprotein 1b, and it binds and stabilizes FVIII in the circulation. VWD, which is caused by deficient or defective plasma VWF, is the most common inherited bleeding disorder, affecting as much as 0.1% to 1% of the population.[31–33] The most common bleeding symptoms reflect a defect in primary hemostasis: mucocutaneous bleeding. In severe cases, FVIII levels may be sufficiently decreased that the aPTT is prolonged and the bleeding phenotype overlaps with that of mild to moderate hemophilia, with delayed bleeding into joints and soft tissue. VWD classification[34] comprises 3 subtypes:

- Type 1 VWD is a partial quantitative deficiency of essentially normal VWF
- Type 2 VWD is a qualitative defective VWF
- Type 3 VWD is a virtually complete quantitative deficiency of VWF.

The 2 main treatments are DDAVP, which results in an increase of Von Willebrand multimers in plasma, and clotting factor concentrates containing both VWF and FVIII (VWF/FVIII concentrate). Other treatment options include antifibrinolytics (tranexamic acid) and hormone therapy (OCP).

Ehlers Danlos Syndrome (EHD)

EDS compromises a heterogeneous group of connective tissue disease sharing clinical manifestations in skin, ligaments and joints, blood vessels, and internal organs. Most subtypes are caused by mutations in structural collagen genes or in genes coding for enzymes involved in their posttranslational modification. Main features are skin hyperextensibility, joint hypermobility, easy bruising, and generalized connective tissue fragility.[20] Prevalence is approximately 1/5000 births, with no racial predisposition.[35] No specific therapy exists for EDS. Interventions for bleeding/bruising may include supplementation of ascorbic acid, a cofactor for cross-linking of collagen fibrils, which can improve bruising symptoms, and DDAVP perioperatively.[20,36]

Thrombocytopenia

Thrombocytopenia is easily diagnosed with a CBC. A repeat CBC and morphologic review of the PBS should be performed to rule out platelet clumping. Also, the mean platelet volume, platelet size, and morphology, as well as additional abnormalities in the other cell lines, may be helpful in narrowing the differential diagnosis. There are several congenital platelet disorders in which thrombocytopenia and platelet dysfunction coexist (**Table 7**). In these cases, the bleeding phenotype seems more severe than expected from the thrombocytopenia alone. Causes, investigations, and treatment of thrombocytopenia are not reviewed here.

Platelet Function Disorders (PFD)

The PFDs compromise a heterogeneous group of inherited causes of abnormal bleeding (**Table 8**). The overall prevalence of PFDs is unknown, but prospective studies of individuals presenting with mucocutaneous symptoms indicate that approximately one-fifth of patients are diagnosed with a mild PFD.[8,37,38] Most of the well-described inherited disorders of platelet function, such as Bernard-Soulier syndrome, Glanzmann thrombasthenia, or the MYH9 mutations, are rare and have been reviewed in detail elsewhere.[38,39] However, it is the incompletely characterized platelet secretion and signal transduction defects that are the most frequently diagnosed inherited PFDs.[8,38] Given the need for specialized testing and experience with interpretation, it is preferable to refer patients with suspected PFDs to a specialist. Acquired PFDs are common and may be a result of drugs, cirrhosis, uremia, myeloma, or myeloproliferative disorders. The diagnosis of platelet dysfunction secondary to drugs or medical illness is typically made based on the history of exposure and onset of symptoms.[7,40] In the case of drug-induced PFD, testing for an underlying PFD after discontinuation of the offending drug helps exclude an underlying disease that may have been unmasked by the drug.

Inherited Coagulation Disorders

Hemophilia

HA and HB, which are deficiencies in FVIII and FIX, respectively, are the 2 most common severe inherited coagulation factor bleeding disorders, with an incidence of 1:10,000 and 1:60,000, respectively, in the general population.[29] HA and HB are X-linked recessive disorders, and thus predominately affect males. More than

Table 7
Congenital PFDs associated with thrombocytopenia

Diagnosis	Peripheral Blood Finding	Associated Findings
Bernard-Soulier syndrome	Giant platelets	None
Platelet-type VWD	Large platelets	None
Wiskott-Aldrich syndrome	Small platelets	Immunodeficiency, eczema, lymphoma,
Gray platelet syndrome	Large platelets with no α-granules	Myelofibrosis
MYH9-related diseases (e.g. May-Hegglin, Epstein, and Sebastian syndromes)	Large platelets, leukocyte inclusions	Deafness, nephritis, cataracts
Mediterranean macrothrombocytopenia	Giant platelets	None
Quebec platelet disorder		
RUNX1 mutations (familial thrombocytopenia)	Myelodysplasia	Propensity for leukemia
Congenital amegakaryocytic thrombocytopenia	Severe thrombocytopenia at birth	Progressive aplasia
Thrombocytopenia and absent radii	None	Absent/shortened radii
GATA-1 related thrombocytopenia with dyserythropoiesis	Dyserythropoiesis, anemia, large platelets	May be associated with β-thalassemia in some patients

Data from Nurden P, Nurden AT. Congenital disorders associated with platelet dysfunctions. Thromb Haemost 2008;99:253–63; Handin RI. Inherited platelet disorders. Hematology Am Soc Hematol Educ Program 2005;396–2.

one-third of diagnoses of hemophilia are caused by de novo mutations of either the *F8* or the *F9* gene and therefore lack a family history.[41] Females may be affected with low levels of coagulation factor and a bleeding diathesis in the following situations[42]:

- Extreme lyonization resulting in skewed inactivation of the nonhemophilia-bearing X chromosome
- Chromosomal abnormalities such as Turner syndrome or translocation
- Homozygosity for the *F8* or *F9* gene mutations (cases of consanguinity) or compound heterozygous mutations affecting both *F8* and *F9* genes

The clinical manifestations of HA or HB are dependent on the level of coagulant activity:

- Severe hemophilia, defined by a factor level less than 1%, is marked by recurrent spontaneous hemarthrosis and deep tissue bleeding, presents in infancy, and requires regular treatment with factor replacement, known as prophylaxis, to avoid long-term sequelae such as debilitating joint damage.
- Mild and moderate hemophilia, defined by a factor level greater than 5%, and between 1% and 5%, respectively, is marked by increased and delayed bleeding with injury or postoperatively; factor replacement is required only with injuries or in anticipation of an invasive procedure.
- In addition, women with hemophilia may suffer from menorrhagia.

Table 8
Examples of the diversity of PFDs. Congenital PFDs can be divided grossly into defects affecting surface proteins and intracellular defects

Defects	Resultant Abnormalities
Surface Defects	
Bernard-Soulier syndrome (mutation of GP1b)	Lack of adhesion to VWF and abnormal response to thrombin
Glanzmann thrombasthenia (mutation to GPαIIbβ3)	Lack of platelet to platelet aggregation
Scott syndrome	Decreased thrombin formation
Platelet-type VWD (GP1bα)	Spontaneous binding of VWF to GP1bα
Mutations to surface receptors (GP6, P2RY12, TBXA2R)	Decreased responses to agonists such as collagen, ADP, TXA$_2$
Intracellular Defects	
Metabolic disorders	Glycogen storage disease or defects in the production of ATP
Mutations of cytoskeleton proteins	*MYH9*-related disorders (e.g. May-Hegglin syndrome)
Abnormalities of dense granules	Hermansky-Pudlak syndrome, Chediak-Higashi syndrome
Abnormalities of α-granules	Gray platelet syndromes, Quebec platelet syndrome
Abnormalities of enzymes	For example, TXA$_2$ synthetase, cyclooxygenase

Abbreviations: ADP, adenosine diphosphatase; ATP, adenosine triphosphate; GP, glycoprotein; TXA$_2$, thromboxane.
Data from Nurden A, Nurden P. Advances in our understanding of the molecular basis of disorders of platelet function. J Thromb Haemost 2011;9 Suppl 1:76–91.

Treatment generally includes indirect therapies such as tranexamic acid, and DDAVP (in the case of mild HA), as well as direct therapies such as replacement of the factor with recombinant products.

Recessive inherited coagulation disorders

The remaining coagulation disorders (frequently referred to as recessive inherited coagulation disorders) such as deficiencies of FII, V, VII, X, XI, XII, or XIII are rare, autosomal-recessive diseases that are more common in consanguineous families.[43] The first-line coagulation screening tests, PT and aPTT, identify most of these clinically significant deficiencies but not deficiencies of FXIII, α_2-antiplasmin, and PAI-1. Factor levels are not severely decreased in heterozygous individuals, but up to 40% of these patients may be symptomatic.[44] The associated bleeding disorders range from mild to severe, and levels of the factor do not always correlate with plasma levels, as in the case of FXI deficiency. Clinical manifestations overlap with those of hemophilia, such as hemarthrosis, muscular hematomas, and excessive bleeding after invasive procedures and injury, but also include mucosal bleeds (epistaxis and menorrhagia), prolonged umbilical cord stump bleeding, and recurrent hemoperitoneum with ovulation.[43]

α_2-Antiplasmin deficiency[45] and PAI-1 deficiency[46] are rare and testing should be considered only in situations in which a significant bleeding disorder is present and testing has otherwise been negative.

Acquired Bleeding Disorders

Acquired disorders of coagulation or platelet function are more common than congenital disorders and generally obvious after a thorough history, physical examination, and screening blood work (**Table 9**) for a list of potential causes. The underlying pathophysiology depends on the cause of the disorder.

Causes of acquired coagulation disorders include:

- Vitamin K deficiency, caused by malabsorption as a result of gastrointestinal disease, antibiotics, and malnutrition, or vitamin K antagonism, by the anticoagulant warfarin, resulting in decreased FII, FVII, FIX, FX, and protein C and S
- Medications (eg, heparin, direct thrombin inhibitors)
- Advanced cirrhosis, which impairs the synthesis of coagulation factors
- Amyloidosis, which may be associated with decreased FX, because amyloid light-chain fibrils in the liver and spleen absorb this factor[47]; in addition, bleeding symptoms may be exacerbated by vascular fragility.

Causes of acquired platelet dysfunction include:

- In paraproteinemias (particularly IgM), coating of platelets by antibodies can be either nonspecific or specifically bind to platelet glycoproteins and result in clinically significant bleeding.[47]
- A bleeding diathesis associated with valproate use may include thrombocytopenia and abnormal platelet function, as well as acquired VWD.[48]
- Both uremia[49] and severe liver disease[50] impair platelet function.
- Medications (ASA, NSAIDs, clopidogrel) impair platelet function by inhibiting certain pathways.

Table 9
Examples of causes of acquired bleeding disorders

Cause of Bleeding Symptoms	Underlying Cause
Platelet dysfunction	Drugs: ASA, NSAIDs
	Renal disease
	Cirrhosis
	Paraproteinemias
	Myeloproliferative neoplasms
Factor deficiencies	Drugs
	Amyloid
	Cirrhosis
VWF deficiency/defect (AVWS)	Valves
	Arteriovenous malformation
	Hypothyroidism
	Drugs (valproic acid)
Inhibitors	Drugs
	Pregnancy
	Malignancy
	Paraproteinemias
	Autoimmune disease
Vessel wall	Amyloid
	Vasculitis

Two acquired disorders warrant special mention: acquired coagulation inhibitors and acquired Von Willebrand syndrome (AVWS).

Acquired Coagulation Inhibitors

Acquired inhibitors against coagulation proteins result in a severe and acute presentation of bleeding. Although inhibitors to FV, IX, X, XI, and XIII have been described, the most common acquired inhibitor is to FVIII, with an incidence of 1 to 4 per million per year.[51] Prompt diagnosis and treatment are important because up to 90% of patients experience a severe bleed, and mortality ranges from 8% to 22%. The incidence increases with age, with most cases occurring between the ages of 68 and 80 years. However, there is a small peak in the age distribution in women during childbearing years associated with inhibitor development during the postpartum period. Acquired FVIII inhibitors may be associated with autoimmune disease, underlying hematologic or solid tumor malignancy, infections, or medications.[51] However, up to 50% of cases are idiopathic. The clinical manifestations of acquired FVIII inhibitor include bleeding into the skin, muscles, soft tissues, and mucous membranes. The laboratory findings of an inhibitor include prolongation of aPTT or PT, depending on which factor is affected. A mixing study fails to correct to a normal aPTT/PT. In cases of an acquired FVIII inhibitor, the mixing study may be time and temperature dependent. Factor assays will identify the affected factor. The inhibitor activity is confirmed by an inhibitor assay (Bethesda assay with Nijmegen modification). Treatment of active bleeding involves the infusion of large amounts of factor, or bypassing agents such as activated prothrombin complex concentrates and recombinant activated FVII. Eradication of the inhibitor may involve the use of prednisone, cyclophosphamide, intravenous immunoglobulin, or rituximab.

Acquired Von Willebrand Syndrome (AVWS)

This acquired mild to moderate bleeding disorder is a result of deficient or defective VWF as a result of a variety of conditions.[52–54] The prevalence of AVWS has not been established, and AVWS was believed to be an uncommon disorder. However, increasing awareness, and several cohort studies suggest that the prevalence may be significantly underestimated. For example, when select patient populations were screened, approximately 10% of patients with hematological disorders,[55] ~79% with aortic stenosis,[56] and up to 100% with left ventricular assist devices were diagnosed with AVWS.[57–59] The median age of diagnosis is 62 years but it may occur in any age group (range 2–96 years).[60] AVWS has diverse causes and may result from:

- Autoantibodies, which may interfere with VWF function or increase VWF clearance (systemic lupus erythematous or lymphoproliferative or plasma cell proliferative disorders)
- Sequestration of the larger, more hemostatically active VWF multimers because of absorption to platelets (essential thrombocythemia or other myeloproliferative disorders) or malignant cells (Wilms tumor or certain lymphoproliferative disorders)
- Proteolytic cleavage of VWF after shear stress-induced unfolding (aortic valvular stenosis and ventricular septal defect)
- Decreased synthesis (hypothyroidism and drugs including valproic acid).

Testing for AVWS involves the same investigations as for VWD: VWF:Ag, VWF:Rco, and FVIII:C. The treatment goals can be divided into 2 categories: to treat or prevent bleeding or to achieve long-term remission. The agents used in the treatment of active bleeding or in perisurgical prophylaxis settings include DDAVP or VWF-containing concentrates, recombinant factor VIIa, antifibrinolytics, intravenous immunoglobulin for AVWS associated with IgG-MGUS (monoclonal gammopathy of uncertain significance), and plasmapheresis for AVWS associated with IgM-MGUS.[61] To achieve hemostasis, often a combination of these agents must be used. Whenever possible, treatment of the underlying disorder should be considered and may result in remission of AVWS. Treatment modalities depend on the underlying disorder and include chemotherapy for lymphoproliferative disorders, cytoreduction for myeloproliferative neoplasms, correction of the underlying cardiac defect, removal of causative medications, or thyroid replacement therapy.

Treatment

The management of a patient with a bleeding disorder can be divided into 4 main categories, and depends on the specific underlying diagnosis:

1. Initial evaluation and education of the patient
2. Localized measures to stop or minimize bleeding
3. Pharmacologic agents that provide indirect hemostatic benefit
4. Treatments that directly increase the plasma levels of the hemostatic defect.

Initial evaluation and education of the patient

Once a bleeding disorder has been confirmed, the following evaluations and educational points should be discussed with the patient:

- Screening for hepatitis B and C as well as human immunodeficiency virus if the individual received blood products or plasma-derived clotting factor concentrates before 1985 (this screening should be followed by vaccinations for hepatitis A and B[53])
- A gynecologic evaluation for women with menorrhagia[62]
- Instructions to avoid any medications that may exacerbate bleeding tendencies, such as ASA and NSAIDs and certain complementary and alternative medications
- Encouragement to seek medical care promptly with any significant bleeding symptoms.

Localized measures

The importance of localized measures to control bleeding such as the application of direct pressure to a site of bleeding should not be understated. Biting down on a piece of gauze may halt bleeding from a tooth socket, and application of a compression bandage and cold pack to an injured limb may reduce subsequent hematoma formation. Management of nosebleeds can be particularly problematic and some patients may benefit from a stepwise action plan that escalates from initial direct pressure to packing after a certain period, and includes guidelines regarding how long to wait before seeking medical attention. In selected cases, nasal cautery may be required for prolonged or excessive epistaxis if localized lesions can be identified on examination.

Indirect Therapies

Several therapies can be used with significant benefit in patients with bleeding disorders, particularly at the time of minor surgery and dental procedures or to treat menorrhagia.

Fibrinolytic inhibitors (ie, tranexamic acid), which inhibit the conversion of plasmin-ogen to plasmin, can be helpful for treatment or prevention of bleeding episodes and have been shown to be useful in a wide range of clinical situations, including both inherited bleeding disorders such as HA[63] and VWD,[64] as well as acquired bleeding disorders, such as warfarin therapy[65] and uremia.[49] This agent can be used either as the sole therapy or as an adjunct in combination with DDAVP, factor replacement, or platelet transfusions, and may be particularly useful for control of bleeding in areas of high fibrinolytic activity such as the oral cavity and gastrointestinal or genitourinary tracts. Common adverse events to tranexamic acid include gastrointestinal side effects and headache. Tranexamic acid is contraindicated in disseminated intravas-cular coagulation and bleeding from the upper urinary tract, which may lead to urinary tract obstruction secondary to large clots.

Hormonal treatments (ie, OCP) can be particularly effective for the treatment of menorrhagia. Nonmedical treatments including the levonorgestrel-releasing intra-uterine system (Mirena IUD [Bayer Healthcare Pharmaceuticals Inc., Wayne, NJ, USA]) or endometrial ablation may be useful in selected patients. A consensus docu-ment on the management of abnormal gynecologic or obstetric bleeding in women with bleeding disorders has recently been published.[62]

The mechanism of action of DDAVP is incompletely understood. It seems that DDAVP induces secretion of VWF from endothelial cells, and results in an increase of VWF and FVIII. Thus, the best-defined indications for DDAVP are VWD[66,67] and HA[68]; in cases of mild to moderate disease, DDAVP promotes release of stored protein and increases levels 3- to 10-fold, thereby providing adequate hemostatic coverage for most invasive procedures. A test dose of DDAVP, followed by serial measurements of VWD or FVIII, is recommended before its clinical use to ensure DDAVP responsiveness. In addition to HA and VWD, DDAVP has been found to be clinically useful in several mild bleeding disorders, including but not limited to PFDs,[39] FXI deficiency,[69] bleeding secondary to connective tissue disease[22] and uremia.[49] Its peak effect is achieved within 30 and 90 minutes with the intravenous and intranasal routes, respectively. The usual parenteral dose is 0.3 µg/kg (maximum dose 20 µg) infused intravenously in ~50 mL of normal saline over ~30 minutes. The dose of the highly concentrated intranasal preparation is 150 µg for children less than 50 kg, and 300 µg for larger children. Common mild side effects include facial flushing and headache. Tachycardia, light-headedness, and mild reductions in blood pressure can occur. The most serious side effects that can develop are severe hyponatremia and seizures.[70] Therefore, desmopressin should be used with caution, particularly in those younger than 2 years because of a higher risk of hyponatremia. Desmopressin is contraindicated in individuals with arteriovascular disease and in those older than 70 years. DDAVP should be avoided in α_2-antiplasmin deficiency,[45] in which its effect of increasing plasma levels of tissue plasminogen activator may exacerbate the enhanced fibrinolysis.

Direct/Replacement Therapies

A variety of products are available as a replacement for the treatment of bleeding disorders. For details regarding the indications, dosing, and side effects of these replacement products, the reader should refer to the appropriate disease-specific guidelines or reviews.[39,43,63] Examples of available products are:

- Recombinant products (rFVIII, rFIX)
- Plasma-derived concentrates (VWF/FVIII, XIII, fibrinogen)
- Prothrombin complex concentrates (which contain FII, VII, IX, and X)

- Cryoprecipitate (which contains a more concentrated amount of VWF/FVIII, FXIII and fibrinogen, compared with frozen plasma)
- Frozen plasma (which contains all of the factors) may be used in situations in which a concentrate is not available (FV deficiency) or associated with adverse events (FXI deficiency and increased risk of thrombosis)
- Platelet transfusion.

In the case of refractory bleeding or an inhibitor, the following bypassing agents may be considered:

- rFVIIa
- FEIBA (FVIII bypassing agent), which is an activated prothrombin complex concentrate.

Bleeding of Unknown Cause (BUC)

Approximately 60% of patients have BUC despite extensive laboratory testing, with up to one-fifth having a prolonged bleeding time.[8] These patients are indistinguishable clinically from patients with known bleeding disorders and experience the same level of morbidity secondary to bleeding symptoms. The approach to patients with BUC is controversial. There is some evidence that tranexamic acid and DDAVP may be useful in treating bleeding symptoms in this population.[71,72] At our center, individuals with BUC are registered and followed in the Inherited Bleeding Disorders Clinic, where they are reviewed annually and have access to specialized physician and nursing care. Treatment of bleeding symptoms or before surgery to prevent abnormal bleeding is tailored to the individual and the presenting complaint, but generally includes a combination of tranexamic acid and DDAVP. If bleeding is refractory to these agents, then second-line intervention includes a trial of platelet transfusion.

SUMMARY

The assessment of a patient complaining of mild to moderate bleeding symptoms is complicated by several factors:

- Bleeding symptoms are common within the normal population.
- The differential diagnosis is broad, including some rare diagnoses, such as FVII deficiency and PAI-1 deficiency.
- Laboratory testing is not standardized and subjected to significant preanalytical and analytical variables (eg, PFD).

The clinician must rely on a thorough clinical history and tools such as the BATs to determine if bleeding symptoms are outside the normal range and warrant investigations. In these cases, patients must be informed that despite extensive investigations, up to 60%[8] may not be diagnosed. This large number highlights the need for ongoing research.

The treatment depends on the specific bleeding disorder and the symptoms of the patient and includes:

- Local measures, such as compression and nasal cautery
- Indirect therapies, such as tranexamic acid, DDAVP, and OCP
- Direct therapies, such as factor replacement with recombinant products, pooled plasma products, or frozen plasma
- Bypassing products, such as rFVIIa.

Referral of these patients to a specialized center may be useful for initial investigations to establish the diagnosis, to outline an approach to the patient's bleeding symptoms, and for longitudinal care.

REFERENCES

1. Silwer J. Von Willebrand's disease in Sweden. Acta Paediatr Scand Suppl 1973; 238:1–159.
2. Lak M, Peyvandi F, Mannucci P. Clinical manifestations and complications of childbirth and replacement therapy in 385 Iranian patients with type 3 von Willebrand disease. Br J Haematol 2000;111:1236–9.
3. Rodeghiero F, Castaman G, Tosetto A, et al. The discriminant power of bleeding history for the diagnosis of type 1 von Willebrand disease: an international, multicenter study. J Thromb Haemost 2005;3:2619–26.
4. Srámek A, Eikenboom JC, Briët E, et al. Usefulness of patient interview in bleeding disorders. Arch Intern Med 1995;155:1409–15.
5. Federici AB. Clinical diagnosis of von Willebrand disease. Haemophilia 2004; 10(Suppl 4):169–76.
6. Favaloro EJ. Rethinking the diagnosis of von Willebrand disease. Thromb Res 2011;2:17–21.
7. Hayward CP. Diagnostic evaluation of platelet function disorders. Blood Rev 2011;25:169–73.
8. Quiroga T, Goycoolea M, Panes O, et al. High prevalence of bleeders of unknown cause among patients with inherited mucocutaneous bleeding. A prospective study of 280 patients and 299 controls. Haematologica 2007;92: 357–65.
9. Warner PE, Critchley HO, Lumsden MA, et al. Menorrhagia I: measured blood loss, clinical features, and outcome in women with heavy periods: a survey with follow-up data. Am J Obstet Gynecol 2004;190:1216–23.
10. Ang-Lee M, Moss J, Yuan C. Herbal medicines and perioperative care. JAMA 2001;286:208–16.
11. Nosek-Cenkowska B, Cheang MS, Pizzi NJ, et al. Bleeding/bruising symptomatology in children with and without bleeding disorders. Thromb Haemost 1991;65:237–41.
12. Drews CD, Dilley AB, Lally C, et al. Screening questions to identify women with von Willebrand disease. J Am Med Womens Assoc 2002;57:217–8.
13. Tosetto A, Rodeghiero F, Castaman G, et al. A quantitative analysis of bleeding symptoms in type 1 von Willebrand disease: results from a multicenter European study (MCMDM-1 VWD). J Thromb Haemost 2006;4:766–73.
14. Bowman M, Mundell G, Grabell J, et al. Generation and validation of the condensed MCMDM-1 VWD bleeding questionnaire for von Willebrand disease. J Thromb Haemost 2008;6:2062–6.
15. Rodeghiero F, Tosetto A, Abshire T, et al. ISTH/SSC bleeding assessment tool: a standardized questionnaire and a proposal for a new bleeding score for inherited bleeding disorders. J Thromb Haemost 2010;8:2063–5.
16. Biss TT, Blanchette VS, Clark DS, et al. Quantitation of bleeding symptoms in children with von Willebrand disease: use of a standardized pediatric bleeding questionnaire. J Thromb Haemost 2010;8:950–6.
17. Biss TT, Blanchette VS, Clark DS, et al. Use of a quantitative pediatric bleeding questionnaire to assess mucocutaneous bleeding symptoms in children with a platelet function disorder. J Thromb Haemost 2010;8:1416–9.

18. Beighton P, Solomon L, Soskolne CL. Articular mobility in an African population. Ann Rheum Dis 1973;32:413–8.
19. Mishra P, Naithani R, Dolai T, et al. Intracranial haemorrhage in patients with congenital haemostatic defects. Haemophilia 2008;14:952–5.
20. De Paepe A, Malfait F. Bleeding and bruising in patients with Ehlers-Danlos syndrome and other collagen vascular disorders. Br J Haematol 2004;127: 491–500.
21. Malfait F, Wenstrup RJ, De Paepe A. Clinical and genetic aspects of Ehlers-Danlos syndrome, classic type. Genet Med 2010;12:597–605.
22. Malfait F, De Paepe A. Bleeding in the heritable connective tissue disorders: mechanisms, diagnosis and treatment. Blood Rev 2009;23:191–7.
23. Quiroga T, Goycoolea M, Munoz B, et al. Template bleeding time and PFA-100 have low sensitivity to screen patients with hereditary mucocutaneous hemorrhages: comparative study of 148 patients. J Thromb Haemost 2004; 2:892–8.
24. Podda GM, Bucciarelli P, Lussana F, et al. Usefulness of PFA-100 testing in the diagnostic screening of patients with suspected abnormalities of hemostasis: comparison with the bleeding time. J Thromb Haemost 2007;5: 2393–8.
25. Favaloro EJ. Laboratory monitoring of therapy in von Willebrand disease: efficacy of the PFA-100 and von Willebrand factor:collagen-binding activity as coupled strategies. Semin Thromb Hemost 2006;32:566–76.
26. Castaman G, Tosetto A, Goodeve A, et al. The impact of bleeding history, von Willebrand factor and PFA-100(®) on the diagnosis of type 1 von Willebrand disease: results from the European study MCMDM-1 VWD. Br J Haematol 2010;151:245–51.
27. Cattaneo M, Hayward CP, Moffat KA, et al. Results of a worldwide survey on the assessment of platelet function by light transmission aggregometry: a report from the platelet physiology subcommittee of the SSC of the ISTH. J Thromb Haemost 2009;7:1029.
28. Hayward CP, Moffat KA, Raby A, et al. Development of North American consensus guidelines for medical laboratories that perform and interpret platelet function testing using light transmission aggregometry. Am J Clin Pathol 2010; 134:955–63.
29. Mannucci PM, Tuddenham EG. The hemophilias–from royal genes to gene therapy. N Engl J Med 2001;344:1773–9.
30. Asakai R, Chung DW, Davie EW, et al. Factor XI deficiency in Ashkenazi Jews in Israel. N Engl J Med 1991;325:153–8.
31. Rodeghiero F, Castaman G. Epidemiological investigation of the prevalence of von Willebrand's disease. Blood 1987;69:454–9.
32. Werner EJ, Broxson EH, Tucker EL, et al. Prevalence of von Willebrand disease in children: a multiethnic study. J Pediatr 1993;123:893–8.
33. Bowman M, Hopman WM, Rapson D, et al. The prevalence of symptomatic von Willebrand disease in primary care practice. J Thromb Haemost 2010;8:213–6.
34. Sadler JE, Budde U, Eikenboom JC, et al. Update on the pathophysiology and classification of von Willebrand disease: a report of the subcommittee on von Willebrand factor. J Thromb Haemost 2006;4:2103–14.
35. Callewaert B, Malfait F, Loeys B, et al. Ehlers-Danlos syndromes and Marfan syndrome. Best Pract Res Clin Rheumatol 2008;22:165–89.
36. Stine KC, Becton DL. DDAVP therapy controls bleeding in Ehlers-Danlos syndrome. J Pediatr Hematol Oncol 1997;19:156–8.

37. Quiroga T, Goycoolea M, Matus V, et al. Diagnosis of mild platelet function disorders. Reliability and usefulness of light transmission platelet aggregation and serotonin secretion assays. Br J Haematol 2009;147:729–36.

38. Hayward CP, Pai M, Liu Y, et al. Diagnostic utility of light transmission platelet aggregometry: results from a prospective study of individuals referred for bleeding disorder assessments. J Thromb Haemost 2009;7:676–84.

39. Bolton-Maggs PH, Chalmers EA, Collins PW, et al. A review of inherited platelet disorders with guidelines for their management on behalf of the UKHCDO. Br J Haematol 2006;135:603–33.

40. Hassan AA, Kroll MH. Acquired disorders of platelet function. Hematology Am Soc Hematol Educ Program 2005;403–8.

41. Oldenburg J, Ananyeva NM, Saenko EL. Molecular basis of haemophilia A. Haemophilia 2004;10(Suppl 4):133–9.

42. Pavlova A, Brondke H, Müsebeck J, et al. Molecular mechanisms underlying hemophilia A phenotype in seven females. J Thromb Haemost 2009;7: 976–82.

43. Mannucci PM, Duga S, Peyvandi F. Recessively inherited coagulation disorders. Blood 2004;104:1243–52.

44. Acharya SS, Coughlin A, Dimichele DM. Rare bleeding disorder registry: deficiencies of factors II, V, VII, X, XIII, fibrinogen and dysfibrinogenemias. J Thromb Haemost 2004;2:248–56.

45. Carpenter SL, Mathew P. Alpha2-antiplasmin and its deficiency: fibrinolysis out of balance. Haemophilia 2008;14:1250–4.

46. Mehta R, Shapiro AD. Plasminogen activator inhibitor type 1 deficiency. Haemophilia 2008;14:1255–60.

47. Eby C. Pathogenesis and management of bleeding and thrombosis in plasma cell dyscrasias. Br J Haematol 2009;145:151–63.

48. Acharya S, Bussel JB. Hematologic toxicity of sodium valproate. J Pediatr Hematol Oncol 2000;22:62–5.

49. Galbusera M, Remuzzi G, Boccardo P. Treatment of bleeding in dialysis patients. Semin Dial 2009;22:279–86.

50. Escolar G, Cases A, Viñas M, et al. Evaluation of acquired platelet dysfunctions in uremic and cirrhotic patients using the platelet function analyzer (PFA-100): influence of hematocrit elevation. Haematologica 1999;84:614–9.

51. Franchini M, Lippi G. Acquired factor VIII inhibitors. Blood 2008;112:250–5.

52. Sucker C, Michiels JJ, Zotz RB. Causes, etiology and diagnosis of acquired von Willebrand disease: a prospective diagnostic workup to establish the most effective therapeutic strategies. Acta Haematol 2009;121:177–82.

53. Nichols WL, Rick ME, Ortel TL, et al. Clinical and laboratory diagnosis of von Willebrand disease: a synopsis of the 2008 NHLBI/NIH guidelines. Am J Hematol 2009;84:366–70.

54. Federici AB. Acquired von Willebrand syndrome: an underdiagnosed and misdiagnosed bleeding complication in patients with lymphoproliferative and myeloproliferative disorders. Semin Hematol 2006;43:S48–58.

55. Mohri H, Motomura S, Kanamori H, et al. Clinical significance of inhibitors in acquired von Willebrand syndrome. Blood 1998;91:3623–9.

56. Vincentelli A, Susen S, Le Tourneau T, et al. Acquired von Willebrand syndrome in aortic stenosis. N Engl J Med 2003;349:343–9.

57. Geisen U, Heilmann C, Beyersdorf F, et al. Non-surgical bleeding in patients with ventricular assist devices could be explained by acquired von Willebrand disease. Eur J Cardiothorac Surg 2008;33:679–84.

58. Uriel N, Pak SW, Jorde UP, et al. Acquired von Willebrand syndrome after continuous-flow mechanical device support contributes to a high prevalence of bleeding during long-term support and at the time of transplantation. J Am Coll Cardiol 2010;56:1207–13.

59. Meyer AL, Malehsa D, Bara C, et al. Acquired von Willebrand syndrome in patients with an axial flow left ventricular assist device. Circ Heart Fail 2010;3: 675–81.

60. Federici AB, Rand JH, Bucciarelli P, et al. Acquired von Willebrand syndrome: data from an international registry. Thromb Haemost 2000;84:345–9.

61. Tiede A, Rand JH, Budde U, et al. How I treat the acquired von Willebrand syndrome. Blood 2011;117:6777–85.

62. James AH, Kouides PA, Abdul-Kadir R, et al. Von Willebrand disease and other bleeding disorders in women: consensus on diagnosis and management from an international expert panel. Am J Obstet Gynecol 2009;201:12.e1–8.

63. Santagostino E, Mannucci PM, Bianchi Bonomi A. Guidelines on replacement therapy for haemophilia and inherited coagulation disorders in Italy. Haemophilia 2000;6:1–10.

64. Nichols WL, Hultin MB, James AH, et al. von Willebrand disease (VWD): evidence-based diagnosis and management guidelines, the National Heart, Lung, and Blood Institute (NHLBI) Expert Panel report (USA). Haemophilia 2008;14:171–232.

65. Ansell J, Hirsh J, Hylek E, et al. Prevention of venous thromboembolism: American College of Chest Physicians evidence-based clinical practice guidelines (8th edition). Chest 2008;133:381S–453S.

66. Castaman G, Lethagen S, Federici AB, et al. Response to desmopressin is influenced by the genotype and phenotype in type 1 von Willebrand disease (VWD): results from the European study MCMDM-1 VWD. Blood 2008;111:3531–9.

67. Federici AB. The use of desmopressin in von Willebrand disease: the experience of the first 30 years (1977–2007). Haemophilia 2008;14(Suppl 1):5–14.

68. Franchini M, Zaffanello M, Lippi G. The use of desmopressin in mild hemophilia A. Blood Coagul Fibrinolysis 2010;21:615–9.

69. Franchini M, Manzato F, Salvagno GL, et al. The use of desmopressin in congenital factor XI deficiency: a systematic review. Ann Hematol 2009;88:931–5.

70. Greaves M, Watson HG. Approach to the diagnosis and management of mild bleeding disorders. J Thromb Haemost 2007;5(Suppl 1):167–74.

71. Edlund M, Blomba M, Fried G. Desmopressin in the treatment of menorrhagia in women with no common coagulation factor deficiency but with prolonged bleeding time. Blood Coagul Fibrinolysis 2002;13:225–31.

72. Lethaby A, Farquhar C, Cooke I. Antifibrinolytics for heavy menstrual bleeding. Cochrane Database Syst Rev 2000;4:CD000249.

Venous Thromboembolism Overview

Elisabeth M. Battinelli, MD, PhD*, Devon L. Murphy, BS,
Jean M. Connors, MD

KEYWORDS

• Deep vein thrombosis • Pulmonary embolism • Anticoagulation

Thrombosis and its associated complications are a common cause of death throughout the world. Each year, more than 200,000 new cases of venous thromboembolism (VTE) are diagnosed and 30% of these patients die in the first 30 days after diagnosis. In addition, many patients suffer long-term physical consequences from the thrombotic event, resulting in an adverse quality of life and millions of dollars spent for health care.

The pathogenesis of thrombosis results from abnormalities in many components of the vascular and coagulation systems. In 1856, Virchow first described the pathogenesis of thrombosis as the result of defects in the vessel wall, platelets, and coagulation proteins. The interplay of these 3 factors became known as the Virchow triad. Thrombi that form within the venous system are rich in fibrin, resulting from disruption in the coagulation process in areas of blood stasis.

In normal circumstances, the endothelial lining of blood vessels is not a thrombotic surface. Surveillance and maintenance by cellular components of blood interact with the endothelial cells to inhibit thrombus formation. Blood cells, such as platelets, release several antithrombotic factors, such as thrombomodulin and plasmin, which regulate the tissue factor pathway inhibitor system as well as the antithrombin systems. As this is occurring, the platelets limit their own coagulation response with aggregation directly inhibited by prostacyclins and nitric oxide.

When the endothelial surface becomes damaged, the platelets become activated and they no longer guard the endothelium but instead perpetuate the coagulation response. Exposure of vascular collagen in the damaged endothelium also leads to activation of the normal mechanisms of hemostasis, including the coagulation cascade, through exposure of tissue factor leading to hemostasis in the wrong place.

The coagulation cascade is the main mediator of this process. Both the tissue factor–mediated pathway (extrinsic) and the contact-mediated pathway (intrinsic pathway)

The authors have no relationships to disclose.
Hematology Division, Brigham and Women's Hospital/Dana Farber Cancer Institute, Harvard Medical School, 75 Francis Street, Boston, MA 02115, USA
* Corresponding author.
E-mail address: ebattinelli@partners.org

Hematol Oncol Clin N Am 26 (2012) 345–367
doi:10.1016/j.hoc.2012.02.010

are based on the systematic activation of inactive enzyme precursors known as serine proteases, which then reflexively lead to activation of the next coagulation factor protein within the coagulation cascade in a chain reaction mechanism (**Fig. 1**). The final steps lead to cross-linking of fibrin with stabilization of the emerging platelet plug culminating in the formation of a thrombus. The extrinsic and intrinsic pathways are essential to this process, with the main mediator being tissue factor. When tissue factor is released as a result of vascular endothelial injury, factor VII is activated and complexes with tissue factor, setting off the cascade. The steps of coagulation are now set into place with this complex, which next initiates activation of factor X and factor IX. Activation of factor X is essential for conversion of prothrombin (factor II) to thrombin through the prothrombinase complex on activated platelets.

The activated platelets are key players in the thrombotic response and act as the glue that mediates the coagulation cascade. They release many procoagulant proteins, including tissue factor, resulting in uncontrolled hemostasis at the site of vascular injury.[1] The release of these coagulation factors initiates a self-renewing process as the activated platelets recruit additional platelets to the area of injury, establishing the site of thrombus formation. These platelets further activate and become tethered together by binding to exposed glycoprotein Ib-V-IX in damaged collagen through interaction with Von Willebrand factor. More platelets are recruited to the growing thrombus through another receptor present on the platelet surface, GPIIb/IIa, which becomes activated upon platelet activation and undergoes a conformational change leading to increased affinity for fibrinogen, which leads to fibrin deposition. The culmination of this process is internal activation of platelets leading to release of even more proteins including, adenosine diphosphate (ADP), serotonin, and thromboxane A_2, all of which are essential for recruitment of more platelets to the growing thrombus.

Coagulation is initiated at the molecular level but rapidly progresses to the cellular level, then microvascular level, and ultimately the macrovascular level. Large thrombi can be organ damaging and life threatening. This article reviews the presentation and

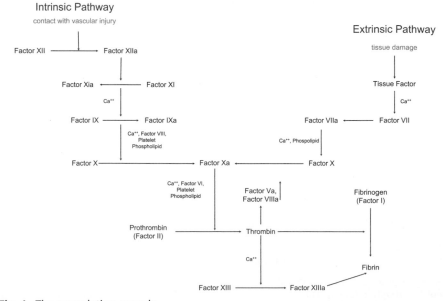

Fig. 1. The coagulation cascade.

diagnosis of VTE. Initial treatment of acute VTE is straightforward, noncontroversial, and is covered briefly here. Areas that are less well defined and for which data are limited and conflicting are reviewed in greater detail. These areas include duration of anticoagulation, bridging anticoagulation, treatment of superficial venous thrombosis, and VTE prophylaxis for travel. Two other areas covered in this article include new oral anticoagulants and testing for thrombophilias.

VENOUS THROMBOEMBOLISM (VTE): PRESENTATION

Patients who develop all 3 components of the Virchow triad of vascular stasis with endothelial damage and hypercoagulability, as described earlier, can form thrombus in a deep vein of sufficient size to result in clinical symptoms. Development of deep venous thrombosis (DVT) alone is roughly twice as common as pulmonary embolism (PE), although the incidence of PE may be underestimated.[2] Those patients who present with classic symptoms of DVT or PE in the context of situations in which the index of clinical suspicion is increased can be readily diagnosed with appropriate testing. **Table 1** shows the percentages of patients experiencing clinical signs and symptoms of DVT and PE.[3]

VENOUS THROMBOEMBOLISM (VTE): DIAGNOSIS

Many of these signs and symptoms, especially those associated with PE, can be the result of other pathologic processes. Making the diagnosis of VTE requires both

Table 1 Clinical signs and symptoms of DVT and PE	
Signs and Symptoms	**Percentage of Patients Experiencing Symptoms**
Clinical Signs and Symptoms of DVT	
Swelling	88
Pain	56
Tenderness	55
Warmth	42
Erythema	34
Homan sign	13
Palpable cord	6
Clinical Signs and Symptoms of PE	
Dyspnea	77
Chest pain	55
Hemoptysis	13
Syncope	10
Sudden death	Rare
Tachypnea	70
Tachycardia	43
Hypoxia	18
Hypotension	10

Data from Anderson FA, Wheeler HB, Goldberg RJ, et al. A population based perspective of the hospital incidence and case fatality rates of deep vein thrombosis and pulmonary embolism. The Worcester DVT study. Arch Int Med 1991;151:933–8.

clinical assessment and appropriate diagnostic testing, because clinical diagnosis alone is frequently wrong. Radiographic imaging is required. Missing a diagnosis of DVT or PE can lead to unnecessary morbidity and mortality. However, of the estimated 1 million patients who undergo diagnostic vascular ultrasound each year, only 12% to 25% have positive results.[4] Strategies to decrease the cost burden of negative tests have been studied. Clinical prediction models to determine pretest probability, many of which incorporate use of D-dimer testing and diagnostic algorithms, have been developed to decrease radiographic testing. These models have not yet been validated in large randomized control trials.[5–12] Detailed reviews of the strategies for diagnosing DVT and PE are covered elsewhere.[13,14] This article briefly reviews the approach to diagnosis of DVT and PE.

When an extremity DVT is suspected based on clinical presentation and examination, compression duplex ultrasound should be the first diagnostic test. This noninvasive test has high sensitivity (89%–100%) and specificity (86%–100%), especially for proximal DVT (97% and 94% respectively).[13–15] Venography is rarely used because it requires iodine-based contrast dye, is invasive, and can be technically difficult to perform because of the challenge of obtaining adequate venous access. Magnetic resonance venography (MRV) is excellent for visualization of the pelvic veins and can image proximal veins in the groin and thigh but has high cost and is less commonly available. MRV should not be considered as a first-line test for diagnosis of DVT in an extremity.

Making the diagnosis of PE can be more complex because the list of differential diagnoses associated with presenting signs and symptoms is extensive and imaging to evaluate for PE is more invasive and costly. Helical computed tomography pulmonary angiography (CTA) for diagnosis of PE is the most commonly used test. It has replaced VQ scanning and conventional pulmonary angiography, both of which are significantly more time consuming and cumbersome to perform and provide less information about alternative diagnoses. A definitive diagnosis of another disorder can be made in 50% to 60% of those cases in which PE is not present on CTA.[16] Computed tomography (CT) requires iodine contrast dye and alternative methods must be used in patients with iodine allergy or significant renal failure. MRV is an excellent alternative for those with iodine allergy. As discussed elsewhere, the positive and negative predictive values of CTA vary with the pretest probability of PE.[17]

VTE can occur in other vascular beds including the cerebral sinuses and abdominal vessels. VTE in these locations are often diagnosed with imaging studies for the evaluation of acute onset of headache or abdominal pain. Routine intravenous (IV) contrast CT scanning can usually detect thrombus; however, dedicated CT may be required to adequately define the extent of thrombosis. Patients who have thrombosis in these locations should undergo thorough evaluation for precipitating factors and prothrombotic conditions, including antiphospholipid antibodies and myeloproliferative neoplasms.

VENOUS THROMBOEMBOLISM (VTE): INITIAL TREATMENT

Anticoagulation therapy should be initiated once a diagnosis of VTE has been made. The initial goal of therapy is to prevent thrombus propagation and embolization, and to allow for natural fibrinolysis to occur. In a small number of clinical situations, such as in patients with significant hemodynamic compromise or limb-threatening acute venous occlusion, thrombectomy and catheter-directed thrombolysis should be considered. Many groups have made detailed and comprehensive guidelines for use of initial anticoagulant therapy for VTE, including the American College of Chest Physicians (ACCP), American College of Physicians, and American Academy of Family

Physicians. The ninth edition of the ACCP Antithrombotic Therapy and Prevention of Thrombosis Guidelines were released on February 8, 2012.[18] These guidelines are derived by consensus agreement after review of available data. The quality and strength of the data are reflected in the grade of the recommendation. The ACCP guidelines are an excellent review of the current data and give evidence-based recommendations for management of antithrombotic therapy; however, individual patient circumstances may dictate modifications of these recommendations for appropriate and successful treatment.

All patients diagnosed with acute VTE should be treated with rapid-onset anticoagulant therapy. In the United States, the only rapid-onset or immediate-onset agents are parenteral. In the European Union in December 2011, rivaroxaban, a new oral direct Xa inhibitor, was the first new oral anticoagulant approved for up-front monotherapy of DVT. The parenteral agents include IV unfractionated heparin (UFH) titrated to partial thromboplastin time (PTT), subcutaneous (SC) UFH, which is monitored with PTT, SC weight-based dose UFH without monitoring, SC low-molecular-weight heparin (LMWH), or SC fondaparinux (a synthetic pentasaccharide Xa inhibitor that works through antithrombin). Although high-quality data from well-controlled studies support the use of any of these agents, LMWH and fondaparinux are preferred agents compared with any type of administration of UFH, as discussed later.

Appropriately selected patients can be treated as outpatients, with no need for hospital admission. The largest number of well-run studies of initial outpatient therapy for DVT have been conducted using LMWHs. These studies show that a variety of types of LMWH are as effective and safe as IV UFH administered in a hospital setting. The use of outpatient therapy significantly affects cost-effectiveness analyses in favor of LMWH and outpatient treatment. For many reasons, initial use of LMWH has become standard of care for treatment of VTE, and is endorsed as such by the ACCP ninth edition guidelines. The hematology consultant needs to consider several factors when recommending the preferred anticoagulant and inpatient versus outpatient management. These factors include the severity of symptoms, the patient's hemodynamic stability, the risk for major bleeding, the ability to comply with directions, and the availability of outpatient medical support. The availability of the brand of LMWH in local outpatient pharmacies affects the decision about which LMWH is prescribed.

Warfarin can be started on the same day as diagnosis of VTE and initiation of parenteral heparin therapy in those patients who will be treated with warfarin. Parenteral therapy must be continued for at least 5 days, even if the International Normalization Ratio (INR) is in the therapeutic range of 2.0 to 3.0, because it can take this long for levels of prothrombin to decline to reach the full anticoagulant effect of warfarin. Warfarin can also cause a transient hypercoagulable state due to a rapid decline in protein C and protein S levels, rarely leading to warfarin-induced skin necrosis.[19]

DURATION OF ANTICOAGULATION THERAPY

The initiation of anticoagulation therapy for acute VTE addresses the primary goal of preventing clot propagation and embolization. The secondary goal of preventing recurrent VTE then needs to be considered. The duration of anticoagulation therapy to prevent recurrent VTE is controversial. Conflicting guidelines from different medical societies have been developed with variable fixed time periods recommended. As new data from well-designed studies are presented, evidence-based guidelines are emerging, however, decision making for an individual patient is a complex, risk-benefit analysis. The consultant needs to consider the benefit of continued anticoagulation to mitigate the patient's risk of recurrent VTE versus the patient's risk of bleeding on anticoagulation therapy. One of the biggest determinants in the assessment of an individual patient's possibility for recurrent VTE is whether the VTE event was provoked by a transient or reversible risk factor or whether it was unprovoked or idiopathic. Unprovoked and idiopathic are used interchangeably during this discussion. These terms refer to VTE events in patients in whom a provoking or causative risk factor is not identified. Generally accepted transient risk factors for VTE include bed rest or hospitalization for 3 or more consecutive days within 12 weeks; surgery or general anesthesia within 12 weeks; trauma within 12 weeks; casting or immobilization, especially of the lower extremity; prolonged travel, greater than 4 to 6 hours; combined estrogen and progesterone oral contraceptive use; and pregnancy and the postpartum state.[20] For patients who are in either category of provoked or unprovoked VTE, the assessment of risk and decision for duration of anticoagulation can be straightforward. However, many patients are not in these provoked or unprovoked categories and require individualized assessment.

Consensus guidelines support 3 to 6 months of anticoagulation therapy for a provoked VTE.[18,21–23] Studies show that 6 weeks is an insufficient duration of therapy because of a high risk of recurrent VTE. The VTE recurrence rate at 2 years is nearly doubled for 6 weeks compared with 6 months of anticoagulation therapy (18.1% vs 9.5%).[24] A meta-analysis of well-conducted randomized clinical trials shows that the risk of VTE recurrence at 12 months is 40% lower in patients treated for 12 to 24 weeks compared with those treated for 3 to 6 weeks, with no significant difference in major bleeding risk.[25] In this analysis, patients who have only transient risk factors for VTE also benefit from longer anticoagulation treatment; however, the benefit of longer anticoagulation is greater in patients with idiopathic VTE.[25] The risk of recurrent VTE in patients with transient risk factors is estimated at 4% to 5.8% in the first year, and declines after that time period.[14,26] The annual risk of major bleeding while on warfarin therapy is 1% to 3%.[27] The risk/benefit ratio in a patient with provoked VTE and no other risk factors favors discontinuation of anticoagulation after 3 to 6 months.

For patients with persistent risks associated with recurrent VTE and for those with idiopathic VTE, the optimal duration of anticoagulation therapy after the first 3 to 6 months of treatment is harder to define.[28,29] In one randomized trial, patients with idiopathic VTE were anticoagulated for 3 versus 24 months. The VTE recurrence rate was higher in the shorter duration treatment group (27.4% vs 1.3% per patient year). This study was stopped at 10 months after interim analysis revealed this significant difference in VTE recurrence rates. Major nonfatal bleeding rate was 3.8% (3 of 79 patients over 10 months of anticoagulation).[30] Similar studies and meta-analyses all suggest that longer duration of anticoagulation therapy decreases recurrence rates; however, the benefit seems to be gained only while the patient is on anticoagulation therapy. In one study of prolonged duration of anticoagulation, final analysis at 3 years revealed no difference in recurrence rate for those patients with idiopathic PE treated for 3 to 6 months versus 12 months (11.2% vs 9.1%).[31] This group found similar results in a study of 3 months versus 12 months of anticoagulation for idiopathic DVT. At 1 year, the recurrent DVT rate was 8.3% for the 3-month arm and 0.7% for the 12-month arm. At 3 years, the DVT recurrence rates were equal at 15.8% and 15.7%.[32]

The decreased risk of recurrent VTE with anticoagulation therapy must be weighed against the risk of bleeding. Many factors affect bleeding risk. Advanced age, renal failure, diabetes, cerebrovascular disease, malignancy, and concomitant use of antiplatelet therapy increase bleeding risk.[33,34] Bleeding risk is the highest at initiation of anticoagulation, 0.8% per day with UFH in one study.[33] In one registry, risk of major bleeding was 2.4% during the first 3 months of warfarin therapy.[35] As noted previously, the estimated annual risk of bleeding with oral vitamin K antagonist (VKA) therapy is 3%.[27] Fatal bleeding events have been reported to occur in 20% of major bleeds, with annual case fatality of 0.6%. In a study of patients with recurrent VTE, indefinite duration of anticoagulation prevented 0.43 episodes of recurrent thromboembolism per month per 100 patients, but at a rate of 0.20 major hemorrhages per month.[14,36] A recent large meta-analysis of major bleeding in patients on anticoagulation longer than 3 months found a rate of 2.7 major bleeds per 100 patient years, with a case fatality rate of 9.1%.[37]

Patients with very high risk for recurrent VTE and an unprovoked event clearly benefit from an indefinite duration of anticoagulation because the risk and consequences of recurrence are significantly greater than the risk of bleeding. High-risk patient populations include those patients with multiple recurrent idiopathic events who have failed off anticoagulation therapy; patients with antiphospholipid syndrome; patients with active cancer and VTE; patients with high-risk inherited thrombophilia and unprovoked VTE, including those with protein S, protein C, and antithrombin deficiencies, homozygous factor V Leiden; or compound factor V Leiden/prothrombin gene G20210A heterozygotes. Strong data for VTE recurrence rates in the inherited thrombophilias are lacking; however, risk is extrapolated from data for risk for first VTE event.[14] Individual patient assessment of bleeding risk may affect the decision for indefinite anticoagulation despite the high risk of recurrent VTE in any of these patient groups, especially in those with malignancy. In one study, the 1-year incidence of recurrent thrombosis was 21% for patients with cancer compared with 6.8% for patients without cancer; however, the 12-month cumulative incidence of major bleeding was 12.4% in patients with cancer and 4.9% in other patients.[38]

Many patients with VTE do not clearly fit into the categories of provoked or unprovoked with high risk of recurrence. They often have a unique combination of risks that give them an intermediate risk of recurrence that can be difficult to quantify or to place neatly into the category of provoked VTE and no need for further anticoagulation or the unprovoked category with high risk that benefits from anticoagulation despite bleeding risk. Many balk at the idea of lifelong anticoagulation therapy. Risk for major bleeding events is a substantial concern but also the economic and psychological burden of testing and impact on lifestyle are significant concerns. Rather than trying to rigidly categorize patients into groups favoring or not favoring indefinite anticoagulation therapy, individual risk assessments should be performed. A detailed patient history, as well as family history, events surrounding the development of VTE, severity of symptoms at presentation, and clot burden should be reviewed. Patient preference for ongoing anticoagulation is also a significant factor that is incorporated in the decision-making process. Some patients are willing to take the risk of approximately 10% to 12% per year of recurrent VTE and forgo anticoagulation, whereas for others the risk and concern for developing fatal PE is too high.

Strategies to help determine individual risk of recurrence have been developed and evaluated. Testing D-dimer levels and use of flexible duration of anticoagulation instead of a fixed time period have been studied. Clinical prediction tools to better quantify individual risk of recurrence and of bleeding risk have been designed and are being validated. Trials of lower intensity anticoagulation have also been performed. The development of new oral anticoagulants that do not require monitoring might significantly affect the risk-benefit analysis for some patients.

D-dimer levels have been used to risk stratify patients with idiopathic VTE into groups with high risk and low risk of recurrence. In most studies, patients with idiopathic VTE complete a specified course of anticoagulant therapy and then have D-dimer levels measured, often 1 month after discontinuation of anticoagulation.

Several studies and meta-analyses have been performed confirming that patients with increased D-dimer levels have a significantly higher risk of recurrent VTE than those with normal levels. In one randomized study, patients with positive levels who remained on anticoagulation had a recurrence rate of 2%. Those who had normal levels and came off anticoagulation had a recurrence rate of 4.4%. Those with positive levels allocated to no anticoagulation had an annual recurrence rate of 10.9%.[39–41]

A recent meta-analysis of 1818 patients with unprovoked VTE showed that the timing of D-dimer testing after stopping anticoagulation, patient age, and threshold D-dimer level for positive results (250 μg/L vs 500 μg/L) did not affect the ability of the D-dimer level to distinguish risk for recurrent VTE.[42] In a prospective cohort study, the PROLONG II study, serial D-dimer levels were evaluated in patients with an unprovoked VTE who had a normal D-dimer level 1 month after stopping anticoagulation. Patients who developed positive D-dimer levels during the ensuing year had increased risk of recurrence compared with those whose D-dimer levels remained normal. A newly positive test at 3 months that remained positive conferred a hazard ratio of 7.9 for recurrence (27 per 100 patient years vs 2.9 per 100 patient years). Patients who developed a positive result after 3 months had an intermediate risk of recurrence at 11.1 per 100 patient years.[43]

Another approach to determining risk for recurrence is to repeat imaging studies to assess for recanalization. Residual thrombosis at the time of discontinuation of anticoagulant therapy is a risk for recurrent VTE, with a hazard ratio of 2.4.[44] A randomized trial was performed by the same investigators to assess fixed duration of anticoagulation versus flexible duration of anticoagulation based on serial ultrasound assessments of DVT. Patients assigned to fixed-duration treatment received 3 months for provoked DVT and 6 months for unprovoked DVT. Those assigned to flexible duration had anticoagulation stopped at 3 months if there was complete recanalization of veins, or continued for up to 9 months for provoked DVT and 21 months for unprovoked. The numbers of patients in each group were insufficient to detect effectiveness and risk of major bleeding. Overall, the rates of recurrent DVT were significantly lower at 11.9% in those receiving flexible-duration treatment versus 17.2% receiving fixed-duration treatment.[45]

Clinical prediction rules have been designed that incorporate these and other factors that have been shown to increase the risk of recurrence in patients with an unprovoked VTE. These factors include (1) male gender, (2) increased body mass index (>30 kg/m^2), and (3) initial presentation with symptomatic PE versus proximal DVT versus isolated calf vein thrombosis.[28,29,46] Two scoring systems have recently been developed to predict risk of recurrence after idiopathic VTE. The Vienna Prediction Model uses a nomogram to obtain a number value to predict individual risk. Several potential risk factors, including biochemical markers of thrombosis, were assessed. The factors that most strongly predicted recurrence included (1) male sex, (2) PE, and (3) increased D-dimer level after stopping anticoagulation. Another clinical scoring system that goes by the mnemonic men and HERDOO2 (male sex and signs of postthrombotic syndrome, including hyperpigmentation of the lower extremities, edema or redness of either leg, a D-dimer level >250 μg/L, obesity [body mass index >30 kg/m^2], and older age [>65 years]) has been developed based on prospective data. It is currently being validated in a larger patient population.[47,48]

The use of a lower INR target, or lower intensity warfarin anticoagulation therapy, has been assessed in 2 large, double-blind, randomized studies. The proposed benefits of lower intensity are similar reduction in recurrent VTE risk but with lower risk of bleeding, and need for less frequent INR testing. In the PREVENT (Prevention of Recurrent Venous Thromboembolism) trial, a target INR of 1.5 to 2.0 was compared with placebo in patients with idiopathic VTE after a median of 6.5 months of full-intensity warfarin treatment. There was a 64% reduction in risk of recurrent VTE events in the 255 patients assigned to low-intensity warfarin (7.2 per 100 patient years) compared with 253 patients assigned to placebo (2.6 per 100 patient years, hazard ratio 0.36, 95% confidence interval 0.19–0.67). The rates of major bleeding were not statistically different at 0.4 per 100 patient years in the placebo group and 0.9 per 100 patient years in the low-intensity warfarin arm. In the ELATE (Extended Low-intensity Anticoagulation for Unprovoked Venous Thromboembolism) trial, patients completed 3 or more months of standard anticoagulant therapy and were then randomized to low-intensity warfarin with a target range of 1.5 to 2.0 or conventional intensity with the standard 2.0 to 3.0 range. The low-intensity arm had a recurrent VTE rate of 1.9 events per 100 patient years; the conventional arm had 0.7 recurrent VTE events per 100 patient years. There was no difference in rates of major bleeding between the 2 arms. The low-intensity group had 1.1 major bleeds per 100 patient years and the conventional-intensity group had 0.9 per 100 patient years. A criticism of the ELATE trial is the unexpectedly low bleeding risk compared with most previously published results in the 2.0 to 3.0 arm. INR tests were performed every 24 days in the conventional warfarin arm and every 26 days in the low-intensity arm. Time in therapeutic range values were reported and were 63% for the low-intensity arm and 69% for the conventional-intensity arm. Although these values are high, they are now routinely reported by many dedicated anticoagulation management services and may be attainable in a community setting. Compared with no long-term anticoagulant therapy, the low-intensity groups from both studies experienced a 76% risk reduction for recurrent VTE; the conventional-intensity arm had a greater than 90% risk reduction.[49,50]

The WARFASA (Warfarin vs Aspirin) study was presented at the American Society of Hematology conference in 2011. Four-hundred and two carefully selected patients with idiopathic VTE were randomized to receive aspirin 100 mg daily or placebo after 6 months of warfarin treatment. Patients on treatment with aspirin had a recurrent VTE rate of 5.9% per patient year compared with 11.0% per patient year in the placebo-treated group (hazard ratio 0.57). Bleeding rates were the same in each group and were extremely low. Risk reduction with aspirin was 40%. In some patients with idiopathic VTE, such as those with high risk of bleeding with conventional anticoagulation, those with a first idiopathic event and otherwise low-risk assessment, and those who do not want to comply with anticoagulation treatment, aspirin could offer some level of protection against recurrence; however, further analysis, longer follow-up, and head-to-head comparison with warfarin is required before this approach can be fully endorsed.[51]

Patients who have had an unprovoked VTE have an increased risk of recurrent VTE if anticoagulation therapy is stopped. Current consensus is to treat for a minimum of 6 months with full-intensity anticoagulation therapy, usually with warfarin. Extending treatment past 6 months with full-intensity warfarin therapy results in the most significant decrease in risk for recurrent events, but with the costs of increased bleeding risk, monitoring, and impact on quality of life. For patients in whom the risk-benefit analysis of continued duration of anticoagulation is not straightforward, an individualized risk-benefit assessment using a variety of the strategies described earlier is performed by most clinicians in the decision-making process. Patient preference is also considered. Although many of these approaches, such as vascular reimaging and use of D-dimer algorithms, have not been rigorously validated, they are widely practiced. Because of the lack of definitive data, none of these practices has been endorsed by any major society's guidelines. Clinicians in practice need to make decisions despite the sometimes conflicting results of trials and the differences of expert opinions. The use of D-dimer testing, repeat vascular imaging, and use of clinical prediction rules or scoring systems can help the clinician decide on an appropriate treatment course for the individual patient. This decision should be reevaluated as new data emerge that better define the true risk of recurrent VTE for an individual patient.

NEW ORAL ANTICOAGULANTS

New oral anticoagulants have been developed with the goal of replacing warfarin, the only oral anticoagulant available for more than 50 years. Warfarin is associated with many unfavorable characteristics, including slow onset of action, slow return to normal hemostasis, narrow therapeutic window, many significant drug and dietary interactions, and need for frequent testing, that make it cumbersome to manage. These new agents have been developed to improve on these limitations of warfarin. They all target either Xa or thrombin (see **Fig. 1**). They bind directly to the coagulation factor and prevent its activity, whereas warfarin impairs vitamin K epoxide activity, resulting in abnormal hepatic synthesis of several coagulation factors that are not able to be activated (II, VII, IX, X). The direct binding of these new oral agents to their targets results in rapid onset of anticoagulant activity within 2 to 3 hours of ingestion. The new oral agents have a wide therapeutic window in comparison with warfarin.

Dabigatran and rivaroxaban are 2 new oral anticoagulants currently available in the United States, Canada, Europe, and Australia. Apixaban has completed, or is nearing completion, of phase III studies for multiple use indications and will be seeking approval in the near future. Dabigatran is a direct thrombin inhibitor. Rivaroxaban and apixaban target Xa. Both dabigatran and rivaroxaban have been approved in the United States for stroke prevention in patients with nonvalvular atrial fibrillation, and for VTE prophylaxis following elective knee and hip replacement.[52,53] Many more new anticoagulants are in various stages of development in the highly competitive anticoagulant arena.

Investigational study design has played a critical role in assessing the results of the trials of these new agents. Both primary efficacy and safety event rates are low, requiring the enrollment of large numbers of patients to satisfy statistical significance. For example, 18,000 patients were enrolled in the study of dabigatran in patients with nonvalvular atrial fibrillation.[54] Each of the 3 study arms was assigned 6000 patients. In the study of apixaban in nonvalvular atrial fibrillation, more than 18,000 patients were randomized to 2 treatment arms with 9000 in each arm.[55] Demonstrating equivalency, or noninferiority, for a new agent compared with warfarin has been the first step in assessing efficacy. Comparison of safety profiles, or rates of major and nonmajor bleeding, is important. Bleeding risk is the most significant risk factor associated with warfarin use, and nonmajor bleeding is a specific reason for decreased quality of life for patients on warfarin.[56] Dabigatran, rivaroxaban, and apixaban have been shown to be noninferior or superior to warfarin in efficacy, with similar or decreased rates of major bleeding across all use indications. Regulatory approval has hinged on demonstration of superiority in either efficacy, safety, or both. Due to limitations and differences in study design, patient populations, rigorousness of warfarin management, and lack of head-to-head trials, the efficacy of the new oral anticoagulants cannot be directly compared with each other.

The new oral anticoagulants promise to improve on the efficacy, safety, and lifestyle issues associated with warfarin. They have yet to be approved for treatment of acute VTE in the United States; however, rivaroxaban was approved for this indication in the European Union in December 2011. Its approval was based on a carefully designed study using rivaroxaban as monotherapy (ie, without the need for a parenteral agent) from the time of diagnosis of acute DVT. It showed noninferiority to warfarin in acute VTE treatment with no difference between rivaroxaban and warfarin in major bleeding. Rivaroxaban was superior to placebo in preventing DVT recurrence after the initial 6 months of treatment.[57] Dabigatran was started after 5 days of parenteral anticoagulation with LMWH. Dabigatran was also noninferior to warfarin in efficacy, with a similar safety profile.[58] A phase III trial of apixaban in acute VTE has not yet been completed.

In the next few years, the treatment of acute VTE and the prevention of recurrent VTE may change significantly if these new oral anticoagulants become available for this use indication. Overall, they all have at least similar efficacy and similar safety profiles compared with warfarin. Further data from longer duration of use in broader patient populations, including postmarketing data derived from patients with atrial fibrillation, will provide more information on safety. Differences in metabolism and clearance must be considered when determining which agent to use. Dabigatran is primarily cleared by the kidneys, whereas apixaban is cleared by the liver, and rivaroxaban by both. Differences in frequency of administration and side effect profiles will also allow clinicians to choose the agent that best fits the individual patient's needs. Improvements in the management of warfarin therapy, with home testing, self-dosing, and improved patient education, make warfarin a continued option, especially for those with renal or hepatic insufficiency. Rigorous cost-effectiveness analyses of new agents versus warfarin need to be performed and need to include all costs associated with anticoagulant management, and not just drug cost, before decisions and policies are made that determine the role of these agents in VTE treatment. Although warfarin is inexpensive compared with the costs of these new agents, the costs associated with the management of warfarin dose by trained staff may equal or exceed the costs of a new agent. Accessibility to test facilities, cost of home monitors and test strips, and other patient-centered costs also need to be considered. The rate of major bleeding and adverse outcomes with potential lifelong sequelae requiring more intensive medical care should also factor into the analyses. The treatment of VTE will become personalized medicine with duration of anticoagulation determined by individualized risk assessments and with a wider range of choice of oral anticoagulants that offer improvement compared with current therapy.

SUPERFICIAL VENOUS THROMBOSIS

One of the more common presentations of thrombotic disorders is superficial VTE (SVT). Although it is not considered as serious an event as a DVT, it still causes substantial adverse consequences and is a risk factor for development of DVT.[59,60] It has been estimated that approximately 125,000 people in the United States will suffer from SVT in the next year.[61] Just as for DVT, the same risk factors seem to be important in development of SVT, including prolonged periods of immobilization, trauma, obesity, underlying hypercoagulable state, oral contraceptives or hormone use, malignancy, and autoimmune disorders.[59] In addition, the presence of varicose veins seems to provide a structural nidus that increases the clotting risk, resulting in higher rates of SVT.

The main focus of SVT management is the prevention of progression to other VTE. It has been estimated that 6.8% to 40% of SVT cases progress to deep vein thrombotic events.[62] As is evident from this wide range, it is difficult to estimate what percentage of patients with SVT will go on to other VTE. Studies that measure the risk of DVT progression from SVT are plagued with poor design strategies including differences in the tests used to make the diagnosis, standardization of patient characteristics, description of SVT event itself, as well as flawed statistical analysis.

To determine what factors might increase the risk of developing a DVT, a large prospective investigation was performed.[63] The goal of the study was to find risk factors that help to establish which patients would be at risk for having a concurrent DVT at the time of presentation with the SVT. In the study, 788 patients with SVT were followed. Risk factors that increased the chance of having a simultaneous DVT included (1) age greater than 75 years, (2) active cancer, and (3) inpatient status at the time of presentation. The presence of a varicosity was not associated with increased risk of having a concurrent DVT. The risk of subsequent DVT development in patients with varicosities was not addressed. The study did investigate the overall rate of developing a VTE by 3 months, and male gender and inpatient status were risk factors.

Others have suggested that location of the SVT is important for identifying which patients are at risk of developing VTE. Most SVTs occur in the saphenous vein (60%–80%). There are 3 ways in which an SVT can progress to a DVT. The clot can progress from the saphenofemoral junction (SFJ) into the common femoral vein; traverse through the knee perforators into the popliteal vein; or travel through the ankle perforators into the tibial and peroneal veins. Initial studies by Chengelis and colleagues[64] showed that 90% of the events occur through the SFJ. In a study by Verlato and colleagues,[65] SVT in the thigh provided substantial risk for adverse events. The presence of SVT in the saphenous vein has been associated with the highest likelihood of becoming DVTs, and full anticoagulation should be considered.[64] Some have tried to look at the proximity of the clot to the SFJ to base decisions on who needs to be considered for aggressive treatment because of the risk of conversion to DVT. Initial studies by Lohr and colleagues[66] suggested that a cutoff of 3 cm near the SFJ should be considered significant and warrant surgical intervention. Sullivan and colleagues,[67] in a meta-analysis, proposed that all incidences of SVT occurring above the knee in the great saphenous vein should be treated with anticoagulation.

Further support of the aggressive nature of clots near the SFJ came from the randomized control trial by Prandoni and colleagues,[68] which showed that patients with SVT within 2 to 3 cm of the SFJ were at risk for clot progression even if they received anticoagulation therapy. Although there was a decrease in the rate of SVT progression in the therapeutic group, the difference was minimal with progression occurring in 8.6% of those who received prophylactic anticoagulation and 7.2% of those on the therapeutic dosing regimen. This study further supports the importance of location in risk stratifying which patients are at increased risk of clot progression. In our experience, an aggressive approach using treatment in this patient population is warranted and, for this reason, we agree with consideration of anticoagulation in those at risk of progression.

SVT has traditionally been treated conservatively with methods aimed at reducing pain and suffering, including warm compresses, nonsteroidal antiinflammatory agents, and compression stockings. This disorder is difficult to treat because it does not consist of just thrombosis alone; it is associated with an inflammatory state as well. The development of an SVT usually occurs in areas of trauma to the external skin or direct damage to the endothelial layer of the blood vessel, leading to inflammation within the vessel through leukocyte activation and edema, increasing the risk of thrombosis. An area of varicosity is more likely to have diminished blood flow that may be associated with increased risk of thrombosis through venous stasis changes. Another factor that can lead to endothelial injury and subsequent thrombosis is intravenous catheter placement. In patients with malignancy, a migratory form of SVT can occur in which repeated thrombosis develops within the superficial venous system. This type of VTE was originally described by Trousseau and can be a harbinger for impending cancer diagnosis and worsening disease burden.

However, recent studies have suggested that, at least for some cases, a more aggressive approach may be warranted. Because there is little consensus within the medical community regarding appropriate treatment of this condition, the range of available treatment modalities is diverse, including everything from no treatment to nonsteroidal antiinflammatory drugs or full-intensity anticoagulation.[69,70] However, this problem has been compounded by a lack of adequately controlled randomized trials. These studies have left many questions regarding dosing of anticoagulation and length of treatment. Initial work by Belcaro and colleagues[62] established the important role of anticoagulation as a means of decreasing the rate of progression of SVT. In this open study, patients with SVT were randomized to conservative treatment versus treatment with anticoagulants. In the control group who received no anticoagulation, the incidence of DVT was as high as 7.7%, whereas no patient who received anticoagulation progressed to DVTs. Marchiori and colleagues[59] studied low and high doses of heparin to treat VTE and there was less progression in those who received the high-dose regimens. However, this trial has been criticized for its small patient numbers. A more rigorous trial was performed by Quenet and colleagues.[71] This was a double-blind study in which 436 patients were randomized to placebo group, prophylactic dosing of LMWH, or therapeutic dosing of LMWH. Although there was no statistically significant difference observed between the groups after 10 days of treatment, the rate of recurrence of SVT was lower in those who had been treated versus those in the placebo group.

The most rigorous trial to address this issue, and the most compelling evidence for treatment of SVT, was presented by the CALISTO (Comparison of Arixtra in Lower Limb Superficial Vein Thrombosis with Placebo) trial in which the efficacy of fondaparinux (Arixtra) for reducing symptomatic VTE complications was addressed.[72] In this study, patients with SVT received prophylactic doses of fondaparinux at 2.5 mg once daily for 45 days. This study showed that the rate of PE or DVT was 85% lower in the group that received the fondaparinux compared with the placebo group, at least up to 77 days after the initial event. The incidence of adverse events such as bleeding was negligible. The investigators concluded that treatment with fondaparinux at a dose of 2.5 mg per day for 45 days was an effective means of decreasing the chance of an SVT leading to a DVT or PE, and that the side effects of this treatment were minimal.

Although these studies clearly establish the benefit of anticoagulation in patients with SVT, questions still remain regarding the length of anticoagulation, dosing regimen, and the agent of choice. It is our experience that patients presenting with SVT at risk of progression should be managed with anticoagulation and repeated ultrasound to monitor efficacy of treatment and to guide decisions regarding length of treatment.

TRAVEL-RELATED VENOUS THROMBOSIS

The mechanism underlying the increased risk of thrombotic events in association with air travel is not well elucidated. The most compelling argument for associated risk seems to be from the venous stasis that occurs during the immobility that is required for air travel.[73] The overall estimate is that air travel for a prolonged period of time confers a 2-fold to 4-fold increased risk of having a VTE.[74–76] The risk can be substantial, with one group reporting that the risk of DVT increases by 26% for every 2-hour increment of air travel.[20] The period of vulnerability to development of VTE extends from time of travel out to 8 weeks after returning from the trip.[77]

It is generally thought that those who have a higher propensity for clotting events are the most at risk for air travel–related thrombosis. For this reason, individual risk assessments need to be performed on patients to determine whether or not any interventions are needed to decrease their overall risk burden during travel. Preexisting risk factors for developing VTE include recent surgery, active malignancy, previous spontaneous VTE, previous travel-related VTE, or underlying hypercoagulable state.[78,79] Others have suggested that presence of other comorbidities, including congestive heart failure and stroke, also increase the risk of developing a thrombotic event.[80] Having more than 1 risk factor is also suspected to have a cumulative effect in terms of overall risk assessment according to an Australian study.[81]

Preventing these thrombotic events should be the main goal for all air travelers. There are several conservative measures that can be taken to help diminish the occurrence. These measures include adequate mobility; avoidance of constrictive clothing; focused exercises to improve flow to lower extremities; avoidance of any agents that increase sedentary state, such as alcohol or sedating drugs; and use of compressing stockings.[82,83]

For those patients with perceived higher risk of VTE, such as those with prior events, anticoagulation therapy is a reasonable option. However, few studies have been performed in this population to validate the use of anticoagulation and to confirm agent of choice, dosing, and timing interval of administration. In our practice, based on experience and minimal clinical data, we generally advise our patients with higher overall risk of VTE to use LMWH prophylactically with dosing a few hours before flying as a single dose. The use of aspirin is not effective in this population to prevent venous-related events.[84] Recent guidelines from ACCP 9th edition provided some guidance for patients with risk factors for travel-related VTE. For patients traveling a long distance who have an increased risk of VTE, such as previous history of VTE, recent surgery or trauma, an active malignancy, estrogen use, or known thrombophilic disorder, they recommend aggressive prevention through increased ambulation and calf muscle exercises and the use of compression stockings during travel (grade 2C). They recommend against the regular use of aspirin or anticoagulants for prevention of VTE, including in those with asymptomatic thrombophilia.[18]

HYPERCOAGULABLE WORK-UP

Several heritable and acquired risk factors negatively affect a patient's risk of developing a VTE. Genetic risk factors that are associated with increased risk of VTE include mutations in factor V (Leiden) and prothrombin 20210, as well as mutations leading to deficiencies in antithrombin, protein C, and protein S. Acquired risk factors include the development of antiphospholipid antibodies and their associated anticardiolipins. The use of tests to assess the presence of these factors to establish overall thrombotic risk is controversial.

Approximately 5% of the white population has at least 1 mutation for factor V Leiden, and 15% to 20% of patients who carry this mutation develop a VTE.[85–88] This point mutation prevents protein C from effectively acting on factor V to limit its activity, leading to hypercoagulability. Another common genetic mutation associated with VTE is the prothrombin gene (G2021A) mutation, which is carried by approximately 2% of the population and may be present in approximately 5% to 15% of persons with VTE.[89] Patients with this mutation have a higher level of prothrombin than normally found because of decreased ability to degrade the protein precursor messenger

RNA. Patients who carry both of these mutations simultaneously are referred to as compound heterozygotes. These patients are particularly vulnerable to clotting, with a 20-fold increased risk of having a clotting event.

Deficiencies in normally present anticoagulant proteins also can account for the hypercoagulable state. Antithrombin III deficiency, which is associated with a frequency of 1 in 300 in the general population, and in 3% to 5% of those with thrombotic events, leads to a 50-fold increased risk in severe cases. The population frequencies of mutations in other genes that are responsible for other coagulation factors, such as in protein C or protein S, are estimated to be 1 in 500 individuals. Deficiency of these proteins is associated with a 10-fold increased thrombotic risk. It was previously thought that genetic mutations in the genes important for methylene tetrahydrofolate reductase and hyperhomocysteinemia increased the risk of venous thromboembolic events; however, this causation has been shown to be less likely.[90] The incidence of increased factor VIII, IX, and XI being associated with thrombotic risk is controversial. Deficiencies in fibrinolytic proteins may also contribute to the overall hypercoagulable state leading to disfibrinolysis disorders such as congenital plasminogen deficiency, deficiency of tissue plasminogen activator, or congenital plasminogen activator increases.

The main acquired risk factor associated with the hypercoagulable state that is known to be important in both venous and arterial thrombosis is the acquisition of antiphospholipid antibodies. These antibodies represent a family of antibodies against phospholipids, such as cardiolipins, and phospholipid binding proteins, such as β 2 glycoprotein I. The mechanisms responsible for thrombosis remain to be elucidated, with some proposed mechanism for hypercoagulability including inhibition of protein C, antithrombin, and annexin A5 expression; binding and activation of platelets; enhanced endothelial cell tissue factor expression; and activation of the complement cascade.[91] For a diagnosis of antiphospholipid syndrome to be made, the presence of both clinical events and laboratory evidence of the presence of antiphospholipid antibodies must be present.[92] In addition, the cutoff values for levels of anticardiolipins have been established for diagnosing this syndrome.

The issue of who to undertake a hypercoagulable work-up on is always controversial. In general, random screening for thrombophilias is not recommended because this does not always directly affect treatment decisions. Screening asymptomatic individuals is even more controversial because, although prophylactic anticoagulation could be offered during high-risk situations, there are no data to support the long-term use of prophylactic anticoagulation in asymptomatic patients. Others would state that having the knowledge of an inherited thrombophilia can directly affect patients' ability to be more proactive about their health care and make informed decisions.

In some situations, it is advisable to screen for thrombophilia. Until more clinical data are available, individual risk assessments need to direct which individuals undergo a thrombophilia work-up. There is an advantage to knowing about homozygous carrier states as well as the presence of multiple genetic defects that overall increase the risk of having a clotting-related event. Also, antithrombin deficiency can have serious impact on thrombotic risk, especially in women who are pregnant. These women should be offered anticoagulation for the duration of their pregnancy, which greatly diminishes their thrombotic risk.

BRIDGING: ANTICOAGULATION BRIDGING FOR INVASIVE PROCEDURES

At some point, almost every patient on long-term anticoagulation requires an invasive procedure that necessitates stopping anticoagulation to prevent excess procedure-related bleeding. For patients on short-acting parenteral LMWH or fonda-parinux, or the new short-acting oral direct Xa or thrombin inhibitors, stopping the anticoagulant before the procedure is simply a matter of holding for the appropriate amount of time so that enough half-lives have passed for the anticoagulant effect to reverse; usually 24 to 72 hours. However, warfarin has such a long duration of effect on coagulation factors that it must be stopped for 5 days before the procedure to reach baseline hemostasis. Bridging is the term used when a short-acting anticoagulant, usually a parenteral LMWH, is used both in the few days before the procedure after stopping warfarin, and often after the procedure, until therapeutic anticoagulation is again achieved with warfarin.

The number of patients on warfarin anticoagulation for primary stroke prevention in cardiovascular disorders, such as in atrial fibrillation or with mechanical heart valves, or for secondary VTE prophylaxis, has increased significantly in the last 2 decades. Bridging strategies have developed in tandem with the increasing numbers of patients on warfarin and with the advent of LMWH, making it easier to bridge in the outpatient setting rather than admit for IV UFH. These strategies have developed without the benefit of data from randomized controlled trials. The use of bridging anticoagulation was based on perceived thromboembolic risk in the absence of anticoagulation, especially in patients with mechanical heart valves. Current critical review and new data raise many questions about the use of bridging anticoagulation.

The intent of bridging is to minimize periprocedural thromboembolic events and bleeding risks. The primary indication for anticoagulation drives the VTE risk, whereas the type of procedure defines the risk of bleeding. Many studies published in the last 10 to 12 years were cohort studies that did not use tight bridging protocols. Results were often conflicting, with some studies reporting low rates of thrombotic events at 0.7% in a selected patient population with perceived moderate risk of thrombotic event in which warfarin was stopped without LMWH bridging. In a similar patient population, the estimated thrombotic event risk of 0.016% was considered too high; hence, warfarin was continued for certain selected dermatologic procedures with no documented increase in bleeding.[93,94]

The largest study on anticoagulation bridging published to date was from a prospective registry study of 1293 patients.[93] The most common indications for long-term anticoagulation in this registry were atrial fibrillation (n = 550), VTE (n = 144), and mechanical prosthetic heart valves (n = 132). The most common procedures were colonoscopy (n = 324), dental (n = 323), or cataract surgery (n = 116). Only 108 of the 1293 patients (8.3%) were bridged. Most patients were simply instructed to omit warfarin for up to 5 days before surgery and to resume warfarin on postoperative day zero. Thromboembolism occurred in none of the bridged patients but in 0.6% of the nonbridged patients. In contrast, major hemorrhage occurred in 3.7% of the bridged patients but in only 0.2% of the nonbridged patients. Based on the low observed risk of thrombotic event, the investigators suggested that bridging may be unnecessary for most patients. The investigators also suggested that routine bridging increases the bleeding risk, leading to more risk than benefit.

Despite the lack of high-quality data from randomized controlled trials, efforts have been made to develop practice guidelines to help the clinician determine optimal management for the individual patient. These guidelines are adapted from risk-stratification schemes that estimate risk of stroke or VTE and are used in the nonperioperative setting (CHADS$_2$ [congestive heart failure, hypertension, age >75 years, diabetes, prior stroke or transient ischemic attack] and CHA$_2$DS$_2$VASc [congestive heart failure; hypertension; age $\geq$75 years; diabetes mellitus; prior stroke, transient ischemic attack, or thromboembolism; vascular disease; age 65–74 years; sex category, ie, female gender]).[95,96] Patients who may benefit from bridging include those with recent thrombosis or with history or risk factors that suggest a high risk of repeat thrombosis when not fully anticoagulated, such as patients with mechanical mitral valve replacement, prior stroke, active cancer diagnosis, new DVT or PE within 3 months of procedure, or prior thromboembolism during perioperative warfarin interruption.[18] In these patients, warfarin is held for 5 days before surgery and generally an LMWH at full dose is started 4 days before surgery. The last dose of LMWH is given 24 hours before surgery. Anticoagulation with LMWH is then generally resumed 24 to 72 hours after surgery, depending on when hemostasis is thought to be satisfactory and on the bleeding risk associated with the type of surgery. In some patients at extremely high risk for thrombotic event or VTE, or at extremely high risk of bleeding, IV UFH with its short half-life can be used to bridge the patient. It is started when the INR is at 2.0 and stopped 4 to 6 hours before surgery. In addition to its shorter half-life compared with LMWH, it can be fully reversed with protamine and its anticoagulant effect readily monitored by PTT testing.

Guidelines for risk of bleeding are based on type of surgery, with general consensus developed for those procedures deemed high, intermediate, and low risk for bleeding. In patients who undergo surgery with high risk of bleeding, postoperative LMWH is often not restarted or is resumed at a later time such as 48 to 72 hours after surgery, and often with a prophylactic dose. Surgical procedures with high bleeding risk include major cardiac surgery, intracranial surgery, intraspinal surgery, major vascular surgery, major orthopedic surgery, and major cancer surgery.[18,97] Urogenital surgery, including prostate and bladder resection surgeries, have an increased risk of bleeding caused by local endogenous urokinase activity. Some minor surgeries and nonsurgical procedures have been deemed high risk for bleeding given anatomic or local factors. These procedures include colon polypectomy if the polyp stalk is greater than 1 cm, prostate or kidney biopsy, and cardiac pacemaker or defibrillator placement.[97]

There are many questions about bridging that have yet to be answered, including which patients truly benefit from bridging and whether a full or prophylactic dose of LMWH should be used. A randomized controlled trial of bridging sponsored by the National Institutes of Health is currently being conducted in the United States. The BRIDGE (Bridging Anticoagulation in Patients who Require Temporary Interruption of Warfarin for an Elective Procedure or Surgery) trial is enrolling patients with chronic atrial fibrillation who require temporary interruption of warfarin treatment, and will attempt to answer some of these questions.

Patients with newly diagnosed VTE should have surgical procedures deferred until 12 weeks after the VTE diagnosis, if possible, because these patients are at high risk for recurrent VTE if anticoagulation is interrupted.[18] If the surgery cannot be postponed, bridging strategies should be used. Anticoagulation should be resumed at 24 hours after surgery or as soon as deemed safe from a bleeding standpoint, with the goal of reaching full-dose anticoagulation as quickly as possible. Patients with a more remote history of VTE should be assessed for need for bridging based on the information provided earlier, taking into account all VTE and thrombotic event risks as well as risk for bleeding.[98]

SUMMARY

Patients with VTE present with a wide range of findings and factors that affect management. Decision making in VTE management is a fluid process that should be reevaluated as new data emerge and individual circumstances change. There is now more focus on VTE management than there was even a decade ago. Diagnostic algorithms, identification of newly identified risk factors, refinement in understanding of the pathogenesis of thrombosis, and identification of new anticoagulants with more favorable risk-benefit profiles will all ultimately contribute to improved patient care.

REFERENCES

1. Alfirevic Z, Alfirevic I. Hypercoagulable state, pathophysiology, classification and epidemiology. Clin Chem Lab Med 2010;48(Suppl 1):S15–26.
2. White H. The epidemiology of venous thromboembolism. Circulation 2003;107: I4–8.
3. Anderson FA, Wheeler HB, Goldberg RJ, et al. A population based perspective of the hospital incidence and case fatality rates of deep vein thrombosis and pulmonary embolism. The Worcester DVT study. Arch Int Med 1991;151:933–8.
4. Kearon C, Julian JA, Math M, et al. Noninvasive diagnosis of deep vein thrombosis. McMaster Diagnostic Imaging Practice Guidelines Initiative. Ann Intern Med 1998;128:663–77.
5. Wells PS, Hirsh J, et al. Accuracy of clinical assessment of deep-vein thrombosis. Lancet 1995;345:1326–30.
6. Wells PS, Anderson DR, Bormanis J, et al. SimpliRED D-dimer can reduce the diagnostic tests in suspected deep vein thrombosis. Lancet 1998;351:1405–6.
7. Wells PS, Anderson DR, Bormanis J, et al. Value of assessment of pretest probability of deep-vein thrombosis in clinical management. Lancet 1997;350:1795–8.
8. Tick LW, Ton E, van Voorthuizen T, et al. Practical diagnostic management of patients with clinically suspected deep vein thrombosis by clinical probability test, compression ultrasonography, and D-dimer test. Am J Med 2002;113:630–5.
9. Anderson DR, Wells PS, Stiell I, et al. Thrombosis in the emergency department: use of a clinical model to safely avoid the need for urgent radiological investigation. Arch Intern Med 1999;159:477–82.
10. Wells PS, Anderson DR, Bormanis J, et al. Application of a diagnostic clinical model for the management of hospitalized patients with suspected deep-vein thrombosis. Thromb Haemost 1999;81:493–7.
11. Anderson DR, Kovacs MJ, Kovacs G, et al. Combined use of clinical assessment and D-dimer to improve the management of patients presenting to the emergency department with suspected deep vein thrombosis (the EDITED Study). J Thromb Haemost 2003;1:645–51.
12. Wells PS, Anderson DR, Rodger M, et al. Evaluation of D-dimer in the diagnosis of suspected deep-vein thrombosis. N Engl J Med 2003;349:1227–35.
13. Brenda KZ. Diagnosis of venous thromboembolism: ultrasonography and diagnosis of venous thromboembolism. Circulation 2004;109:I9–14.
14. Hirsh J, Lee AY. How we diagnose and treat deep vein thrombosis. Blood 2002; 99:3102–10.
15. Tapson VF, Carroll BA, Davidson BL, et al. The diagnostic approach to acute venous thromboembolism. Clinical practice guideline. American Thoracic Society. Am J Respir Crit Care Med 1999;160:1043–66.
16. Remy-Jardin M, Remy J, Deschildre F, et al. Diagnosis of pulmonary embolism with spiral CT: comparison with pulmonary angiography and scintigraphy. Radiology 1996;200(3):699–706.
17. Stein PE, Fowler SE, Goodman LR, et al. Multidetector computed tomography for acute pulmonary embolism. N Engl J Med 2006;354:2317–27.

18. Antithrombotic Therapy and Prevention of Thrombosis, 9th edition: American College of Chest Physicians Evidence-Based Clinical Practice Guidelines. Chest 2012;141:7S–47S.

19. Chan YC, Valenti D, Mansfield AO. Warfarin induced skin necrosis. Br J Surg 2000;87(3):266–72.

20. Chandra D, Parisini E, Mozaffarian D. Meta-analysis: travel and risk for venous thromboembolism. Ann Intern Med 2009;151(3):180–90.

21. Segal JB, Streiff MB, Hofmann LV, et al. Management of venous thromboembolism: a systematic review for a practice guideline. Ann Intern Med 2007;146: 211–22.

22. McRae SJ, Ginsberg JS. Initial treatment of venous thromboembolism. Circulation 2004;110:I3–9.

23. Kearon C, Kahn SR, Agnelli G, et al. American College of Chest Physicians. Chest 2008;133(Suppl 6):454S.

24. Schulman S, Rhedin AS, Lindmarker P, et al. A comparison of 6 weeks with 6 months of oral anticoagulant therapy after a first episode of venous thromboembolism. Duration of Anticoagulation Trial Study Group. N Engl J Med 1995;332: 1661.

25. Pinede L, Duhaut P, Cucherat M, et al. Comparison of long versus short duration of anticoagulant therapy after a first episode of venous thromboembolism: a meta-analysis of randomized, controlled trials. J Intern Med 2000;247:553–62.

26. Iorio A, Kearon C, Filippucci E, et al. Risk of recurrence after a first episode of symptomatic venous thromboembolism provoked by a transient risk factor: a systematic review. Arch Intern Med 2010;170:1710–6.

27. Levine MN, Raskob G, Landefeld S, et al. Hemorrhagic complications of anticoagulant treatment. Chest 2001;119:108S–21S.

28. Kyrle PA, Minar E, Bialonczyk C, et al. The risk of recurrent venous thromboembolism in men and women. N Engl J Med 2004;350:2558–63.

29. Eichinger S, Hron G, Bialonczyk C, et al. Overweight, obesity, and the risk of recurrent venous thromboembolism. Arch Intern Med 2008;168:1678–83.

30. Kearon C, Gent M, Hirsh J, et al. A comparison of three months of anticoagulation therapy with extended anticoagulation for a first episode of idiopathic venous thromboembolism. N Engl J Med 1999;340:901–7.

31. Agnelli G, Prandoni P, Becattini C, et al, for the Warfarin Optimal Duration Italian Trial Investigators. Extended oral anticoagulant therapy after a first episode of pulmonary embolism. Ann Intern Med 2003;139:19–25.

32. Agnelli G, Prandoni P, Santamaria MG, et al, for the Warfarin Optimal Duration Italian Trial Investigators. Three months versus one year of oral anticoagulant therapy for idiopathic deep venous thrombosis. N Engl J Med 2001;345:165–9.

33. Landefeld CS, Beyth RJ. Anticoagulant related bleeding: clinical epidemiology, prediction, and prevention. Am J Med 1993;95:315–28.

34. Nieuwenhuis HK, Albada J, Banga JD, et al. Identification of risk factors for bleeding during treatment of acute venous thromboembolism with heparin or low molecular weight heparin. Blood 1991;78:2337–43.

35. Ruiz-Gimenez N, Suarez C, Gonzalez R, et al. Predictive variables for major bleeding events in patients presenting with documented acute venous thromboembolism. Findings from the RIETE Registry. J Thromb Haemost 2008;100: 26–31.

36. Schulman S, Granqvist S, Holmstrom M, et al, for the Duration of Anticoagulation Trial Study Group. The duration of oral anticoagulant therapy after a second episode of venous thromboembolism. N Engl J Med 1997;336:393–8.

37. Linkins LA, Choi PT, Douketis JD. Clinical impact of bleeding in patients taking oral anticoagulant therapy for venous-thromboembolism: a meta-analysis. Ann Intern Med 2003;139:893.

38. Prandoni P, Lensing AW, Piccioli A, et al. Recurrent venous thromboembolism and bleeding complications during anticoagulant treatment in patients with cancer and venous thrombosis. Blood 2002;100:3484–8.

39. Palareti G, Cosmi B, Legnani C, et al. D-dimer testing to determine the duration of anticoagulation therapy. N Engl J Med 2006;355:1780–9.

40. Bruinstroop E, Klok FA, Van De Ree MA, et al. Elevated D-dimer levels predict recurrence in patients with idiopathic venous thromboembolism: a meta-analysis. J Thromb Haemost 2009;7:611–8.

41. Verhovsek M, Douketis JD, Yi Q, et al. Systematic review: D-Dimer to predict recurrent disease after stopping anticoagulant therapy for unprovoked venous thromboembolism. Ann Intern Med 2008;149:481.

42. Douketis J, Tosetto A, Marcucci M, et al. Patient-level meta-analysis: effect of measurement timing, threshold, and patient age on ability of D-dimer testing to assess recurrence risk after unprovoked venous thromboembolism. Ann Intern Med 2010;153(8):523–31.

43. Cosmi B, Legnani C, Tosetto A, et al. Usefulness of repeated D-dimer testing after stopping anticoagulation for a first episode of unprovoked venous thromboembolism: the PROLONG II prospective study. Blood 2010;115(3):481–8.

44. Prandoni P, Lensing AW, Prins MH, et al. Residual vein thrombosis as a predictive factor of recurrent venous thromboembolism. Ann Intern Med 2002;137:955.

45. Prandoni P, Prins MH, Lensing AW, et al. Residual thrombosis on ultrasonography to guide the duration of anticoagulation in patients with deep venous thrombosis: a randomized trial. Ann Intern Med 2009;150:577–85.

46. Eichinger S, Weltermann A, Minar E, et al. Symptomatic pulmonary embolism and the risk of recurrent venous thromboembolism. Arch Intern Med 2004;164:92–6.

47. Eichinger S, Heinze G, Jandeck LM, et al. Risk assessment of recurrence in patients with unprovoked deep vein thrombosis or pulmonary embolism: the Vienna Prediction Model. Circulation 2010;121:1630–6.

48. Rodger MA, Kahn SR, Wells PS, et al. Identifying unprovoked thromboembolism patients at low risk for recurrence who can discontinue anticoagulant therapy. CMAJ 2008;179:417–26.

49. Ridker PM, Goldhaber SZ, Danielson E, et al. Long-term, low-intensity warfarin therapy for prevention of recurrent venous thromboembolism. N Engl J Med 2003;348:1425–34.

50. Kearon C, Ginsberg JS, Kovacs MJ, et al, for the Extended Low-Intensity Anticoagulation for Thrombo-Embolism Investigators. Comparison of low-intensity warfarin therapy with conventional-intensity warfarin therapy for long-term prevention of recurrent venous thromboembolism. N Engl J Med 2003;349:631–9.

51. Becattini C, Giancarlo A, Renzo P, et al. After oral anticoagulants for prevention of recurrence in patients with unprovoked venous thromboembolism. The WARFA-SA study. 53rd ASH Annual Meeting. San Diego (CA), December 10-13, 2011.

52. Pradaxa [package insert]. Available at: http://www.pradaxa.com/Boehringer. Ridgefield, CT 06877: Ingelheim Pharmaceuticals, Inc., USA.

53. Xarelto (rivaroxaban) [package insert]. Available at: http://www.xarelto.com/ Janssen . Titusville, NJ 08560: Pharmaceuticals, Inc., USA.

54. Connolly SJ, Ezekowitz MD, Yusuf S, et al. Dabigatran versus warfarin in patients with atrial fibrillation. N Engl J Med 2009;361:1139–51.

55. Granger CB, Alexander JH, McMurray JJV, et al. Apixaban versus warfarin in patients with atrial fibrillation. N Engl J Med 2011;365:981–92.
56. Lancaster TR, Singer DE, Sheehan MA, et al. The impact of long-term warfarin therapy on quality of life: evidence from a randomized trial. Arch Intern Med 1991;151:1944–9.
57. The EINSTEIN Investigators. Oral rivaroxaban for symptomatic venous thromboembolism. N Engl J Med 2010;363:2499–510.
58. Schulman S, Kearon C, Kakkar AK, et al. Dabigatran versus warfarin in the treatment of acute venous thromboembolism. N Engl J Med 2009;361(24): 2342–52.
59. Marchiori A, Mosena L, Prandoni P. Superficial vein thrombosis: risk factors, diagnosis, and treatment. Thromb Haemost 2006;32(7):737–43.
60. Decousus H, Quere I, Presles E, et al. Superficial venous thrombosis and venous thromboembolism: a large, prospective epidemiologic study. Ann Intern Med 2010;152(4):218–24.
61. Litzendorf ME, Satiani B. Superficial venous thrombosis: disease progression and evolving treatment approaches. Vasc Health Risk Manag 2011;7:569–75.
62. Belcaro G, Nicolaides AN, Errichi BM, et al. Superficial thrombophlebitis of the legs: a randomized, controlled, follow up study. Angiology 1999;50(7):523–9.
63. Galanaud JP, Genty C, Sevestre MA, et al. Predictive factors for concurrent deep-vein thrombosis and symptomatic venous thromboembolic recurrence in case of superficial venous thrombosis. The OPTIMEV study. Thromb Haemost 2011; 105(1):31–9.
64. Chengelis DL, Bendick PJ, Glover JL, et al. Progression of superficial venous thrombosis to deep vein thrombosis. J Vasc Surg 1996;24(5):745–9.
65. Verlato F, Zucchetta P, Prandoni P, et al. An unexpectedly high rate of pulmonary embolism in patients with superficial thrombophlebitis of the thigh. J Vasc Surg 1999;30(6):1113–5.
66. Lohr JM, McDevitt DT, Lutter KS, et al. Operative management of greater saphenous thrombophlebitis involving the saphenofemoral junction. Am J Surg 1992; 164(3):269–75.
67. Sullivan V, Denk PM, Sonnad SS, et al. Ligation versus anticoagulation: treatment of above-knee superficial thrombophlebitis not involving the deep venous system. J Am Coll Surg 2001;193(5):556–62.
68. Prandoni P, Tormene D, Pesavento R. High vs. low doses of low-molecular-weight heparin for the treatment of superficial vein thrombosis of the legs: a double-blind, randomized trial. Thromb Haemost 2005;3(6):1152–7.
69. Kearon C, Kahn SR, Agnelli G, et al. Antithrombotic therapy for venous thromboembolic disease: American College of Chest Physicians Evidence-Based Clinical Practice Guidelines (8th edition). Chest 2008;133(Suppl 6):454S–545S.
70. Cesarone MR, Belcaro G, Agus G, et al. Management of superficial vein thrombosis and thrombophlebitis: status and expert opinion document. Angiology 2007;58(Suppl 1):7S–14S [discussion: 14S, 15S].
71. Quenet S, Laporte S, Décousus H, et al. Factors predictive of venous thrombotic complications in patients with isolated superficial vein thrombosis. J Vasc Surg 2003;38(5):944–9.
72. Decousus H, Prandoni P, Mismetti P, et al. Fondaparinux for the treatment of superficial-vein thrombosis in the legs. N Engl J Med 2010;363(13):1222–32.
73. Delis KT, Knaggs AL, Sonecha TN, et al. Lower limb venous haemodynamic impairment on dependency: quantification and implications for the "economy class" position. Thromb Haemost 2004;91(5):941–50.

74. Perez-Rodriguez E, Jimenez D, Diaz G, et al. Incidence of air travel-related pulmonary embolism at the Madrid-Barajas airport. Arch Intern Med 2003;163(22): 2766–70.
75. Kelman CW, Kortt MA, Becker NG, et al. Deep vein thrombosis and air travel: record linkage study. BMJ 2003;327(7423):1072.
76. Giangrande PL. Air travel and thrombosis. Br J Haematol 2002;117(3):509–12.
77. Watson HG, Baglin TP. Guidelines on travel-related venous thrombosis. Br J Haematol 2011;152(1):31–4.
78. Arya R, Barnes JA, Hossain U, et al. Long-haul flights and deep vein thrombosis: a significant risk only when additional factors are also present. Br J Haematol 2002;116(3):653–4.
79. Hughes RJ, Hopkins RJ, Hill S, et al. Frequency of venous thromboembolism in low to moderate risk long distance air travellers: the New Zealand Air Traveller's Thrombosis (NZATT) study. Lancet 2003;362(9401):2039–44.
80. Brenner B. Travel-related thrombosis: is this a problem? Isr Med Assoc J 2006; 8(12):859–61.
81. Kuipers S, Cannegieter SC, Doggen CJ, et al. Effect of elevated levels of coagulation factors on the risk of venous thrombosis in long-distance travelers. Blood 2009;113(9):2064–9.
82. Geerts WH, Pineo GF, Heit JA, et al. Prevention of venous thromboembolism: the Seventh ACCP Conference on Antithrombotic and Thrombolytic Therapy. Chest 2004;126(Suppl 3):338S–400S.
83. Chee YL, Watson HG. Air travel and thrombosis. Br J Haematol 2005;130(5): 671–80.
84. Cesarone MR, Belcaro G, Nicolaides AN, et al. Venous thrombosis from air travel: the LONFLIT3 study–prevention with aspirin vs low-molecular-weight heparin (LMWH) in high-risk subjects: a randomized trial. Angiology 2002;53(1):1–6.
85. Prandoni P. Acquired risk factors for venous thromboembolism in medical patients. Hematology Am Soc Hematol Educ Program 2005;458–61.
86. Rosendaal FR. Venous thrombosis: the role of genes, environment, and behavior. Hematology Am Soc Hematol Educ Program 2005;1–12.
87. Cushman M. Inherited risk factors for venous thrombosis. Hematology Am Soc Hematol Educ Program 2005;452–7.
88. Vossen CY, Conard J, Fontcuberta J, et al. Risk of a first venous thrombotic event in carriers of a familial thrombophilic defect. The European Prospective Cohort on Thrombophilia (EPCOT). J Thromb Haemost 2005;3(3):459–64.
89. Kottke-Marchant K. Genetic polymorphisms associated with venous and arterial thrombosis: an overview. Arch Pathol Lab Med 2002;126(3):295–304.
90. Ray JG. Hyperhomocysteinemia: no longer a consideration in the management of venous thromboembolism. Curr Opin Pulm Med 2008;14(5):369–73.
91. Lim W. Antiphospholipid antibody syndrome. Hematology Am Soc Hematol Educ Program 2009;233–9.
92. Cohen D, Berger SP, Steup-Beekman GM, et al. Diagnosis and management of the antiphospholipid syndrome. BMJ 2010;340:c2541.
93. Garcia DA, Regan S, Henault LE, et al. Risk of thromboembolism with short-term interruption of warfarin therapy. Arch Intern Med 2008;168(1):63–9.
94. Kovich O, Otley CC. Thrombotic complications related to discontinuation of warfarin and aspirin therapy perioperatively for cutaneous operation. J Am Acad Dermatol 2003;48:233–7.
95. Lip GY, Nieuwlaat R, Pisters R, et al. Refining clinical risk stratification for predicting stroke and thromboembolism in atrial fibrillation using a novel risk

factor-based approach: the euro heart survey on atrial fibrillation. Chest 2010; 137(2):263–72.

96. Gage BF, Waterman AD, Shannon W, et al. Validation of clinical classification schemes for predicting stroke: results from the National Registry of Atrial Fibrillation. JAMA 2001;285(22):2864–70.

97. Douketis JD, Berger PB, Dunn AS, et al. The perioperative management of antithrombotic therapy: American College of Chest Physicians Evidence-Based Clinical Practice Guidelines (8th edition). Chest 2008;133(Suppl 6):299S–339S.

98. Douketis JD. Perioperative management of patients who are receiving warfarin therapy: an evidence-based and practical approach. Blood 2011;117(19): 5044–9.

Does My Patient Have a Life- or Limb-Threatening Thrombocytopenia?

Nathan T. Connell, MD[a],*, Joseph D. Sweeney, MD[b]

KEYWORDS

- Thrombocytopenia • Heparin-induced thrombocytopenia
- Thrombotic microangiopathy • Preeclampsia

The consulting hematologist is often faced with the evaluation of patients with low platelet counts, many times of less than 10×10^9/L (single-digit thrombocytopenia). These consults require quick action for both diagnosis and treatment because the consequences of a severe thrombocytopenia may include life-threatening bleeding, especially intracerebral hemorrhage, or, paradoxically because of accompanying thrombosis, limb-threatening ischemia. The major causes of these severe thrombocytopenias are heparin-induced thrombocytopenia (HIT), the thrombotic microangiopathies, catastrophic antiphospholipid syndrome, and posttransfusion purpura. Immune thrombocytopenia purpura (ITP) is also a cause of severe thrombocytopenia but is described elsewhere in this issue and is not addressed here. This article covers the basic definitions, pathophysiology, and management strategies for these life-threatening and limb-threatening thrombocytopenias. More detailed discussions of each individual topic can be found in the cited primary literature and reviews.

DISEASE ENTITIES

Heparin-Induced Thrombocytopenia

HIT is divided into 2 major types. Type 1 HIT is benign and self-limited, and is characterized by a mild drop in the platelet count within 2 days of heparin administration that partially or completely self-corrects with continued heparin administration. This form of HIT is due to platelet clumping and is also known to occur in vitro in heparinized specimens.[1] Type 2 HIT, however, is more serious and requires intervention on the

Funding sources: None.

Conflict of interest: None.

[a] Department of Medicine, Rhode Island and The Miriam Hospitals, Alpert Medical School of Brown University, 593 Eddy Street, Providence, RI 02903, USA

[b] Department of Pathology & Laboratory Medicine, Rhode Island and The Miriam Hospitals, Alpert Medical School of Brown University, 593 Eddy Street, Providence, RI 02903, USA

* Corresponding author.

E-mail address: Nathan_Connell@brown.edu

part of the clinician to avoid serious harm to the patient. Type 2 HIT is the result of the formation of antibodies directed against epitopes on the antigen complex of heparin combined with platelet factor 4 (PF4).[2] It is more likely to occur in women, in those receiving unfractionated heparin as opposed to low molecular weight heparin, and in surgical patients as opposed to medical patients.

The diagnosis of HIT requires clinical suspicion and is triggered by a decreasing platelet count in the setting of heparin administration. Patients with HIT classically develop thrombocytopenia 5 to 10 days after initiation of heparin therapy, and they have a drop in platelet count by greater than 50% from their baseline and a nadir between 20 and 100 × 10^9/L. Lesser degrees of platelet drop or a nadir of less than 10 × 10^9/L are uncommon with HIT. The major risk associated with HIT is thrombosis; in retrospective analyses, upwards of 75% of patients with HIT may develop thrombosis. Thrombosis may be the presenting sign leading to the diagnosis of HIT.[3]

Because many of the tests used to diagnose HIT have a long turnaround time (TAT), defined as greater than 24 hours, a clinical prediction model known as the 4 Ts was created in 2006 to assist clinicians in determining the probability of HIT. This model has been prospectively validated.[4]

1. **T**hrombocytopenia: Two points are awarded if the platelet count decrease is greater than 50% and the nadir is 20 × 10^9/L or more. One point is awarded for a drop in platelet count between 30% and 50% or if the nadir is between 10 and 19 × 10^9/L. No points are included for a platelet count decrease less than 30% or nadir of less than 10 × 10^9/L.
2. **T**iming: Two points are awarded if there is clear onset between days 5 and 10 or by day 1 if there is previous heparin exposure in the past 30 days. One point is awarded for a decrease that appears to be between days 5 and 10 but is not entirely clear; if the onset is after day 10 or the decrease is less than 1 day after initiation of heparin administration but the prior heparin exposure was 30 to 100 days before. No points are awarded for platelet count decreases before 4 days without recent heparin exposure.
3. **T**hrombosis: New thrombosis or skin necrosis is awarded 2 points, whereas progressive or recurrent thrombosis is awarded 1 point. No points are awarded for the absence of thrombosis.
4. O**T**her causes for thrombocytopenia: If no other apparent cause can be found, 2 points are awarded. If there is a possible cause, 1 point is awarded and if another definite cause can be determined, no points are awarded in this category.

A composite score is calculated by awarding points in each category and then tabulating the sum. High clinical probability is defined as 6 to 8 points, intermediate clinical probability is 4 to 5 points, and low clinical probability is 3 points or less. Determination of this score allows the consulting hematologist to make recommendations for further workup and management. The calculated score has a high negative predictive value, with only 1.6% of patients with a low clinical probability having clinically significant HIT antibodies in the validation study referenced here. The positive predictive value varied in the validation study depending on the clinical context, including experience of the clinician in applying the score to an individual patient and the frequency of which unfractionated versus low molecular weight heparin is used in an institution.

For patients with a high clinical probability (score 6–8), all heparin products should be discontinued; this should include all heparin flushes and heparin-coated catheters. Thrombosis remains a risk, and patients diagnosed with HIT should be started on a direct thrombin inhibitor (DTI) such as argatroban, bivalirubin, or lepirudin. Argatroban is cleared by the liver while lepirudin and bivalirudin are cleared by the kidney, so the clinician should take liver and kidney disease into account when making treatment decisions.

For patients with an intermediate clinical probability (score 4–5), further diagnostic testing should be conducted to either confirm or exclude the diagnosis. In the interim, all heparin products should be discontinued and a DTI initiated. Two major diagnostic tests commonly in use are a screening enzyme-linked immunosorbent assay (ELISA) to look for antibodies against the heparin-PF4 complex and a functional assay using serotonin release.[5] If the screening ELISA is positive, a confirmatory test should be performed using neutralization with heparin or a more specific immunoglobulin (Ig)G HIT ELISA. If this confirmatory test is also positive, the patient should be considered to have HIT and treatment continued as such. A more specific serotonin release assay (SRA) can be useful, but in practice this is only performed by reference laboratories and may be limited in clinical practice because of a long TAT. A summary of the diagnostic tests for HIT are shown in **Table 1**.[6] The screening ELISA detects antibodies of all isotypes (IgM, IgG, IgA) against the heparin-PF4 complex, but only IgG antibodies are able to activate platelets by binding to the platelet FcγRIIA receptor and cause HIT. **Fig. 1** shows that ELISA optical densities less than 1.0 can be shown to be negative by IgG HIT ELISA in about 50% of samples, thus avoiding the use of a parenteral DTI.

Patients with a low clinical probability (scores $\leq$3) are unlikely to have HIT and, in most cases, heparin can be safely continued. Testing in this context is controversial, but a more specific test such as the IgG HIT ELISA or SRA should be used to prevent a false positive. A caveat is that there should be an ongoing assessment until a firm alternative diagnosis is made. Recalculation of the clinical probability score should be made on a daily basis with diagnostic and therapeutic interventions made as appropriate. Seemingly defying the known pathophysiology, it is possible for HIT to occur in a delayed fashion, sometimes between 9 and 40 days.[7] Clinicians should be aware of this timing difference and consider the diagnosis.

KEY POINTS: DIAGNOSIS AND MANAGEMENT OF HEPARIN-INDUCED THROMBOCYTOPENIA

- Pretest probability is determined using the 4 Ts: degree of Thrombocytopenia, Timing, Thrombosis, and oTher.

- Diagnostic tests include the screening (all-isotype) ELISA to detect a heparin-PF4 complex and the more specific IgG HIT ELISA or SRA.

- Patients considered to have HIT are at high risk for development of thrombosis if continued on heparin, so all heparin administrations should be discontinued and patients started on a DTI.

[Tags: heparin-induced thrombocytopenia, HIT, heparin, platelet-factor 4, PF4, heparin-PF4 complex, serotonin release assay, direct thrombin inhibitor].

Thrombotic Microangiopathies

Disseminated intravascular coagulation

Disseminated intravascular coagulation (DIC) is a process whereby there is an imbalance in the coagulation and fibrinolytic systems of the body, leading to inappropriate thrombin generation. It is the result of an underlying clinical condition such as sepsis, malignancy, or trauma, and determination of the underlying cause is crucial to treatment.[8] As this process continues unregulated, there is a depletion of coagulation factors, leading to bleeding. Formation of thrombi and then uncontrolled bleeding

Table 1	
Diagnostic tests for heparin-induced thrombocytopenia	
Test	**Characteristics**
HIT ELISA	Detects immunoglobulins that bind to the heparin-PF4 complex
	These immunoglobulins may be IgG, IgA, or IgM
	IgG is the antibody that clinically causes HIT, and a more specific IgG HIT ELISA can avoid false positives
	Is more sensitive but less specific than the SRA
SRA	Patient plasma is incubated with 2 concentrations of heparin and platelets from selected normal healthy humans. If the HIT antibody is present, the platelets are activated at the lower heparin concentration (but not the higher) and release serotonin
	Considered the gold standard test for HIT

Abbreviations: ELISA, enzyme-linked immunosorbent assay; HIT, heparin-induced thrombocytopenia; Ig, immunoglobulin; PF4, platelet factor 4; SRA, serotonin release assay.

leads to end-organ damage. Thrombocytopenia is common in acute DIC and is associated with characteristic changes in clotting factors (**Fig. 2**). Note the extremely low fibrinogen, factor VIII:C, and factor V, which required more than 24 hours to return to normal.

The platelet count in acute DIC is commonly less than 100×10^9/L and is associated with microangiopathic changes (ie, schistocytes) seen on the peripheral blood smear. Activation of the coagulation system can be determined with widely available coagulation tests, such as decreased levels of fibrinogen, and by elevation of cross-linked fibrin degradation products, such as the D-dimer.

The most important aspect in the treatment of DIC is the identification and reversal of the underlying cause. The acute DIC process will continue until this occurs even in the setting of aggressive supportive care. Patients with a fibrinogen count of less than 150 mg/dL should have cryoprecipitate transfused because this will provide fibrinogen. There are no good data to support one serum fibrinogen target level in preference to another, and clinical scenarios should guide transfusion practice. If the prothrombin time (PT) or activated partial thromboplastin time (aPTT) is prolonged greater than 1.5 times the normal limit, fresh frozen plasma (FFP) can be transfused to

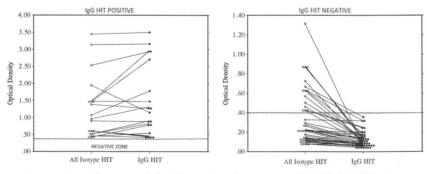

Fig. 1. Comparison of enzyme-linked immunosorbent assays (ELISAs) for all-isotype versus IgG heparin-induced thrombocytopenia (HIT). (*Left*) The optical density for the all-isotype ELISA generally correlates with the optical density for the IgG if the IgG is positive. (*Right*) Whereas the ELISA for all isotypes may be positive, not all are positive for IgG. HIT is only clinically apparent in patients with IgG antibodies (ie, optical density >0.4).

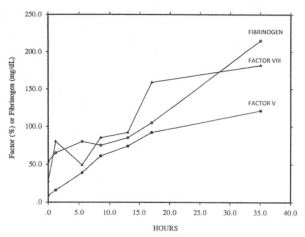

Fig. 2. Levels of fibrinogen, factor VIII, and factor V in a patient with disseminated intravascular coagulation secondary to an ABO-incompatible red cell transfusion. Profound hypofibrinogenemia is present as well as severe decreases in factors V and VIII:C; these normalize spontaneously within 24 hours.

replete coagulation factors. Platelets can be transfused at thresholds of 20 × 10⁹/L and red blood cells transfused to manage anemia. These criteria for blood-component transfusion are arbitrary and are intended as a guideline rather than an evidence-based approach. Clinical judgment should be used in conjunction with these laboratory tests.

Some work has been done to evaluate use of interventions such as heparin, recombinant activated protein C, thrombomodulin, tissue factor pathway inhibitor, or activated factor VII in the treatment of DIC.[9,10] It should be noted, however, that there are no data to support use of these products in the pregnant patient.[11] For women who are pregnant, standard of care remains transfusion of blood components as noted earlier.

KEY POINTS: DIAGNOSIS AND MANAGEMENT OF DISSEMINATED INTRAVASCULAR COAGULATION

- DIC is the result of an imbalance in coagulation and fibrinolysis and has several causes.
- Treatment involves supportive care with blood components until the underlying cause can be identified and reversed.

[Tags: disseminated intravascular coagulation, DIC, fresh frozen plasma, FFP, cryoprecipitate, schistocytes, thrombin, thrombosis, fibrin, fibrinolysis].

Thrombotic thrombocytopenic purpura

Thrombotic thrombocytopenic purpura (TTP) is the result of a deficiency or inactivation of ADAMTS13, a metalloproteinase that cleaves large multimers of Von Willebrand factor (VWF).[12] Its deficiency leads to the presence of abnormal ultrahigh molecular weight VWF, which causes platelets to aggregate in small arterioles with resulting end-organ ischemia. A consumptive severe thrombocytopenia results, not uncommonly with a platelet count of less than 10 × 10⁹/L.

Patients often present with varying degrees of neurologic dysfunction, and on physical examination may have fever and evidence of petechiae or purpura. On laboratory evaluation there is severe thrombocytopenia, and hemolytic anemia accompanied by extreme elevations in lactate dehydrogenase (LDH). As seen in **Fig. 3**, examination of the peripheral blood smear shows thrombocytopenia along with schistocytes, demonstrating a microangiopathic process. One review showed that the full pentad of microangiopathic hemolytic anemia, fever, thrombocytopenia, renal failure, and neurologic dysfunction is rare in TTP, found in only 3% of patients at presentation.[13] Activity of ADAMTS13 can be determined and is often less than 5%, but given the TAT for this test, it is of limited clinical utility at this stage in the assessment.

While most cases of TTP are idiopathic, some are drug-associated whereas others occur in the setting of infection, pregnancy, or concurrent autoimmune disorders. In a review of the Oklahoma TTP-HUS registry, severe ADAMTS13 deficiency was found more often in women, African Americans, and those who were obese.[14]

Treatment of TTP involves therapeutic plasma exchange (TPE) with either FFP, plasma frozen within 24 hours of phlebotomy (FP24), or cryoreduced plasma as the exchange fluid. This therapy should be initiated as early as possible, but in all cases within 24 hours of the diagnosis. Plasma exchange should continue daily until the platelet count and LDH return to the normal reference interval. The benefit of plasma exchange over plasma infusion was demonstrated in 2 randomized trials showing a 6-month survival of 78% with plasma exchange and only 50% with plasma infusion.[15] Patients diagnosed at centers without TPE capabilities should be transferred to centers where this can be accomplished in a timely manner. If there is any delay, FFP infusion may be initiated to temporarily begin treatment until TPE can be initiated.[16] The role of steroids, antiplatelet agents, and immunomodulatory therapies such as rituximab (Rituxan)[17] is not clear at this point, although they are commonly used in patients who appear refractory to TPE. These agents may be best used in combination with TPE for particular clinical scenarios, but should not be used in place of TPE until more data are available.[18]

KEY POINTS: DIAGNOSIS AND MANAGEMENT OF THROMBOTIC THROMBOCYTOPENIC PURPURA

- TTP is due to a deficiency of ADAMTS13, which is responsible for cleaving of the large multimers of VWF.
- Classically described as a pentad of thrombocytopenia, microangiopathic hemolytic anemia, renal dysfunction, neurologic symptoms, and fever, many cases do not include all 5 features and severe renal failure is not a feature.
- Treatment involves TPE, and immunosuppressive agents may be useful adjuncts.

[Tags: thrombotic thrombocytopenic purpura, TTP, ADAMTS13, fresh frozen plasma, FFP, cryoprecipitate, schistocytes, plasma exchange, Von Willebrand factor, VWF].

Hemolytic uremic syndrome

Often difficult to differentiate from TTP, the hemolytic uremic syndrome (HUS) also presents with thrombocytopenia and hemolytic anemia, with renal failure as a more prominent clinical feature. HUS can be divided into 2 major clinical forms, classic HUS and atypical HUS, differentiated by their pathophysiology.

Classic HUS results from an infection with *Escherichia coli*, and there is release of a shigalike toxin. This toxin can lead to endothelial dysfunction, neutrophil

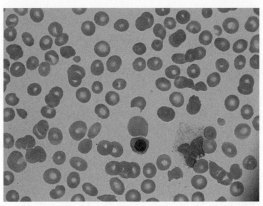

Fig. 3. Peripheral blood smear of a patient with thrombotic thrombocytopenic purpura. Numerous schistocytes are present as well as a nucleated red blood cell and polychromatophilic cells, indicating bone marrow response to the hemolytic anemia.

accumulation, and cytokine release. The endothelial dysfunction does not allow ADAMTS13 to break down the ultralarge multimers of VWF. Glycolipid Gb3 is expressed on the surface of renal endothelial cells and has a particular binding preference for the circulating shigalike toxin.[19] Patients often have a preceding diarrheal illness, which may worsen if treated with antibiotics.

By contrast, patients with atypical HUS (aHUS) typically do not have diarrhea or evidence of *E coli* infection, and aHUS is thought to be the result of mutations in complement proteins, either plasma or cell bound, such as C3, factor H, factor I, or membrane cofactor protein.

Treatment of classic HUS is the same as that for TTP, and involves TPE. By contrast, atypical HUS patients do not generally respond to plasma exchange, and this treatment failure provides an indication that the patient has deficiency of the complement protein inhibitors. Eculizumab (Soliris), a monoclonal antibody to C5, has been shown to block the terminal complement cascade and to be effective in the treatment of aHUS.[20] The use of eculizumab has been associated with life-threatening meningococcal infections, and patients should be monitored carefully and vaccinated in all cases.[21]

KEY POINTS: DIAGNOSIS AND MANAGEMENT OF THE HEMOLYTIC UREMIC SYNDROME

- Classic HUS is the result of a shigalike toxin produced by *E coli* entering the blood stream and inactivating ADAMTS13.
- aHUS is the result of defects in the complement protein inhibitors, factor H, membrane cofactor protein (CD46), and factor I.
- Treatment is generally supportive and may need to include dialysis. Antibiotics should be avoided in classic HUS, as this may induce toxin formation and worsen clinical status.
- Some data support the use of the anti-C5 monoclonal antibody eculizumab in the treatment of aHUS.

[Tags: hemolytic uremic syndrome, HUS, *Escherichia coli*, shigalike toxin, ADAMTS13, atypical hemolytic uremic syndrome, factor H, membrane cofactor protein, CD46, factor I, eculizumab].

Preeclampsia/HELLP

For further discussion on preeclampsia/HELLP the reader is referred to the article "Special Hematologic Issues in the Pregnant Patient" by Rizack and Rosene-Montella elsewhere in this issue.

Thrombocytopenia is common in pregnancy (incidence 5%–7%) and is most commonly due to incidental (gestational) thrombocytopenia; more severe forms are caused by ITP, preeclampsia, eclampsia, and the other thrombotic microangiopathies including TTP-HUS.

The HELLP syndrome is an acronym for **H**emolysis, **E**levated **L**iver enzymes, and **L**ow **P**latelet count. The relationship between HELLP and preeclampsia is not completely understood, and there may be overlap in many patients. Its highest incidence is in the third trimester or early puerperium, but it may occur at other times during the pregnancy.

The peripheral blood smear shows schistocytes, indicating a microangiopathic hemolytic anemia, and laboratory markers demonstrate elevated LDH along with an unconjugated hyperbilirubinemia and decreased haptoglobin. The platelet count is often less than 100×10^9/L.

Differentiating between HELLP and TTP-HUS may be difficult for the consulting hematologist, but doing so is important because of differences in treatment. Timing is important, with TTP occurring more commonly in the first and second trimester and HELLP in the third trimester. Preeclampsia and HELLP do not occur before 20 weeks' gestation. The peripheral blood smear may be helpful, as the percentage of schistocytes in HELLP is often less than 1% and higher in TTP.[22] ADAMTS13 activity will differentiate TTP from HELLP because activity is less than 5% in TTP. As mentioned previously, the long TAT for this test means that this is more useful in confirming the diagnosis at a later time.

Thrombocytopenia in HELLP syndrome should be managed in a coordinated fashion with the obstetrician and anesthesiologist. In addition to delivery of the fetus, if delivery can be performed safely, platelet transfusion is indicated if there is evidence of maternal bleeding or if the platelet count is less than 20×10^9/L. Delivery by cesarean section or use of neuraxial anesthesia may necessitate higher platelet counts such as 50 to 80×10^9/L for safety, although the threshold platelet count for safe delivery is not well established.

KEY POINTS: DIAGNOSIS AND MANAGEMENT OF HELLP

- HELLP syndrome stands for Hemolytic anemia, Elevated Liver enzymes, and Low Platelet count.
- HELLP syndrome may be difficult to differentiate from TTP-HUS, and the key to distinguishing the two is a combination of timing and other laboratory parameters.
- Along with delivery of the fetus, platelet transfusion may be necessary if there is evidence of maternal bleeding or severely low platelet counts.

[Tags: HELLP, preeclampsia, TTP, pregnancy].

Malignant hypertension

Extremely high blood pressure can lead to vascular endothelial injury, resulting in activation of coagulation, especially in the microvasculature. Similar to all thrombotic microangiopathies, the result is hemolysis along with the consumption of platelets.[23] Platelet transfusion is rarely indicated, as the degree of thrombocytopenia is not associated with spontaneous hemorrhage. Both the hemolytic anemia and thrombocytopenia resolve with treatment of the hypertensive emergency.

KEY POINTS: DIAGNOSIS AND MANAGEMENT OF MALIGNANT HYPERTENSION

- Malignant hypertension may present with a microangiopathic hemolytic anemia and associated thrombocytopenia.
- Treatment of the hypertensive crisis generally results in reversal of the hematologic changes.

[Tags: hypertension, malignant hypertension, hypertensive crisis, hypertensive emergency].

Catastrophic antiphospholipid-antibody syndrome

Thrombocytopenia is just one of many hematologic manifestations of the antiphospholipid-antibody syndrome (APS), and generally is mild. Affected patients may also present with thrombosis, and a consumptive process may initially be blamed for the thrombocytopenia. The peripheral blood smear may demonstrate schistocytes and may be difficult to distinguish from TTP. Platelet counts may be in the range of 50 to 140 × 10^9/L.

Diagnosis of the APS requires both a clinical event (either thrombosis or pregnancy loss) and laboratory evidence of an antiphospholipid antibody. The laboratory tests can be either antigen tests, such as for anticardiolipin antibodies and anti-β2 GP1, or a functional test such a lupus anticoagulant test. Confirmation of these antibodies must be performed by repeat testing at least 12 weeks apart, as it is possible to have a falsely reactive antibody test shortly after thrombosis.[24]

The clinical presentation of the APS can be varied, ranging from a single thrombotic event to life-threatening thrombosis and stroke. A magnetic resonance image of the brain of a patient with the catastrophic antiphospholipid-antibody syndrome secondary to systemic lupus erythematosus is shown in **Fig. 4**.

Even with thrombocytopenia, patients are at risk for thrombotic events. Treatment of the antiphospholipid-antibody syndrome is similar to the treatment of other thrombotic events. Patients should be started on heparin therapy and then transitioned to warfarin for long-term therapy.[25] If pregnant, patients should be maintained on heparin, as warfarin (Coumadin; Jantoven) is contraindicated in early pregnancy. Newer anticoagulants such as the oral DTIs or oral factor Xa inhibitors may play a role in future therapy, but there are currently no data to support their use outside of a clinical trial.

KEY POINTS: DIAGNOSIS AND MANAGEMENT OF THE CATASTROPHIC ANTIPHOSPHOLIPID SYNDROME

- Diagnosis of the antiphospholipid-antibody syndrome requires both a clinical event (either vascular or loss of pregnancy) and presence of laboratory-confirmed antiphospholipid antibodies.
- Treatment of APS involves heparin therapy initially with transition to warfarin for long-term anticoagulation.

[Tags: antiphospholipid antibody, catastrophic antiphospholipid syndrome, CAS, systemic lupus erythematosus, anticoagulation, anticardiolipin, lupus anticoagulant].

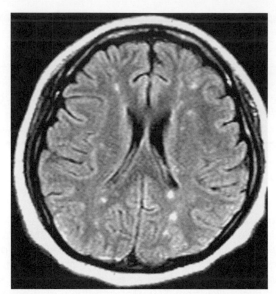

Fig. 4. Magnetic resonance image of the brain of an 18-year-old female patient with the catastrophic antiphospholipid syndrome secondary to systemic lupus erythematosus (SLE). The patient presented with ataxia and weakness progressing to altered mental status. Numerous punctate infarcts were noted in the cerebral hemispheres bilaterally. Neurologic symptoms improved with anticoagulation and immunosuppression to treat her SLE.

Posttransfusion Purpura

On rare occasions patients develop severe thrombocytopenia after transfusion of blood components, most commonly red blood cells. Patients with posttransfusion purpura (PTP) develop antibodies against antigens located on one of the human

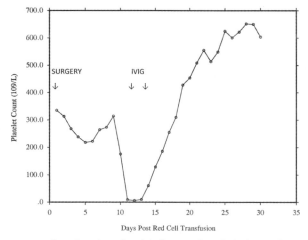

Fig. 5. Platelet counts after 4 units of red cells transfused during colorectal surgery. The initial perioperative decrease in the platelet count is attributable to the dilution effect of red cell transfusion and other crystalloids. On day 10, there was a precipitous drop in platelet count consistent with posttransfusion purpura. Intravenous immunoglobulin (IVIG) was administered twice with a rapid increase in platelet count. Note the rebound thrombocytosis between days 20 and 35 after surgery.

Table 2
Comparison of the key clinical and laboratory features of various life-threatening thrombocytopenias

Entity	Key Clinical Features	Platelet Count	Other Laboratory Tests	Treatment
Heparin-induced thrombocytopenia (HIT)	Antecedent heparin exposure; clinical thrombosis may be present	Usually 20–100 × 10^9/L	ELISAs for antibodies against PF4-heparin complex; serotonin release assay	Cessation of all heparin products; prompt initiation of a direct thrombin inhibitor if clinically suspected
Thrombotic thrombocytopenic purpura (TTP)/hemolytic uremic syndrome (HUS)	Fever, neurologic changes, hemolytic anemia, renal failure	Often <10 × 10^9/L	ADAMTS13; factor I, factor H, membrane cofactor protein for atypical HUS	Therapeutic plasma exchange for TTP; eculizumab for atypical HUS
Disseminated intravascular coagulation	Both thrombosis and bleeding	Variable, but rarely <10 × 10^9/L	Prolonged PT and aPTT, decreased fibrinogen	Supportive care and treatment of underlying cause
Posttransfusion purpura	Within 5–10 days of transfusion	Often <10 × 10^9/L	Testing for platelet-specific alloantibodies	Prompt treatment with IVIG
Catastrophic antiphospholipid syndrome (CAS)	Thrombosis, may be secondary to other conditions	Generally 50–100 × 10^9/L	Prolonged aPTT; anticardiolipin antibodies, lupus anticoagulant, anti-β2 GP1	Anticoagulation; treatment of underlying disorder (ie, immunosuppressants) if secondary CAS
Immune thrombocytopenic purpura	Petechiae or purpura, antecedent viral illness, may be clinically isolated	Often <10 × 10^9/L	Diagnosis of exclusion (need to evaluate for HIV and HCV and rule out other causes of thrombocytopenia)	Steroids, rituximab, eltrombopag, romiplostim, splenectomy

Abbreviations: aPTT, activated partial thromboplastin time; HCV, hepatitis C virus; HIV, human immunodeficiency virus; IVIG, intravenous immunoglobulin; PT, prothrombin time.

platelet antigen systems (HPA), most commonly against HPA-1a. The typical history is of a red cell transfusion approximately 10 days before the (abrupt) onset of thrombocytopenia. The condition is frequently misdiagnosed as acute ITP. PTP can be confirmed by measurement of platelet alloantibodies to any of the aforementioned antigens, but these results typically are only available days after initial, often emergency room, presentation. In the case of anti–HPA-1a, the patients are phenotypically homozygous for HPA-1b and nearly always Class II DR52 positive. The mechanism of destruction of platelets is unclear because they do not display the antigen to which the antibody develops.

The preferred treatment is the infusion of intravenous immunoglobulin (IVIG) at a dose of 400 to 500 mg/kg body weight per day for 5 days. If the patient can tolerate higher-volume transfusion, 1 g/kg daily for 2 days can be used as alternative dosing.[26] Plasma exchange as well as corticosteroids have been used in the past, but the role for either with the availability of IVIG is questionable. **Fig. 5** illustrates the precipitous drop in the platelet count after a red cell transfusion 10 days previously and the rapid recovery (12–36 hours) after treatment with IVIG.

KEY POINTS: DIAGNOSIS AND MANAGEMENT OF POSTTRANSFUSION PURPURA

- PTP is a rare condition mainly affecting women. It may be difficult to distinguish from ITP.
- Treatment is prompt initiation of IVIG.

[Tags: posttransfusion purpura, transfusion, red cell transfusion, intravenous immunoglobulin, IVIG, HPA-1a].

SUMMARY

Each of the described clinical entities overlaps and can be present with severe thrombocytopenia, often but not always with a platelet count of less than 10×10^9/L. The consulting hematologist needs to be aware of the subtle differences between these entities, as treatment strategies differ and early diagnosis and intervention can greatly reduce the associated morbidity and mortality. A summary of the key clinical features, laboratory findings, laboratory tests, and treatment options is summarized in **Table 2**. Clinical clues, such as antecedent events provided in the history or review of the platelet count over time, can help provide a working diagnosis, with subsequent confirmation by laboratory data.

REFERENCES

1. Sweeney JD, Holme S, Heaton WA, et al. Pseudothrombocytopenia in platelet-pheresis donors. Transfusion 1995;35(1):46–9.
2. Rauova L, Zhai L, Kowalska MA, et al. Role of platelet surface PF4 antigenic complexes in heparin-induced thrombocytopenia pathogenesis: diagnostic and therapeutic implications. Blood 2006;107(6):2346–53.
3. Warkentin TE, Kelton JG. A 14-year study of heparin-induced thrombocytopenia. Am J Med 1996;101(5):502–7.
4. Lo GK, Juhl D, Warkentin TE, et al. Evaluation of pretest clinical score (4 T's) for the diagnosis of heparin-induced thrombocytopenia in two clinical settings. J Thromb Haemost 2006;4(4):759–65.

5. Napolitano LM, Warkentin TE, Almahameed A, et al. Heparin-induced thrombocytopenia in the critical care setting: diagnosis and management. Crit Care Med 2006;34(12):2898–911.
6. Prechel M, Walenga JM. The laboratory diagnosis and clinical management of patients with heparin-induced thrombocytopenia: an update. Semin Thromb Hemost 2008;34(1):86–96.
7. Rice L, Attisha WK, Drexler A, et al. Delayed-onset heparin-induced thrombocytopenia. Ann Intern Med 2002;136(3):210–5.
8. Kaneko T, Wada H. Diagnostic criteria and laboratory tests for disseminated intravascular coagulation. J Clin Exp Hematop 2011;51(2):67–76.
9. Kawano N, Yoshida S, Ono N, et al. Clinical features and outcomes of 35 disseminated intravascular coagulation cases treated with recombinant human soluble thrombomodulin at a single institution. J Clin Exp Hematop 2011;51(2):101–7.
10. Levi M, de Jonge E, van der Poll T. New treatment strategies for disseminated intravascular coagulation based on current understanding of the pathophysiology. Ann Med 2004;36(1):41–9.
11. Castaldo DJ, Maurice DV. Shell gland adenosine triphosphatase in hens producing strong and weak egg shells. Br Poult Sci 1990;31(1):225–9.
12. Zhou Z, Nguyen TC, Guchhait P, et al. Von Willebrand factor, ADAMTS-13, and thrombotic thrombocytopenic purpura. Semin Thromb Hemost 2010;36(1):71–81.
13. George JN. How I treat patients with thrombotic thrombocytopenic purpura: 2010. Blood 2010;116(20):4060–9.
14. Vesely SK, George JN, Lammle B, et al. ADAMTS13 activity in thrombotic thrombocytopenic purpura-hemolytic uremic syndrome: relation to presenting features and clinical outcomes in a prospective cohort of 142 patients. Blood 2003;102(1):60–8.
15. Rock GA, Shumak KH, Buskard NA, et al. Comparison of plasma exchange with plasma infusion in the treatment of thrombotic thrombocytopenic purpura. Canadian Apheresis Study Group. N Engl J Med 1991;325(6):393–7.
16. Coppo P, Bussel A, Charrier S, et al. High-dose plasma infusion versus plasma exchange as early treatment of thrombotic thrombocytopenic purpura/hemolytic-uremic syndrome. Medicine 2003;82(1):27–38.
17. Scully M, McDonald V, Cavenagh J, et al. A phase 2 study of the safety and efficacy of rituximab with plasma exchange in acute acquired thrombotic thrombocytopenic purpura. Blood 2011;118(7):1746–53.
18. Noris P, Balduini CL. Investigational drugs in thrombotic thrombocytopenic purpura. Expert Opin Investig Drugs 2011;20(8):1087–98.
19. Obrig TG, Louise CB, Lingwood CA, et al. Endothelial heterogeneity in Shiga toxin receptors and responses. J Biol Chem 1993;268(21):15484–8.
20. Kose O, Zimmerhackl LB, Jungraithmayr T, et al. New treatment options for atypical hemolytic uremic syndrome with the complement inhibitor eculizumab. Semin Thromb Hemost 2010;36(6):669–72.
21. Brodsky RA, Young NS, Antonioli E, et al. Multicenter phase 3 study of the complement inhibitor eculizumab for the treatment of patients with paroxysmal nocturnal hemoglobinuria. Blood 2008;111(4):1840–7.
22. Stella CL, Dacus J, Guzman E, et al. The diagnostic dilemma of thrombotic thrombocytopenic purpura/hemolytic uremic syndrome in the obstetric triage and emergency department: lessons from 4 tertiary hospitals. Am J Obstet Gynecol 2009;200(4):381.e1–6.
23. Zhang B, Xing C, Yu X, et al. Renal thrombotic microangiopathies induced by severe hypertension. Hypertens Res 2008;31(3):479–83.

24. Erkan D, Espinosa G, Cervera R. Catastrophic antiphospholipid syndrome: updated diagnostic algorithms. Autoimmun Rev 2010;10(2):74–9.
25. Dentali F, Crowther M. Antiphospholipid antibodies in critical illness. Crit Care Med 2010;38(Suppl 2):S51–6.
26. Mueller-Eckhardt C, Kiefel V. High-dose IgG for post-transfusion purpura-revisited. Blut 1988;57(4):163–7.

Does My Patient with a Serum Monoclonal Spike have Multiple Myeloma?

Giada Bianchi, MD[a], Irene M. Ghobrial, MD[b],*

KEYWORDS

- Monoclonal spike • MGUS • Multiple myeloma • Progression

EPIDEMIOLOGY OF MONOCLONAL GAMMOPATHY OF UNDETERMINED SIGNIFICANCE

The nomenclature monoclonal gammopathy of undetermined significance (MGUS) was introduced by Kyle[1] in 1978, and, since then, the fundamental characteristics, natural history, and diagnostic criteria of this condition have been extensively revised. According to the most current International Myeloma Working Group consensus, MGUS is defined by the simultaneous presence of 3 criteria: (1) a monoclonal spike (M spike) of less than 3 g/dL on serum protein electrophoresis (SPEP), (2) bone marrow infiltration by monoclonal malignant plasma cells (PCs) of less than 10%, and (3) the absence of any end-organ damage related to multiple myeloma (MM), the so-called CRAB (hypercalcemia, renal failure, anemia, and bone lesions) criteria (**Table 1**).[2] Other diseases that can present with an M spike, such as chronic lymphocytic leukemia, B-cell and T-cell lymphomas, chronic myeloid leukemia, and other PC dyscrasias (amyloid light chain [AL] amyloidosis, Waldenström macroglobulinemia [WM], and heavy chain disease) should also be excluded before making a diagnosis of MGUS. Epidemiologic studies in the Olmsted County have estimated that MGUS affects around 3% of individuals aged 50 years or more, with prevalence increasing with age.[3] These data refer to a cohort heavily skewed toward whites, and the 3% figure does not reflect the 2- to 3-fold increased incidence of MGUS in African Americans and blacks from Africa or the decreased incidence in Asians and Mexicans in comparison with the white population.[4–8] A familial predisposition, with increased risk of MGUS in first-degree relatives of patients with MGUS, has also been observed.[9] MGUS carries a 1%-per-year unremitting, lifelong risk of transformation to hematologic cancer, mainly MM. Clinical research has focused on identifying predictive

[a] Department of Internal Medicine, Mayo Clinic, 200 First Street SW, Rochester, MN 55905, USA
[b] Department of Medical Oncology, Dana-Farber Cancer Institute, Harvard Medical School, 450 Brookline Avenue, Boston, MA 02115, USA
* Corresponding author.
E-mail address: Irene_Ghobrial@DFCI.HARVARD.EDU

Hematol Oncol Clin N Am 26 (2012) 383–393
doi:10.1016/j.hoc.2012.02.009
0889-8588/12/$ – see front matter © 2012 Elsevier Inc. All rights reserved.

Table 1
The most recent diagnostic criteria for PC dyscrasia according to the International Myeloma Working Group

Criteria	M Spike		BM		CRAB[a]	Comments
MGUS	<3 g/dL	AND	<10%	AND	Absent	Diagnosis requires exclusion of other lymphoproliferative diseases
SMM	≥3 g/dL	OR	≥10%	AND	Absent	—
MM	Any concentration on SPEP/UPEP or abnormal FLC ratio	AND	Any percentage or presence of plasmacytoma	AND	Present	Truly nonsecretory MM is an exception because an M spike cannot be identified on SPEP, UPEP, or FLC
PC Leukemia[b]	Absent/present	AND	Absent/present	AND	Absent/present	Defined by the presence of peripheral blood circulating clonal PC >2 × 10⁹/L or 20% of leukocytes
Solitary Plasmacytoma	Absent[c]	AND	Absent	AND	Absent	Defined as a single site of abnormal PC proliferation in the bone (osseous) or soft tissue (extraosseous)

Abbreviations: BM, bone marrow invasion by monoclonal malignant PCs; FLC, free light chain; SMM, smoldering MM; UPEP, urine protein electrophoresis.

[a] Hypercalcemia is defined as a total serum calcium level higher than 11.5 mg/dL; renal insufficiency is defined by a serum creatinine level exceeding 2 mg/dL or an estimated glomerular filtration rate less than 40 mL/min; anemia is defined by a hemoglobin level less than 10 g/dL or less than 2 g/dL the normal reference values; bone lesions include lytic lesions, pathologic fractures, or severely osteopenic bone disease. Hyperviscosity, recurrent infections related to hypogammaglobulinemia, and amyloidosis also represent evidence of end-organ damage.

[b] PC leukemia is further classified as primary, when occurring de novo, or secondary, when it represents the leukemic phase of MM.

[c] A small M spike can occasionally be seen.

factors of progression and risk stratification models to provide appropriate patient counseling and guide follow-up.[10–12]

DIAGNOSIS AND FOLLOW-UP OF PATIENTS WITH MONCLONAL GAMMOPATHY OF UNDETERMINED SIGNIFICANCE (MGUS)

In most instances, MGUS is an incidental diagnosis on blood work performed to investigate a variety of signs and symptoms.[13] The diagnosis is usually made by general practitioners in the ambulatory setting while evaluating complaints that are rather nonspecific, such as fatigue, lack of stamina, or forgetfulness, or symptoms and signs suggestive of MM or amyloidosis, such as back or bone pain, abnormal liver function test results, or neuropathy. The evidence of an M spike on SPEP and/or an abnormal immunofixation (IF) is suggestive of PC dyscrasia, although these findings can occur with other diseases.[14] In the absence of clinical or diagnostic findings suggestive of MM, WM, amyloidosis, or other myeloid or lymphoid neoplasia, an M spike smaller than 3 g/dL on SPEP is pathognomonic of MGUS. The CRAB criteria need to be excluded or, when present, explained by another condition (ie, hypercalcemia secondary to primary hyperparathyroidism, renal failure secondary to diabetic or hypertensive nephropathy, iron deficiency anemia in chronic gastrointestinal [GI] losses).[13] Given its prognostic value, free light chain (FLC) assay is recommended in patients newly diagnosed with MGUS.[11] Bone survey and/or bone marrow aspiration and biopsy are not a mandatory part of the workup of patients with MGUS in the absence of clinical presentations suspicious for active MM or amyloidosis (excruciating or new unremitting bone pain, neurologic symptoms, heart failure) or abnormal laboratory findings. Fat aspiration to exclude amyloidosis should only be performed when clinically indicated (ie, evidence of unexplained liver, heart, peripheral nerve, or GI tract abnormalities).[15]

Although the risk of progression to MM or a related malignancy (WM, amyloidosis) in patients with MGUS is small, it is unremitting and lifelong. In the most updated consensus, the International Myeloma Working Group recommends a repeated SPEP for patients with newly diagnosed MGUS at 6-month follow-up.[2] If the M spike proves stable, complete blood cell counts, kidney function tests, determination of serum calcium levels, and SPEP should be performed yearly in patients with high-risk features (see next section) in an attempt to promptly identify transformation to MM and avoid complications.[16] If clinical conditions are stable, patients with low-risk MGUS could tentatively be assessed with laboratory studies every 2 to 3 years.[2] Patients should be informed to pay special attention to new-onset bone pain, progressive fatigue, or progressive confusion and promptly seek medical attention if such conditions arise. If there is suspicion of interim progression to symptomatic MM, a detailed history taking and complete physical examination should be performed and diagnostic studies, as deemed appropriate, should be recommended to exclude evolution to active disease.

RISK FACTORS FOR PROGRESSION AND STRATIFICATION MODELS FOR PATIENTS WITH MONCLONAL GAMMOPATHY OF UNDETERMINED SIGNIFICANCE (MGUS)

Retrospective epidemiologic studies showed non-IgG immunoglobulin subtypes (IgA, IgD, or IgM), monoclonal component levels of 1.5 g/dL or more, and an abnormal FLC ratio (κ:λ ratio <0.26 or >1.65) to be risk factors for the progression of MGUS to MM.[11]

The Mayo Clinic group has proposed a risk model on the basis of these parameters; patients presenting with all 3 risk factors had a 58% risk of MGUS progression to MM over a period of 20 years. This likelihood was reduced to 37%, 21%, and 5% in patients with MGUS presenting with 2, 1, or no risk factors, respectively.[11]

The Spanish group has proposed a second risk progression model based on the preponderance of aberrant monoclonal PCs in the bone marrow aspirate, evaluated by multiparametric flow cytometry.[12] A percentage of aberrant PCs equal to or exceeding 95% of the total bone marrow PC population and the presence of DNA aneuploidy were established as risk factors for progression to symptomatic MM. Patients with MGUS presenting with both risk factors carried a 46% risk of progression at 5 years versus 10% when only 1 risk factor was present and 2% when both risk factors were absent.

Two recent prospective studies performed by Weiss and colleagues[17] and Landgren and colleagues[18] provided useful information on the natural history of MGUS and outlined the challenges related to predicting progression to MM in the clinical setting. Both studies showed that MM is (almost) inevitably preceded by MGUS. In the study by Landgren and colleagues,[18] only half of the patients whose MGUS progressed to MM presented with a yearly progressive rise in the M spike, whereas the other half had a relatively stable M spike until MM diagnosis, making a rising M spike only a partially reliable marker of disease transformation.

EPIDEMIOLOGY AND DIAGNOSTIC CRITERIA FOR SMOLDERING MULTIPLE MYELOMA (SMM), MULTIPLE MYELOMA (MM), AND PLASMA CELL (PC) DYSCRASIA VARIANTS

MM is further classified as smoldering MM (SMM) and active MM (referred simply as MM from now on). The former is a precancerous condition diagnosed by the presence of an M spike of 3 g/dL or higher and/or a bone marrow invasion by malignant PCs of 10% or more in the absence of end-organ damage (CRAB, see **Table 1**).[2,19] Unlike MGUS, patients with SMM have a risk of progression to active MM or related PC dyscrasia of 10% per year in the first 5 years, 3% per year in the following 5 years, and 1% per year thereafter, with a cumulative probability of progression of more than 70% at 15 years.[20] Bone marrow involvement by MM cells of 10% or more, M spike equal to or greater than 3 g/dL, and an abnormal FLC ratio ($\kappa{:}\lambda \leq 0.125$ or ≥ 8) have been identified as risk factors for progression to active disease.[21] Current guidelines recommend close observation and monitoring with no active treatment of patients with SMM.[22] Yet, the paradigm of PC dyscrasia is evolving, with the timing of active therapy for patients with high-risk SMM being recently questioned and early treatment being advocated, in an attempt to slow disease progression and possibly prolong survival.[23,24]

Three criteria need to be satisfied to diagnose MM: (1) bone marrow invasion by monoclonal PCs or evidence of a plasmacytoma, (2) presence of an M spike on SPEP or urine protein electrophoresis (UPEP) or an abnormal FLC ratio, and (3) evidence of end-organ damage related to the PC clone (any of the CRAB criteria or hyperviscosity, amyloidosis, or recurrent infections) (see **Table 1**).[2] True nonsecretory MM, which represents around 3% of all MM, is an exception to these criteria because an M spike is not identifiable on either SPEP or UPEP with IF.[2,25,26] True solitary plasmacytoma is a variant within PC dyscrasia and occurs in around 3% to 5% of cases.[2,27] It is characterized by a single area of monoclonal PC proliferation either within the bone (osseous plasmacytoma) or in the soft tissues (extraosseous plasmacytoma), tipically of the upper respiratory or GI tract, in the absence of systemic disease and bone marrow involvement.[15] These patients can occasionally present with a small monoclonal component, but generally an M spike cannot be identified on SPEP or UPEP. By definition, in solitary plasmacytoma, CRAB features must not be diagnosed, with the exception of the single plasmacytoma-related lytic lesion for osseous plasmacytoma (see **Table 1**).[15,27] PC leukemia is defined by the presence of peripheral blood–circulating PCs exceeding 2×10^9 per liter or 20% of leukocytes and can be either primary (occurring de novo) or secondary (the leukemic transformation of a preexisting MM) (see **Table 1**).[2] Around 60% of PC leukemia cases are primary.[16,28]

In the Western world, MM accounts for more than 10% of hematologic malignancies and 2% of annual cancer-related deaths. According to the American Cancer Society, almost 22,000 new cases of MM and 10,700 MM-related deaths are expected for 2012.[29] Although the past decade has witnessed a remarkable improvement in prognosis, mostly related to the introduction of novel chemotherapy agents such as thalidomide, lenalidomide, and bortezomib, MM remains incurable and the current 5-year relative survival rate is estimated to be around 40%.[29]

CLINICAL PRESENTATION OF MULTIPLE MYELOMA (MM)

The clinical presentation of patients with MM can be explained by abnormal proliferation of the malignant clone within the bone marrow and/or direct pathogenic effect of monoclonal immunoglobulin or FLC secreted by the PC clone (**Table 2**). The former leads to suppression of normal hematopoiesis and immunoparesis and accounts for fatigue secondary to anemia, hemostasis disorders due to thrombocytopenia, and recurrent infections related to hypogammaglobulinemia or leukopenia.[14] Although cytokine-driven bone reabsorption plays a prominent role, hypercalcemia, punched-out lytic lesions, and pathologic fractures can also be explained by the aberrant proliferation of myeloma cells in the bone marrow (see **Table 2**).[14,30] Monoclonal immunoglobulins and FLC can be directly toxic due to immunodeposition in the kidneys, leading to either tubular or glomerular damage (cast nephropathy and light chain deposition disease, respectively), or due to infiltration of a variety of organs (ie, heart, liver, small intestine, nerves) as in the case of systemic AL amyloidosis. Hyperviscosity syndrome can arise in the case of particularly elevated paraproteinemia, especially IgA or IgM, and can lead to cerebrovascular events and respiratory failure (see **Table 2**).[31] Complications of solitary plasmacytoma include compression fractures and lytic lesions from osseous plasmacytoma or extrinsic compression and/or invasion of vital structures such as bronchial tree, GI tract, or lymph nodes in the extraosseous plasmacytoma.[32–34]

SUSPECTING MULTIPLE MYELOMA (MM) IN A PATIENT WITH A MONOCLONAL SPIKE (M SPIKE)

To diagnose with MM a patient who has an M spike, end-organ damage related to the PC dyscrasia must be present.[15] When the disease is overt, patients seek emergent medical attention because of MM-related complications such as pathologic fractures, severe hypercalcemia, or acute renal failure. In these instances, the disease has declared itself, and achieving a diagnosis in this acute setting may be easier than in the outpatient setting. In most cases, in the ambulatory setting where presenting symptoms of MM transformation are more subtle, physicians are faced with the challenge of identifying patients whose MGUS has progressed to MM. Despite stringent clinical follow-up of patients with MGUS, a recent retrospective analysis showed that only a minority of asymptomatic patients would be diagnosed with MM on the sole basis of abnormal laboratory test results.[35] Most patients are diagnosed either secondary to a major morbidity (ie, pathologic fracture, acute renal failure, or severe hypercalcemia) or on the basis of the workup of self-reported symptoms, typically bone pain or asthenia and lack of stamina.[35] The complaint of new-onset back pain in a patient with MGUS should prompt evaluation for lytic lesions, while asthenia

Table 2
Most frequently occurring signs and symptoms of MM with their pathogenic correlate

Signs and Symptoms	Diagnostic Findings	Pathogenic Mechanisms	Bibliography
Bone/back pain, cord compression, cauda equina	Lytic lesions, pathologic fractures, severe osteopenia	Myelophthisis, increased osteoclastogenesis, osteoblast inhibition, solitary plasmacytoma	30,34
Fatigue, malaise	Anemia	Myelophthisis, decreased EPO, hemolysis	43,44
	Renal failure	Light chain deposition, cast nephropathy, hypercalcemia-induced vasoconstriction, amyloidosis, urate nephropathy	45,46
	Hypercalcemia	Bone reabsorption secondary to myelophthisis and cytokine release	47,48
	Hepatitis, liver failure	Amyloid infiltration, MM cell infiltration	37,49
Recurrent infections	Hypogammaglobulinemia, leukopenia	Myelophthisis	50,51
Neurologic symptoms	Polyradiculopathy, ischemic strokes, altered mental status	Amyloid deposition, cryoglobulinemia type I, hyperviscosity, hypercalcemia, uremia	31,52
Respiratory distress	Infiltrative cardiomyopathy, arrhythmias, pleural effusions, pulmonary edema	Cardiac or pulmonary amyloid, plasmacytoma, malignant pleural effusions, hyperviscosity	31,37,53
Purpura, petechiae, bleeding, acrocyanosis	Cryoglobulinemia type I, thrombocytopenia, hyperviscosity	Light chain deposition, myelophthisis, hyperviscosity	31,54

Abbreviation: EPO, erythropoietin.

and lack of energy are usually secondary to anemia, although uremia and hypercalcemia can also present with similar, nonspecific symptoms.

DIAGNOSTIC INVESTIGATIONS IN PATIENTS WHOSE MONCLONAL GAMMOPATHY OF UNDETERMINED SIGNIFICANCE (MGUS) EVOLVES INTO MULTIPLE MYELOMA (MM)

Complete physical examination and careful history taking are mandatory and crucial in guiding diagnostic workup in patients whose MGUS is suspected to evolve into MM. Plain radiography with dedicated views of the affected area should be obtained in every patient with MGUS complaining of unremitting, excruciating, or rapidly progressive bone pain. If an impending vertebral fracture or spinal cord compromise (ie, cord compression or cauda equina) is suspected, magnetic resonance imaging (MRI) of the spine should be performed to provide emergent radiation therapy or surgical stabilization so that permanent neurologic damage may be avoided. MRI also proves helpful in confirming MM evolution because an abnormal signal on T1- and/or T2-weighted images suggests pathologic bone marrow infiltration. Positron emission tomography/computed tomography (PET/CT) may be used to evaluate new-onset bone pain in patients whose MGUS is suspected to be evolving to MM. Active disease appears as ^{18}F fludeoxyglucose–avid bone marrow uptake.[36] Its use is recommended if a strong suspicion for lytic lesions or pathologic fractures is present but standard radiologic study results are abnormal. MRI and PET/CT are useful techniques to evaluate solitary plasmacytoma, and CT-guided biopsy of these lesions should be performed, whenever possible, to provide a definitive diagnosis.[15] Although patients with true solitary plasmacytoma do not require systemic therapy and treatment is either localized radiation or surgical resection, close follow-up is required, given the higher risk of the plasmacytoma's evolution to systemic MM.[15,33,34]

Progressive worsening symptoms of asthenia and malaise in a patient with known MGUS should be evaluated, at minimum, with complete blood cell counts, peripheral blood smears, and determination of creatinine and calcium levels to exclude anemia, renal failure, or hypercalcemia. In a minority of patients, MGUS progresses to amyloidosis in which symptoms are related to the organ affected by the disease. In cardiac amyloid, both the conduction system and pump function can be affected, resulting in electrophysiologic abnormalities or heart failure. Hepatitis and liver failure related to amyloid deposition can initially present with nonspecific symptoms such as asthenia and unintentional weight loss. GI involvement can present with dysmotility, malabsorption, diarrhea, or recurrent GI bleeding. Peripheral neuropathy, including bilateral carpal tunnel syndrome, can occur frequently in patients with amyloidosis and is typically multifocal.[37]

If evolution to MM is suspected on the basis of clinical presentation and laboratory results, unilateral bone marrow aspiration and biopsy are mandatory to confirm diagnosis and plan adequate treatment. Cytogenetics, fluorescence in situ hybridization (FISH) analysis, and labeling index should be performed on bone marrow aspirate for risk stratification.[15,38] To provide staging and estimate disease burden, lactate dehydrogenase, β_2-microglobulin, albumin, serum FLC ratio, quantification of serum immunoglobulins, SPEP with IF, and 24-hour urine collection with UPEP and IF should be obtained after initial laboratory testing. Two staging systems are currently available for MM: the Durie-Salmon system and the international staging system.[39,40] The former is more intuitive from a clinical standpoint, but at times difficult to objectify, whereas the latter provides useful prognostic information based on 2 commonly available and standardized laboratory values: albumin and β_2-microglobulin. If amyloidosis is suspected, a Congo red stain on fat aspirate and bone marrow is warranted. This stain can be performed on other pathologic specimens, if available, to confirm organ involvement by amyloidogenic light chain deposition.

Newly diagnosed MM patients should be promptly referred to a specialist in hematology/oncology to provide counseling and establish appropriate treatment.

THE IMPORTANCE OF AN EARLY DIAGNOSIS OF MULTIPLE MYELOMA (MM)

Two recent studies, one from the United Kingdom and the other from the United States, showed that diagnosis of MM after evaluation of symptoms such as fatigue or back pain tends to be significantly delayed (>3 months) in the ambulatory setting.[41,42] Although no impact on overall survival was noticed in either study, there was a higher incidence of complications and hospitalizations during the interim time between the first medical evaluation and diagnosis, thus emphasizing a negative impact on the patient's quality of life. Multiple factors were responsible for the delay, including the nonspecific nature of MM-presenting symptoms that are common in the aging population and tend to be prematurely dismissed as benign. Therefore, a preexistent diagnosis of MGUS should serve as an important reminder for both patients and physicians to carefully evaluate any change in current health status, especially if progressive or unremitting.

SUMMARY AND REMARKS

An M spike is a frequent finding in the general population. It is generally an incidental diagnosis of MGUS or SMM and requires no treatment, although both patients and physicians are faced with the medical, psychological and economic consequences of a premalignant diagnosis that is non curable, and the obligation (or lack thereof) for follow up because of a lifelong risk of progression to MM or related malignancies. Despite close laboratory follow-up, most patients with MGUS are diagnosed with MM between medical visits because of new onset of complications, such as pathologic fractures, or symptoms, predominantly bone pain and fatigue. Patients with MGUS should be encouraged to report any new symptom to their physician and promptly seek medical attention to decide whether further diagnostic studies are required. Physicians should carefully evaluate such patients with detailed history taking and physical examination, obtain laboratory and radiologic studies deemed necessary to achieve a diagnosis, and promptly refer them to hematology/oncology specialists for initiation of treatment. A delay in the chain of events that leads to MM diagnosis can be a cause of significant morbidity and poor quality of life for patients, and every effort should be made to diagnose MM early in the course of illness.

REFERENCES

1. Kyle RA. Monoclonal gammopathy of undetermined significance. Natural history in 241 cases. Am J Med 1978;64(5):814–26.
2. International Myeloma Working Group. Criteria for the classification of monoclonal gammopathies, multiple myeloma and related disorders: a report of the International Myeloma Working Group. Br J Haematol 2003;121(5):749–57.
3. Kyle RA, Therneau TM, Rajkumar SV, et al. Prevalence of monoclonal gammopathy of undetermined significance. N Engl J Med 2006;354(13):1362–9.
4. Landgren O, Gridley G, Turesson I, et al. Risk of monoclonal gammopathy of undetermined significance (MGUS) and subsequent multiple myeloma among African American and white veterans in the United States. Blood 2006;107(3):904–6.

5. Landgren O, Katzmann JA, Hsing AW, et al. Prevalence of monoclonal gammopathy of undetermined significance among men in Ghana. Mayo Clin Proc 2007; 82(12):1468–73.

6. Bowden M, Crawford J, Cohen HJ, et al. A comparative study of monoclonal gammopathies and immunoglobulin levels in Japanese and United States elderly. J Am Geriatr Soc 1993;41(1):11–4.

7. Iwanaga M, Tagawa M, Tsukasaki K, et al. Prevalence of monoclonal gammopathy of undetermined significance: study of 52,802 persons in Nagasaki City, Japan. Mayo Clin Proc 2007;82(12):1474–9.

8. Ruiz-Delgado GJ, Gomez Rangel JD. Monoclonal gammopathy of undetermined significance (MGUS) in Mexican mestizos: one institution's experience. Gac Med Mex 2004;140(4):375–9 [in Spanish].

9. Vachon CM, Kyle RA, Therneau TM, et al. Increase d risk of monoclonal gammopathy in first-degree relatives of patients with multiple myeloma or monoclonal gammopathy of undetermined significance. Blood 2009;114(4):785–90.

10. Kyle RA, Rajkumar SV. Monoclonal gammopathy of undetermined significance and smouldering multiple myeloma: emphasis on risk factors for progression. Br J Haematol 2007;139(5):730–43.

11. Rajkumar SV, Kyle RA, Therneau TM, et al. Serum free light chain ratio is an independent risk factor for progression in monoclonal gammopathy of undetermined significance. Blood 2005;106(3):812–7.

12. Perez-Persona E, Vidriales MB, Mateo G, et al. New criteria to identify risk of progression in monoclonal gammopathy of uncertain significance and smoldering multiple myeloma based on multiparameter flow cytometry analysis of bone marrow plasma cells. Blood 2007;110(7):2586–92.

13. Rajkumar SV, Dispenzieri A, Kyle RA. Monoclonal gammopathy of undetermined significance, Waldenström macroglobulinemia, AL amyloidosis, and related plasma cell disorders: diagnosis and treatment. Mayo Clin Proc 2006;81(5):693–703.

14. Munshi NC, Longo DL, Anderson KC. Plasma cell disorders. In: Longo DL, Fauci AS, Kasper DL, et al, editors. Harrison's principles of internal medicine, vol. 1. 18th edition. New York (NY): McGraw-Hill; 2011. p. 936–44.

15. Anderson KC, Alsina M, Bensinger W, et al. Multiple myeloma. J Natl Compr Canc Netw 2011;9(10):1146–83.

16. Kyle RA, Durie BG, Rajkumar SV, et al. Monoclonal gammopathy of undetermined significance (MGUS) and smoldering (asymptomatic) multiple myeloma: IMWG consensus perspectives risk factors for progression and guidelines for monitoring and management. Leukemia 2010;24(6):1121–7.

17. Weiss BM, Abadie J, Verma P, et al. A monoclonal gammopathy precedes multiple myeloma in most patients. Blood 2009;113(22):5418–22.

18. Landgren O, Kyle RA, Pfeiffer RM, et al. Monoclonal gammopathy of undetermined significance (MGUS) consistently precedes multiple myeloma: a prospective study. Blood 2009;113(22):5412–7.

19. Blade J, Dimopoulos M, Rosinol L, et al. Smoldering (asymptomatic) multiple myeloma: current diagnostic criteria, new predictors of outcome, and follow-up recommendations. J Clin Oncol 2010;28(4):690–7.

20. Kyle RA, Remstein ED, Therneau TM, et al. Clinical course and prognosis of smoldering (asymptomatic) multiple myeloma. N Engl J Med 2007;356(25): 2582–90.

21. Dispenzieri A, Kyle RA, Katzmann JA, et al. Immunoglobulin free light chain ratio is an independent risk factor for progression of smoldering (asymptomatic) multiple myeloma. Blood 2008;111(2):785–9.

22. Kyle RA, Buadi F, Rajkumar SV. Management of monoclonal gammopathy of undetermined significance (MGUS) and smoldering multiple myeloma (SMM). Oncology (Williston Park) 2011;25(7):578–86.
23. Rajkumar SV, Dispenzieri A, Fonseca R, et al. Thalidomide for previously untreated indolent or smoldering multiple myeloma. Leukemia 2001;15(8):1274–6.
24. Mateos MV, Lopez-Corral L, Hernández MT, et al. Multicenter, randomized, open-label, phase III trial of lenalidomide-dexamethasone (len/dex) vs therapeutic abstention in smoldering multiple myeloma at high risk of progression to symptomatic MM: results of the first interim analysis. ASH annual meeting abstracts. New Orleans, Louisiana, USA. Blood 2009;114:614.
25. Lorsbach RB, Hsi ED, Dogan A, et al. Plasma cell myeloma and related neoplasms. Am J Clin Pathol 2011;136(2):168–82.
26. Dispenzieri A, Kyle R, Merlini G, et al. International Myeloma Working Group guidelines for serum-free light chain analysis in multiple myeloma and related disorders. Leukemia 2009;23(2):215–24.
27. Kremer M, Ott G, Nathrath M, et al. Primary extramedullary plasmacytoma and multiple myeloma: phenotypic differences revealed by immunohistochemical analysis. J Pathol 2005;205(1):92–101.
28. Albarracin F, Fonseca R. Plasma cell leukemia. Blood Rev 2011;25(3):107–12.
29. American Cancer Society. Cancer facts and figures 2012. Atlanta (GA): American Cancer Society; 2012.
30. Raje N, Roodman GD. Advances in the biology and treatment of bone disease in multiple myeloma. Clin Cancer Res 2011;17(6):1278–86.
31. Mehta J, Singhal S. Hyperviscosity syndrome in plasma cell dyscrasias. Semin Thromb Hemost 2003;29(5):467–71.
32. Alexiou C, Kau RJ, Dietzfelbinger H, et al. Extramedullary plasmacytoma: tumor occurrence and therapeutic concepts. Cancer 1999;85(11):2305–14.
33. Blade J, Fernandez de Larrea C, Rosinol L, et al. Soft-tissue plasmacytomas in multiple myeloma: incidence, mechanisms of extramedullary spread, and treatment approach. J Clin Oncol 2011;29(28):3805–12.
34. Dimopoulos MA, Hamilos G. Solitary bone plasmacytoma and extramedullary plasmacytoma. Curr Treat Options Oncol 2002;3(3):255–9.
35. Bianchi G, Kyle RA, Colby CL, et al. Impact of optimal follow-up of monoclonal gammopathy of undetermined significance on early diagnosis and prevention of myeloma-related complications. Blood 2010;116(12):2019–25 [quiz: 2197].
36. Mena E, Choyke P, Tan E, et al. Molecular imaging in myeloma precursor disease. Semin Hematol 2011;48(1):22–31.
37. Merlini G, Seldin DC, Gertz MA. Amyloidosis: pathogenesis and new therapeutic options. J Clin Oncol 2011;29(14):1924–33.
38. Kumar SK, Mikhael JR, Buadi FK, et al. Management of newly diagnosed symptomatic multiple myeloma: updated Mayo Stratification of Myeloma and Risk-Adapted Therapy (mSMART) consensus guidelines. Mayo Clin Proc 2009; 84(12):1095–110.
39. Durie BG, Salmon SE. A clinical staging system for multiple myeloma. Correlation of measured myeloma cell mass with presenting clinical features, response to treatment, and survival. Cancer 1975;36(3):842–54.
40. Greipp PR, San Miguel J, Durie BG, et al. International staging system for multiple myeloma. J Clin Oncol 2005;23(15):3412–20.
41. Friese CR, Abel GA, Magazu LS, et al. Diagnostic delay and complications for older adults with multiple myeloma. Leuk Lymphoma 2009;50(3):392–400.

42. Kariyawasan CC, Hughes DA, Jayatillake MM, et al. Multiple myeloma: causes and consequences of delay in diagnosis. QJM 2007;100(10):635–40.
43. Ludwig H, Pohl G, Osterborg A. Anemia in multiple myeloma. Clin Adv Hematol Oncol 2004;2(4):233–41.
44. Snowden JA, Ahmedzai SH, Ashcroft J, et al. Guidelines for supportive care in multiple myeloma 2011. Br J Haematol 2011;154(1):76–103.
45. Wirk B. Renal failure in multiple myeloma: a medical emergency. Bone Marrow Transplant 2011;46(6):771–83.
46. Dimopoulos MA, Kastritis E, Rosinol L, et al. Pathogenesis and treatment of renal failure in multiple myeloma. Leukemia 2008;22(8):1485–93.
47. Laubach J, Richardson P, Anderson K. Multiple myeloma. Annu Rev Med 2011; 62:249–64.
48. Oyajobi BO. Multiple myeloma/hypercalcemia. Arthritis Res Ther 2007;9(Suppl 1):S4.
49. Bhandari MS, Mazumder A, Vesole DH. Liver involvement in multiple myeloma. Clin Lymphoma Myeloma 2007;7(8):538–40.
50. Terpos E, Cibeira MT, Blade J, et al. Management of complications in multiple myeloma. Semin Hematol 2009;46(2):176–89.
51. Anderson KC, Carrasco RD. Pathogenesis of myeloma. Annu Rev Pathol 2011;6: 249–74.
52. Drappatz J, Batchelor T. Neurologic complications of plasma cell disorders. Clin Lymphoma 2004;5(3):163–71.
53. Kapoor P, Thenappan T, Singh E, et al. Cardiac amyloidosis: a practical approach to diagnosis and management. Am J Med 2011;124(11):1006–15.
54. Molina-Garrido MJ, Guillen-Ponce C. A revision on cryoglobulinemia associated to neoplastic diseases. Clin Transl Oncol 2007;9(4):229–36.

Why Does My Patient Have Lymphadenopathy or Splenomegaly?

Gabriela Motyckova, MD, PhD, David P. Steensma, MD*

KEYWORDS

- Lymphadenopathy • Splenomegaly • Differential diagnosis
- Hematological malignancy

Enlarged lymph nodes or a palpable spleen tip are exceptionally common physical findings and are not always signs of disease.[1–3] For instance, in one US pediatric practice, 45% of children aged 5 years or less had palpable lymph nodes in the head and neck region.[1] However, lymphadenopathy or splenomegaly may also be the first sign, or even the only sign, of a serious or life-threatening condition, so physicians must be able to judge accurately when lymphadenopathy or splenomegaly are potentially pathologic, and clinicians should be comfortable with contemporary diagnostic approaches to evaluate these findings.

Lymphadenopathy and splenomegaly can be detected in symptomatic or asymptomatic patients. The possible causes of each finding are diverse, with a broad differential diagnosis ranging from nonmalignant conditions, such as inflammatory disorders or acute or chronic infections, to malignant processes, including hematologic malignancies or metastatic carcinomas.[4,5] The sites and characteristics of lymphadenopathy, as well as age of the patient and presence or absence of associated symptoms such as constitutional symptoms, fevers, weight loss, or other physical findings, can help direct evaluation and can point to a specific cause of the lymphadenopathy. In most cases of persistent lymphadenopathy or splenomegaly, pathologic (tissue) diagnosis is necessary to rule out malignant conditions.

MECHANISMS OF LYMPHADENOPATHY

Physical enlargement of a lymph node can occur via several processes. Polyclonal lymphocyte proliferation due to a reaction to a specific group of antigens or monoclonal proliferation from malignant transformation of a lymphoid cell can increase the size and number of lymph node follicles, thereby expanding the node. Enlargement of a lymph node can also occur due to infiltration of the node by nonlymphoid cells,

The authors have no relevant disclosures.
Dana-Farber Cancer Institute, Harvard Medical School, Boston, MA, USA
* Corresponding author. Department of Medical Oncology, Dana-Farber Cancer Institute, Suite D1B30, 450 Brookline Avenue, Boston, MA 02215.
E-mail address: david_steensma@dfci.harvard.edu

Hematol Oncol Clin N Am 26 (2012) 395–408
doi:10.1016/j.hoc.2012.02.005
0889-8588/12/$ – see front matter © 2012 Elsevier Inc. All rights reserved.

such as inflammatory reaction by neutrophils in lymphadenitis, or metastatic spread of cancer cells from a primary site of neoplasia. In addition, systemic processes can cause a release of cytokines resulting in edema of lymph nodes; such cytokine-mediated adenopathy is usually diffuse and not localized to a single node or nodal group. In metabolic storage disorders, engorged macrophages can accumulate in a lymph node, causing enlargement.[4,5]

MECHANISMS OF SPLENOMEGALY

Because the splenic white pulp serves as an active immune organ with efferent lymphatic vessels, the mechanisms by which splenomegaly can occur overlap with the mechanisms that cause lymphadenopathy. Because the spleen is also a phagocytic organ with mechanical filtration capability (eg, for senescent erythrocytes) as well as a potential site of hematopoiesis, there are additional mechanisms for splenomegaly, including brisk hemolysis and extramedullary hematopoiesis. Furthermore, spleno-megaly can also occur due to disruption of venous blood flow from the organ, such as splenic or portal vein thrombosis, or portal hypertension due to intrinsic hepatic disease.

LOCATION OF LYMPHADENOPATHY

The normal peripheral lymph node chains in the body are responsible for drainage of lymphatic fluid from specific anatomic locations (**Table 1**). Drainage patterns of deep/central lymph nodes (eg, mesenteric, retroperitoneal) are less predictable, although

Table 1
Peripheral lymph nodes and associated anatomic sites

Lymph Node Group	Sites
Preauricular	Conjunctiva, anterior and temporal scalp, anterior ear canal
Posterior auricular	Parietal and temporal scalp
Parotid	Forehead, midface, temporal scalp, external ear canal, middle ear, parotid glands, gums
Cervical-superficial	Parotid gland, lower larynx, lower ear canal
Cervical	Larynx, thyroid, palate, esophagus, paranasal sinuses, tonsils, adenoids, posterior scalp and neck, nose
Occipital	Posterior scalp
Submandibular	Nose, lips, tongue, cheek, submandibular gland, buccal mucosa
Submental	Floor of mouth, lower lip
Supraclavicular	Chest and abdomen (left supraclavicular, abdomen; right supraclavicular, mediastinum and lungs)
Axillary	Lower neck, upper extremity, lateral breast, chest wall
Deltopectoral	Upper extremity
Epitrochlear	Upper extremity below the elbow
Inguinal	Lower extremity, genital region, buttock, abdominal wall below the umbilicus
Popliteal	Lower extremity below the knee

Adapted from Henry M, Kamat D. Integrating basic science into clinical teaching initiative series: approach to lymphadenopathy. Clin Pediatr (Phila) 2011;50(8):685, with permission; and Friedmann AM. Evaluation and management of lymphadenopathy in children. Pediatr Rev 2008;29(2):54, with permission.

unilateral hilar lung node enlargement usually reflects a pathologic process in the ipsilateral lung. Enlargement of peripheral lymph nodes in a specific area may point to a regional source of the abnormality, but this is not always reliable. A differential diagnosis of lymphadenopathy according to the sites of pathologic enlargement is shown in **Box 1**. Although a search for enlarged lymph nodes is one of the most important components of a physical examination, discussion of specific physical examination techniques is beyond the scope of this review.

Generalized Lymphadenopathy

Malignant, inflammatory, and infectious causes can all cause generalized lymphadenopathy. Hematologic malignancies (most commonly lymphoid neoplasms: acute lymphoblastic leukemia [ALL], chronic lymphocytic leukemia [CLL], and Hodgkin and non-Hodgkin lymphomas) and infectious processes (infectious mononucleosis and a diverse roster of other viral, bacterial, and fungal processes) can cause a diffuse nodal reaction, as can advanced carcinomas. Rarely, mesenchymal tumors such as rhabdomyosarcoma or neuroblastoma can present with adenopathy. Hypersensitivity reactions to drugs should be considered, especially if rash, fever, or eosinophilia is present.

Cervical and Occipital Lymphadenopathy

Enlargement of cervical lymph nodes is most commonly caused by an infection in the head and neck region; malignancy is the second most common cause. Infectious causes include pharyngitis, otitis (media and external), dental abscesses, and scalp infections; cervical adenopathy may also be the only sign of systemic infections including infectious mononucleosis or infection caused by cytomegalovirus (CMV). Among malignancies, lymphoma (Hodgkin and non-Hodgkin lymphomas) and head and neck cancers are the most common causes of cervical adenopathy. Small preauricular nodes may be palpable in conjunctivitis or ocular lymphoproliferative disorders. Localized lymphadenopathy in the posterior cervical chains can be seen in histiocytic necrotizing lymphadenopathy (Kikuchi disease),[13–16] toxoplasmosis, or rubella.[11] Computed tomographic (CT) and ultrasonographic studies have been reported to help differentiate malignant versus reactive lymph nodes, but their test characteristics in this region remain uncertain and biopsy is often necessary for adenopathy that persists beyond 2 to 3 weeks without known cause.[17–25]

In a study of 155 patients who presented with lymphadenopathy in the cervical region without prior history of malignancy, histologic diagnosis could be made by core needle biopsy in 146 (94%) patients.[18] The pathologic examination results showed 44 cases of reactive hyperplasia, 37 cases of tuberculosis, 25 cases of Kikuchi disease, 16 cases of metastatic malignancies, 16 cases of lymphoma, 1 diagnosis of toxoplasmosis, and normal findings in 7 patients. The study reported sensitivity, specificity, and accuracy of sonographically guided core biopsy of 97.9%, 99.1%, and 97.9%, respectively.[18]

Enlargement of salivary glands can mimic adenopathy. Rheumatologic causes in one series underlied 4% of all cases of cervical lymphadenopathy.[26]

Supraclavicular Lymphadenopathy

Abdominal and thoracic malignancies may metastasize to supraclavicular lymph nodes. Supraclavicular adenopathy, especially unilateral left-sided (ie, Troisier or Virchow sentinel node, named after French pathologist Charles Emile Troisier [1844–1919] or German pathologist Rudolf Virchow [1821–1902]), can be the first sign of a visceral malignancy, including cancer of the gastroesophageal junction or stomach or of other intrathoracic or intra-abdominal organs.[11,27] Infectious causes, as already mentioned, may cause enlargement in several lymph node chains,

---

Box 1
Differential diagnosis of lymphadenopathy according to location

Generalized lymphadenopathy[6]

Infections[5]:

> Viral: common upper respiratory tract infections; infections caused by Epstein-Barr virus, cytomegalovirus, human immunodeficiency virus, varicella-zoster virus, human T cell lymphotropic virus, and adenovirus; measles; rubella typhoid fever; syphilis; plague

> Bacterial: a broad range of bacterial infectious, including those caused by *Bartonella*, tuberculosis, nontubercular mycobacterial infections, syphilis

> Protozoal: toxoplasmosis

> Fungal: coccidioidomycosis

Malignancy: non-Hodgkin lymphoma, Hodgkin lymphoma, chronic lymphocytic leukemia, acute lymphoblastic leukemia

Autoimmune disorders: rheumatoid arthritis, systemic lupus erythematosus

Noninfectious granulomatous disease: sarcoidosis

Atypical lymphoproliferative disorders[7]

Angioimmunoblastic lymphadenopathy[8]

Atypical cellular disorders[9]

Cervical lymphadenopathy

Infections: dental abscess; otitis media and externa; pharyngitis; toxoplasmosis; and infections caused by Epstein-Barr virus, cytomegalovirus, and adenovirus; hepatitis; rubella

Malignancies: non-Hodgkin lymphoma, Hodgkin disease, head and neck cancer

Kikuchi disease[10]

Supraclavicular lymphadenopathy

Malignancy: thoracic, abdominal

Diseases of the thyroid and larynx

Infections: tuberculosis, fungal infection

Axillary lymphadenopathy

Infection: infections caused by *Staphylococcus* and *Streptococcus*, sporotrichosis, cat-scratch disease, tularemia

Malignancies: breast cancer, non-Hodgkin lymphoma

Hilar and mediastinal lymphadenopathy

Hilar unilateral

> Infection: bacterial, mycobacterial, and fungal infections; pertussis; tularemia; psittacosis

> Malignancy: lung, breast, or gastrointestinal cancer; Hodgkin disease; non-Hodgkin lymphoma

> Granulomatous disease

Hilar bilateral, mediastinal

> Infection

> Malignancy: metastatic cancer, Hodgkin disease, non-Hodgkin lymphoma

> Granulomatous disease

Abdominal lymphadenopathy

Malignancy: metastatic gastrointestinal cancer, non-Hodgkin lymphoma, Hodgkin disease, chronic lymphocytic leukemia, urinary transitional cell carcinoma

Infection: tuberculosis

Epitrochlear lymphadenopathy

Connective tissue disorders

Granulomatous disease: sarcoidosis

Dermatologic disease

Syphilis, leishmaniasis, leprosy, rubella

Inguinal lymphadenopathy

Reactive

Malignancy: non-Hodgkin lymphoma, Hodgkin disease, melanoma, squamous cell cancer of the vulva, penis cancer, anal cancer

Infection: cellulitis, sexually transmitted diseases

Adapted from Refs,[5,11,12] with permission.

---

including supraclavicular nodes, which may be the only palpable peripheral nodal group. Less commonly reported causes of supraclavicular lymphadenopathy include silicone breast implants[28] or amyloidosis.[29]

The term Delphian node, evoking the classical oracle at Delphi, Greece, refers to a midline prelaryngeal node that could be a sign of laryngeal or thyroid cancer or inflammatory thyroid disease (eg, Hashimoto thyroiditis).[30]

Axillary Lymphadenopathy

Similar to most other lymph node chain enlargements, infections and malignancies are the 2 most common causes of axillary lymphadenopathy.[31,32] Common malignancies presenting as axillary adenopathy include lymphoproliferative neoplasms and breast carcinoma. Occasionally, a left axillary lymph node may be a metastasis from gastric carcinoma, also called Irish node.[33] Infectious causes of axillary adenopathy include *Staphylococcus* and *Streptococcus* skin infections and other infections of the hand or arm (eg, sporotrichosis, cat-scratch disease due to *Bartonella* organisms).[11,31,32] Patients, especially small children, may not recall a recent hand injury because the incubation period between inoculation and axillary adenopathy may be as long as 2 months.

Mediastinal and Hilar Lymphadenopathy

The causes of intrathoracic lymphadenopathy are particularly diverse[11,34] and include a broad range of infectious, inflammatory, and malignant processes.

Unilateral hilar lymphadenopathy can be seen in inflammatory pneumonitis; infections such as bacterial pneumonia, tuberculosis, and atypical mycobacterial infection; pertussis; or granulomatous diseases such as fungal infections (eg, histoplasmosis or coccidioidomycosis) and sarcoidosis; less common infections such as tularemia or psittacosis should be considered in the appropriate clinical setting. Malignant causes of hilar adenopathy include lung cancer, breast cancer, metastases from the gastrointestinal tract, or involvement by Hodgkin or non-Hodgkin lymphoma.

Bilateral hilar lymphadenopathy can be caused by Hodgkin and non-Hodgkin lymphoma, chronic granulomatous disease (sarcoidosis, berylliosis), or metastatic cancer from a wide variety of primary sites.[11,35] Calcified hilar lymphadenopathy is seen in tuberculosis, silicosis, sarcoidosis, and histoplasmosis.[11]

Mediastinal lymphadenopathy also occurs in a variety of conditions ranging from infectious to malignant, and the differential diagnosis overlaps with that of hilar adenopathy.[11,29,36,37]

Abdominal or Retroperitoneal Lymphadenopathy

Enlargement lymph nodes in the abdomen or retroperitoneum, including periportal, celiac, mesenteric, iliac, and periaortic node clusters, is a recurrent finding during abdominal imaging and is often worrisome for underlying malignancy. Limits on upper limits of normal size for abdominal lymph nodes have been proposed.[38,39] An abnormal lymph node in the umbilical region ("pants button umbilicus," also called the Sister Mary Joseph node, named after surgeon William Mayo's surgical scrub nurse in the 1920s and 1930s at Mayo Clinic in Minnesota) can be associated with intra-abdominal or pelvic malignancy.[40]

Epitrochlear Lymphadenopathy

Epitrochlear adenopathy is less well studied than adenopathy in other nodal groups. In one series of 184 consecutive patients with diseases in which lymphadenopathy occurs, 27% of patients had palpable epitrochlear lymph nodes, compared with 140 healthy controls, all of who did not have palpable epitrochlear lymphadenopathy.[41] In that series, patients with epitrochlear lymphadenopathy in the setting of lymph node enlargement in other regions were most commonly found to have non-Hodgkin lymphoma, CLL, or infections, including human immunodeficiency virus (HIV) infection. Other causes included connective tissue disorders and sarcoidosis.[41]

Popliteal Lymphadenopathy

Popliteal lymph nodes drain the lower extremities and may be a sign of an infection of the heel or foot. Only scarce data are available specifically about popliteal lymphadenopathy. Popliteal swelling due to a Baker cyst or an aneurysm or other vascular disorder is sometimes confused with adenopathy.

Inguinal Lymphadenopathy

Because of the chronic colonization of the anogenital region by bacteria, a small amount of reactive lymphadenopathy in the inguinal/femoral region is not necessarily pathologic and appears commonly in healthy populations. However, inguinal lymphadenopathy can be caused by sexually transmitted diseases, as well as cellulitis, including pedal dermatophytosis.[11] Among metastatic lesions, inguinal metastases can be seen in cancers of skin of the lower extremities, cervix, vulva, skin of the trunk, mucosal surfaces of the rectum and anus, or the ovary or penis.[42] Terminology of inguinal region nodes in the medical literature is inconsistent, with some investigators referring to femoral nodes as those below the inguinal ligament (eg, the node of Cloquet) and inguinal nodes as those above the inguinal ligament, whereas others using less precise terms such as vertical or horizontal nodes.[43]

EVALUATION OF LYMPHADENOPATHY

Although adenopathy due to a cause that is obvious on history taking and physical examination (such as pharyngitis, odontogenic infection, or regional cellulitis) does not merit further evaluation, adenopathy that is of unknown cause and persists for more than a week or two demands further evaluation. Although an expedited evaluation is particularly important if worrisome constitutional symptoms such as fever, night sweats, or weight loss are present, young patients with adenopathy who lack constitutional symptoms may also harbor a serious disorder, including a neoplasm. Still, most patients with adenopathy have a benign condition; in one series of 550 patients who were identified by their primary care physicians as requiring further evaluation of worrisome lymphadenopathy, only 17.5% proved to have a neoplasm.[44]

Simple laboratory studies may help determine the cause of lymphadenopathy in many cases. For example, hematological neoplasms may be suggested by a complete blood cell count with a peripheral smear, whereas in the right clinical setting, serologies for CMV, Epstein-Barr virus, or HIV infection in patients with risk factors may be diagnostic (but HIV positivity can also be associated with other causes of adenopathy, including Kaposi sarcoma, lymphoproliferative neoplasms, and multicentric Castleman disease). Nonspecific laboratory indices of inflammation are less helpful, which include erythrocyte sedimentation rate, C-reactive protein level, or serum fibrinogen level, because abnormal results are very frequent in the presence of adenopathy yet do not point to a particular etiology. Serum lactate dehydrogenase (LDH) levels are also not diagnostically specific but may give a sense of the rate of cell turnover; very high LDH levels suggest a lymphoid neoplasm.

Serum and urine protein electrophoresis and serum free light chains may show an abnormal M spike, which could be associated with multiple myeloma, amyloidosis, lymphomas, or CLL. Decreased serum immunoglobulin levels (hypogammaglobulinemia) and lymphadenopathy can be seen in amyloidosis, CLL, Whipple disease, or common variable immunodeficiency.[45] If malignancy is suspected, body CT or positron emission tomography scanning may be important for staging.

Biopsy of accessible lymph nodes aids the diagnosis of the underlying condition. In a retrospective analysis of 925 patients undergoing lymph node biopsy between 1973 and 1977, 60% of the biopsies showed benign lesions (eg, reactive hyperplasia), 28% revealed carcinoma, and 12% of biopsies demonstrated lymphoma.[46] Malignant findings were most common in peripheral lymph nodes and least common in intrathoracic nodes, possibly reflecting selection bias in which patients underwent biopsies (**Table 2**). In older patients, especially older than 50 years, lymph node biopsies tend to show more carcinomas; therefore age is one of the most important factors to consider in evaluating lymphadenopathy.[46]

The differential diagnosis of lymphadenopathy is highly dependent on clinical context. For instance, a retrospective study evaluating 1724 patients with peripheral lymphadenopathy in India showed that 35.6% of patients had nonspecific lymphadenitis (including benign follicular hyperplasia, reactive hyperplasia, or reactive hyperplasia).[12] Other common causes were tuberculous lymphadenitis (31.3%), which is rare in the United States, and malignancy (25.9%). The study also detected rare diseases such as Kikuchi disease (histiocytic necrotizing lymphadenitis), Kimura

Table 2 Results of lymph node biopsies			
Lymph Node Biopsy Results	Benign (%)	Carcinoma (%)	Lymphoma (%)
Overall	60	28	12
Abdominal	63	33	4
Intrathoracic	73	26	1
Peripheral	56	29	15

Adapted from Lee Y, Terry R, Lukes RJ. Lymph node biopsy for diagnosis: a statistical study. J Surg Oncol 1980;14(1):53–60; with permission.

disease (an idiopathic chronic painless cervical adenopathy that is most common in Asian men), and Rosai-Dorfman disease (sinus histiocytosis with massive lymphadenopathy).[12]

LYMPH NODE CHARACTERISTICS

Key physical features of palpable abnormal lymph nodes include the size of the node, the presence or absence of tenderness, and the consistency and physical conformation of the enlarged node or nodal cluster (eg, firm, rubbery, matted/confluent, shotty). Of these features, the most important diagnostic feature is size, as discussed later. In general, the presence of nodal tenderness suggests an infectious or inflammatory cause, whereas a nontender stony hard lymph node indicates a malignancy, but these features are not reliable enough to alter the diagnostic algorithm.

LYMPH NODE SIZE AND BIOPSY CONSIDERATIONS

The cutoff size of a lymph node above which pathology is likely to be apparent on nodal biopsy is not clear-cut. The prior probability of an abnormal biopsy result is affected by location of lymphadenopathy as well as the patient's history of antigenic exposure, and the size of normal lymph nodes also varies between patients.

A size of 1.5 cm was used to help differentiate malignant lymphadenopathy in one study of 220 lymph node biopsies.[47] Other investigators consider a patient with a persistent dominant lymph node of size 10 mm or more in all lymph node chains except for inguinal as a reasonable candidate for a biopsy. Several different criteria for lymphadenopathy in the cervical,[20] thoracic,[34,36,37] and abdominal[38,39] regions have been published. Malignancy becomes more likely in lymph nodes that are larger than 2 cm.[4]

Some clinicians consider a lymph nodes biopsy only after unsuccessful treatment of the patient with antibiotics or corticosteroids. Because antibiotic and especially glucocorticoid treatment can make nodal biopsy specimens more difficult to interpret, empiric treatment of lymphadenopathy should be avoided.

In patients without prior diagnosis, an excisional biopsy is recommended over fine-needle aspiration (FNA).[48,49] Excisional biopsy was shown to yield a final definitive diagnosis in 63% of cases in a review of 290 samples.[50,51] FNA can provide a diagnosis in some cases such as metastatic carcinoma and may be the only option in a frail or an unstable patient with a deep node detected on CT, but the utility of FNA is limited in hematologic malignancies (especially lymphoma) in which lymph node architecture is critical in making the diagnosis.[52] In some cases, excisional biopsy is simply not possible because of the location of the lesion or suspected complications, but even in these cases a core needle biopsy is preferred to FNA.[18,53–56] The sensitivity and diagnostic yield of FNA may improve in the future by analysis of molecular markers in the FNA sample.[57]

SPLENOMEGALY

In children, the most common causes of splenomegaly are infections (causing increased antigenic stimulation, with viral infection being most common), autoimmune disorders, and destruction of abnormal blood cells (such as brisk hemolysis).[4] Collagen vascular diseases and malignancy, especially lymphomas, ALL, or chronic myelogenous leukemia, and other myeloproliferative disorders, are more common in adults but can rarely present in children, especially ALL. Congestive heart failure and liver cirrhosis can also result in intrahepatic blood flow obstruction and splenomegaly; splenic or portal vein thrombosis may also enlarge the spleen. Common causes of splenomegaly are listed in **Box 2**.

Box 2
Causes of splenomegaly

Excessive antigenic stimulation

    Infection: viral (most common in children), bacterial, protozoal, and fungal

        Common causes include Epstein-Barr virus infection, tuberculosis, malaria

Autoimmune disorders

Collagen vascular disorders

Sarcoidosis

Amyloidosis

Excessive destruction of abnormal blood cells

    Hemolysis (eg, hereditary spherocytosis, thalassemia major)

Chronic myeloproliferative disorders

    Especially myelofibrosis and chronic myelogenous leukemia

Malignancy

    ALL, non-Hodgkin lymphoma, Hodgkin lymphoma, and acute or chronic myelogenous leukemia

Obstruction of venous flow

    Cirrhosis, portal vein thrombosis, congestive heart failure

Storage diseases

    Gaucher disease

    Niemann-Pick disease

Splenic enlargement can occur alone, or less commonly (4.5% of cases in one series) in combination with lymphadenopathy.[47] As discussed earlier, the causes of splenomegaly overlap with causes of lymphadenopathy and also include conditions such as extramedullary hematopoiesis and myeloproliferative disorders,[58,59] lysosomal storage diseases,[60] or hemolysis.

Splenomegaly may be detected on physical examination. A palpable spleen is usually enlarged,[61] and its cause should be investigated even though the diagnostic yield is likely low and some cases of splenomegaly may occur in otherwise normal individuals. In a study of 2200 incoming Dartmouth College studies, 63 (2.9%) had enlarged spleen, but only 5 were not healthy or did not remain healthy for 10 years at follow-up report.[2,3] In another study of postpartum and otherwise healthy women, 12% were found to have palpable splenomegaly.[62]

The normal size of spleen may vary but is usually less than 250 g.[61] The most commonly used cutoff for normal length of spleen by radioisotopic scintiscan is 12 cm. On ultrasonography, splenomegaly is suspected when the longest dimension of the spleen reaches 11 to 13 cm or more. Splenomegaly is also considered when the sonographic width of spleen is greater than 4 cm and the diameter greater than 7 cm.[61,63] The normal splenic volume by CT scan is 214.6 cm^3, with a range from 107.2 to 314.5 cm^3.[64] The upper limit of normal splenic volume of 314.5 cm^3 correlates to a maximum spleen length of 9.76 cm by CT scan.[65] Splenic size also correlates with height.[63]

Biopsies of the spleen are less common than lymph node biopsies because of the risk of hemorrhage, but some investigators have advocated splenic biopsy during

---

Box 3
General differential diagnosis of lymphadenopathy

Autoimmune/rheumatologic disorders, hypersensitivity disorders

Rheumatoid arthritis, juvenile rheumatoid arthritis, Sjögren syndrome, system lupus erythematosus, mixed connective tissue disease, and dermatomyositis

Allergic/hypersensitivity

Drug hypersensitivity such as that to allopurinol, indomethacin, diphenylhydantoin, carbamazepine, and silicone

Serum sickness

Bone marrow disorders (nonmalignant)

Primary myelofibrosis, extramedullary hematopoiesis

Infections

Bacterial: infections caused by *Staphylococcus*, *Streptococcus*, atypical mycobacteria, and *Chlamydia*; TB; syphilis; and cat-scratch fever

Viral: EBV, HIV, CMV, VZV, human T cell lymphotropic virus 1, adenovirus

Fungal: coccidioidomycosis, histoplasmosis, actinomycosis

Other: toxoplasmosis, infection caused by *Rickettsia*, filariasis, lymphogranuloma venereum

Immunodeficiency

AIDS

Hereditary

Familial Mediterranean fever

Lymphoproliferative disorders

Castleman disease, granulomatosis with polyangiitis, angioimmunoblastic lymphadenopathy with dysproteinemia, lymphomatoid granulomatosis

Malignancy

Metastatic cancer such as that of lung, breast, prostate, esophagus, head and neck, and others

Hematologic malignancies: leukemias, Hodgkin disease, non-Hodgkin lymphoma, systemic mastocytosis, multiple myeloma, Waldenström macroglobulinemia

Other

Granulomatous disorders

Uncommon: histiocytic necrotizing lymphadenitis (Kikuchi disease), sinus histiocytosis with massive lymphadenopathy (Rosai-Dorfman disease), inflammatory pseudotumor of lymph nodes

Adapted from Refs.[4,11,70]

---

evaluation of unknown origin or infection causes.[63] In the authors' experience, this is rarely necessary.

The assessment of splenomegaly on physical examination can be performed by percussion and palpation. The detection ability, sensitivity, and specificity of physical examination compared with those of imaging studies have been investigated. Palpation compared with ultrasonography or scintigraphy showed a sensitivity of 20% to 71% depending on whether the investigator was aware of being evaluated. Without prior knowledge of splenomegaly, palpation may have a sensitivity of 20% to 27%

but a high specificity of 98% to 100% compared with an autopsy or scintigraphy standard.[61] Percussion may have a sensitivity of 59% to 82% compared with ultrasonography or scintigraphy.[61] Imaging studies are more sensitive than physical examination in detecting splenomegaly.[61] Splenic enlargement can be readily seen by magnetic resonance imaging.[66,67]

WHEN SHOULD AN ENLARGED SPLEEN BE REMOVED

When the cause of symptomatic splenomegaly is known, the spleen can often be managed by medications or radiotherapy. Splenectomy is usually considered only for select patients who are good surgical candidates in situations in which the diagnosis is either unclear or when other measures have failed to control the spleen enlargement, given the morbidity and mortality risk of the procedure (mortality up to 10% in some series).[68]

Splenectomy is usually not the initial consideration in treatment of malignant causes of splenomegaly but remains an important option in selected cases; disease-by-disease considerations are beyond the scope of this review. Splenectomy may aid in treating hypersplenism due to splenomegaly or in management of symptoms caused by splenomegaly. In some conditions such as myelofibrosis or storage disorders, decisions about splenectomy must also take into consideration the effect of splenomegaly on liver function.

Palliative splenectomy can be used in the treatment of patients with myelofibrosis in whom splenomegaly may be massive and may cause significant discomfort.[68] Other disease settings in which splenectomy for splenomegaly has therapeutic benefit include hairy cell leukemia or splenic marginal zone lymphoma.

Reducing splenic size by chemotherapy or radiation or removal of an enlarged spleen may improve patients' symptoms (early satiety, decreased appetite, or left upper quadrant discomfort and pain). As an alternative to open surgical procedure, splenectomy can be safely performed laparoscopically in many cases, and surgical practice is evolving.[69,70]

SUMMARY

Lymphadenopathy and splenomegaly are important findings that may be noted by the patient, detected on a physical examination, or uncovered during an imaging study. Enlargement of lymph nodes or the spleen has a broad differential diagnosis, including infectious causes, autoimmune and inflammatory disorders, and a variety of hematological malignancies and solid tumors (**Box 3**). Pathologic diagnosis from excisional lymph node biopsy and supplemental laboratory studies are usually necessary to obtain a correct diagnosis. Lymphadenopathy and splenomegaly should be followed up closely and evaluated promptly because most causes, including hematologic malignancies, are treatable and potentially curable.

REFERENCES

1. Herzog LW. Prevalence of lymphadenopathy of the head and neck in infants and children. Clin Pediatr (Phila) 1983;22(7):485–7.
2. McIntyre OR, Ebaugh FG Jr. Palpable spleens in college freshmen. Ann Intern Med 1967;66(2):301–6.
3. Ebaugh FG Jr, McIntyre OR. Palpable spleens: ten-year follow-up. Ann Intern Med 1979;90(1):130–1.
4. Henry M, Kamat D. Integrating basic science into clinical teaching initiative series: approach to lymphadenopathy. Clin Pediatr (Phila) 2011;50(8):683–7.

5. Friedmann AM. Evaluation and management of lymphadenopathy in children. Pediatr Rev 2008;29(2):53–60.
6. Libman H. Generalized lymphadenopathy. J Gen Intern Med 1987;2(1):48–58.
7. Greiner T, Armitage JO, Gross TG. Atypical lymphoproliferative diseases. Hematology Am Soc Hematol Educ Program 2000;133–46.
8. Sallah S, Gagnon GA. Angioimmunoblastic lymphadenopathy with dysproteinemia: emphasis on pathogenesis and treatment. Acta Haematol 1998;99(2):57–64.
9. McClain KL, Natkunam Y, Swerdlow SH. Atypical cellular disorders. Hematology Am Soc Hematol Educ Program 2004;283–96.
10. Prignano F, D'Erme AM, Zanieri F, et al. Why is Kikuchi-Fujimoto disease misleading. Int J Dermatol 2011. [Epub ahead of print].
11. Habermann TM, Steensma DP. Lymphadenopathy. Mayo Clin Proc 2000;75(7): 723–32.
12. Mohan A, Reddy MK, Phaneendra BV, et al. Aetiology of peripheral lymphadenopathy in adults: analysis of 1724 cases seen at a tertiary care teaching hospital in southern India. Natl Med J India 2007;20(2):78–80.
13. Nikanne E, Ruoppi P, Vornanen M. Kikuchi's disease: report of three cases and an overview. Laryngoscope 1997;107(2):273–6.
14. Norris AH, Krasinskas AM, Salhany KE, et al. Kikuchi-Fujimoto disease: a benign cause of fever and lymphadenopathy. Am J Med 1996;101(4):401–5.
15. Tsang WY, Chan JK. Fine-needle aspiration cytologic diagnosis of Kikuchi's lymphadenitis. A report of 27 cases. Am J Clin Pathol 1994;102(4):454–8.
16. Tsang WY, Chan JK, Ng CS. Kikuchi's lymphadenitis. A morphologic analysis of 75 cases with special reference to unusual features. Am J Surg Pathol 1994; 18(3):219–31.
17. Khanna R, Sharma AD, Khanna S, et al. Usefulness of ultrasonography for the evaluation of cervical lymphadenopathy. World J Surg Oncol 2011;9:29.
18. Kim BM, Kim EK, Kim MJ, et al. Sonographically guided core needle biopsy of cervical lymphadenopathy in patients without known malignancy. J Ultrasound Med 2007;26(5):585–91.
19. Lai KK, Stottmeier KD, Sherman IH, et al. Mycobacterial cervical lymphadenopathy. Relation of etiologic agents to age. JAMA 1984;251(10):1286–8.
20. Steinkamp HJ, Cornehl M, Hosten N, et al. Cervical lymphadenopathy: ratio of long- to short-axis diameter as a predictor of malignancy. Br J Radiol 1995; 68(807):266–70.
21. Steinkamp HJ, Maurer J, Cornehl M, et al. Recurrent cervical lymphadenopathy: differential diagnosis with color-duplex sonography. Eur Arch Otorhinolaryngol 1994;251(7):404–9.
22. Sumi M, Ohki M, Nakamura T. Comparison of sonography and CT for differentiating benign from malignant cervical lymph nodes in patients with squamous cell carcinoma of the head and neck. AJR Am J Roentgenol 2001;176(4):1019–24.
23. Wu CH, Chang YL, Hsu WC, et al. Usefulness of Doppler spectral analysis and power Doppler sonography in the differentiation of cervical lymphadenopathies. AJR Am J Roentgenol 1998;171(2):503–9.
24. Ying M, Ahuja A, Metreweli C. Diagnostic accuracy of sonographic criteria for evaluation of cervical lymphadenopathy. J Ultrasound Med 1998;17(7):437–45.
25. Ying M, Ahuja AT, Evans R, et al. Cervical lymphadenopathy: sonographic differentiation between tuberculous nodes and nodal metastases from non-head and neck carcinomas. J Clin Ultrasound 1998;26(8):383–9.
26. Knopf A, Bas M, Chaker A, et al. Rheumatic disorders affecting the head and neck: underestimated diseases. Rheumatology (Oxford) 2011;50(11):2029–34.

27. Morgenstern L. The Virchow-Troisier node: a historical note. Am J Surg 1979; 138(5):703.
28. Shipchandler TZ, Lorenz RR, McMahon J, et al. Supraclavicular lymphadenopathy due to silicone breast implants. Arch Otolaryngol Head Neck Surg 2007; 133(8):830–2.
29. Yong HS, Woo OH, Lee JW, et al. Primary localized amyloidosis manifested as supraclavicular and mediastinal lymphadenopathy. Br J Radiol 2007;80(955): e131–3.
30. Olsen KD, DeSanto LW, Pearson BW. Positive Delphian lymph node: clinical significance in laryngeal cancer. Laryngoscope 1987;97(9):1033–7.
31. Copeland EM, McBride CM. Axillary metastases from unknown primary sites. Ann Surg 1973;178(1):25–7.
32. de Andrade JM, Marana HR, Sarmento Filho JM, et al. Differential diagnosis of axillary masses. Tumori 1996;82(6):596–9.
33. Kobayashi O, Sugiyama Y, Konishi K, et al. Solitary metastasis to the left axillary lymph node after curative gastrectomy in gastric cancer. Gastric Cancer 2002; 5(3):173–6.
34. Sharma A, Fidias P, Hayman LA, et al. Patterns of lymphadenopathy in thoracic malignancies. Radiographics 2004;24(2):419–34.
35. Winterbauer RH, Belic N, Moores KD. Clinical interpretation of bilateral hilar adenopathy. Ann Intern Med 1973;78(1):65–71.
36. Glazer GM, Gross BH, Quint LE, et al. Normal mediastinal lymph nodes: number and size according to American Thoracic Society mapping. AJR Am J Roentgenol 1985;144(2):261–5.
37. Kiyono K, Sone S, Sakai F, et al. The number and size of normal mediastinal lymph nodes: a postmortem study. AJR Am J Roentgenol 1988;150(4):771–6.
38. Dorfman RE, Alpern MB, Gross BH, et al. Upper abdominal lymph nodes: criteria for normal size determined with CT. Radiology 1991;180(2):319–22.
39. Einstein DM, Singer AA, Chilcote WA, et al. Abdominal lymphadenopathy: spectrum of CT findings. Radiographics 1991;11(3):457–72.
40. Abu-Hilal M, Newman JS. Sister Mary Joseph and her nodule: historical and clinical perspective. Am J Med Sci 2009;337(4):271–3.
41. Selby CD, Marcus HS, Toghill PJ. Enlarged epitrochlear lymph nodes: an old physical sign revisited. J R Coll Physicians Lond 1992;26(2):159–61.
42. Zaren HA, Copeland EM 3rd. Inguinal node metastases. Cancer 1978;41(3): 919–23.
43. Wapnick S, MacKintosh M, Mauchaza B. Shoelessness, enlarged femoral lymph nodes, and femoral hernia. A possible association. Am J Surg 1973;126(1):108–10.
44. Chau I, Kelleher MT, Cunningham D, et al. Rapid access multidisciplinary lymph node diagnostic clinic: analysis of 550 patients. Br J Cancer 2003;88(3):354–61.
45. Pruzanski W. Lymphadenopathy associated with dysgammaglobulinemia. Semin Hematol 1980;17(1):44–62.
46. Lee Y, Terry R, Lukes RJ. Lymph node biopsy for diagnosis: a statistical study. J Surg Oncol 1980;14(1):53–60.
47. Pangalis GA, Vassilakopoulos TP, Boussiotis VA, et al. Clinical approach to lymphadenopathy. Semin Oncol 1993;20(6):570–82.
48. Baron BW, Baron JM. The diagnostic value of biopsy of small peripheral lymph nodes in patients with suspected lymphoma. Am J Hematol 2011. [Epub ahead of print].
49. Gupta AK, Nayar M, Chandra M. Reliability and limitations of fine needle aspiration cytology of lymphadenopathies. An analysis of 1,261 cases. Acta Cytol 1991; 35(6):777–83.

50. Margolis IB, Matteucci D, Organ CH Jr. To improve the yield of biopsy of the lymph nodes. Surg Gynecol Obstet 1978;147(3):376–8.
51. Sinclair S, Beckman E, Ellman L. Biopsy of enlarged, superficial lymph nodes. JAMA 1974;228(5):602–3.
52. Pinkus GS. Needle biopsy in malignant lymphoma. J Clin Oncol 1996;14(9): 2415–6.
53. Ben-Yehuda D, Polliack A, Okon E, et al. Image-guided core-needle biopsy in malignant lymphoma: experience with 100 patients that suggests the technique is reliable. J Clin Oncol 1996;14(9):2431–4.
54. Pappa VI, Hussain HK, Reznek RH, et al. Role of image-guided core-needle biopsy in the management of patients with lymphoma. J Clin Oncol 1996;14(9): 2427–30.
55. de Kerviler E, de Bazelaire C, Mounier N, et al. Image-guided core-needle biopsy of peripheral lymph nodes allows the diagnosis of lymphomas. Eur Radiol 2007; 17(3):843–9.
56. de Larrinoa AF, del Cura J, Zabala R, et al. Value of ultrasound-guided core biopsy in the diagnosis of malignant lymphoma. J Clin Ultrasound 2007;35(6): 295–301.
57. Suh YJ, Kim MJ, Kim J, et al. Tumor markers in fine-needle aspiration washout for cervical lymphadenopathy in patients with known malignancy: preliminary study. AJR Am J Roentgenol 2011;197(4):W730–6.
58. Tefferi A. Primary myelofibrosis: 2012 update on diagnosis, risk stratification, and management. Am J Hematol 2011;86(12):1017–26.
59. Tefferi A, Vainchenker W. Myeloproliferative neoplasms: molecular pathophysiology, essential clinical understanding, and treatment strategies. J Clin Oncol 2011;29(5):573–82.
60. vom Dahl S, Mengel E. Lysosomal storage diseases as differential diagnosis of hepatosplenomegaly. Best Pract Res Clin Gastroenterol 2010;24(5):619–28.
61. Grover SA, Barkun AN, Sackett DL. The rational clinical examination. Does this patient have splenomegaly? JAMA 1993;270(18):2218–21.
62. Berris B. The incidence of palpable liver and spleen in the postpartum period. Can Med Assoc J 1966;95(25):1318–9.
63. Benter T, Kluhs L, Teichgraber U. Sonography of the spleen. J Ultrasound Med 2011;30(9):1281–93.
64. Prassopoulos P, Daskalogiannaki M, Raissaki M, et al. Determination of normal splenic volume on computed tomography in relation to age, gender and body habitus. Eur Radiol 1997;7(2):246–8.
65. Bezerra AS, D'Ippolito G, Faintuch S, et al. Determination of splenomegaly by CT: is there a place for a single measurement? AJR Am J Roentgenol 2005;184(5): 1510–3.
66. Stark DD, Moss AA, Goldberg HI. Nuclear magnetic resonance of the liver, spleen, and pancreas. Cardiovasc Intervent Radiol 1986;8(5–6):329–41.
67. Lee J, Kim KW, Lee H, et al. Semiautomated spleen volumetry with diffusion-weighted MR imaging. Magn Reson Med 2011. [Epub ahead of print].
68. Mesa RA. How I treat symptomatic splenomegaly in patients with myelofibrosis. Blood 2009;113(22):5394–400.
69. Koshenkov VP, Nemeth ZH, Carter MS. Laparoscopic splenectomy: outcome and efficacy for massive and supramassive spleens. Am J Surg 2011. [Epub ahead of print].
70. Lavu H. The feasibility and safety of laparoscopic splenectomy for massive splenomegaly: a comparative study. J Surg Res 2011. [Epub ahead of print].

Special Hematologic Issues in the Pregnant Patient

Tina Rizack, MD, MPH[a],*, Karen Rosene-Montella, MD[b]

KEYWORDS

- Hematologic disorder • Blood • Pregnancy
- Physiologic changes

An understanding of hematologic disorders in pregnancy requires knowledge of the normal physiologic changes in pregnancy (**Table 1**). During pregnancy, plasma volume increases by about 50%, rapidly by week 6 of gestation and then more gradually, peaking by week 30. Erythrocyte mass increases by only 18% to 30% during pregnancy, resulting in a dilution effect (hematocrit 30%–32%) referred to as physiologic anemia of pregnancy.[1,2] Other physiologic changes, including an increase in clotting factors, occur as the parturient accommodates a growing uterus and placenta and prepares for the hemostasis needed for delivery.

ANEMIA

In pregnancy, anemia is generally well tolerated. The Centers for Disease Control and Prevention defines anemia in pregnancy as a hemoglobin of less than 11 g/dL in the first and third trimesters and less than 10.5 g/dL in the second trimester.[3] For women with adequate iron stores, the hemoglobin should return to normal around 1 to 6 weeks after delivery.[4] A hemoglobin of less than 10 g/dL should prompt a work-up for a pathologic cause. Severe anemia, defined as a hemoglobin less than 6 g/dL, has been associated with reduced amniotic fluid volume, fetal cerebral vasodilatation, and nonreassuring fetal heart rate tracings.[5] There have also been reports of increased risk of prematurity, spontaneous abortion, low birth weight, and fetal death.[6] A hemoglobin of less than 7 g/dL increases the risk of maternal mortality.[7] Current recommendations are for all pregnant women to have a baseline complete blood count before pregnancy or at the first prenatal visit, and again in the third trimester.

Disclosures: Dr Tina Rizack has no financial relationship to disclose. Dr Karen Rosene-Montella has no financial relationship to disclose.

[a] Women & Infants Hospital, Alpert Medical School of Brown University, 101 Dudley Street, Providence, RI 02905, USA
[b] The Miriam Hospital, Alpert Medical School of Brown University, 164 Summit Avenue, Providence, RI 02906, USA
* Corresponding author.
E-mail address: trizack@wihri.org

Hematol Oncol Clin N Am 26 (2012) 409–432
doi:10.1016/j.hoc.2012.02.004
0889-8588/12/$ – see front matter © 2012 Elsevier Inc. All rights reserved.

hemonc.theclinics.com

Table 1 Normal hematologic values and changes in pregnancy		
Test	**Reference Intervals**	**Change in Pregnancy**
CBC		
WBC	$3.00–10.5 \times 10^9/L$	↑ to $10–16 \times 10^9/L$
Hb	115–155 g/L	↓ 100–130 g/L
Platelet count	$100–400 \times 10^9/L$	↓ near term to as low as $100 \times 10^9/L$
PTT	24–36 s	↔
INR	0.9–1.2	↔
Fibrinogen	>2.0 g/L	↑↑
VWF	Group 0: 0.40–1.75 U/mL Nongroup 0: 0.70–2.10 U/mL	↑
Factor VIII	0.6–1.95 U/mL	↑
D-dimer	<300 µg/L	↑
Protein C	Functional: 0.75–1.60 U/mL Antigen: 0.70–1.20 U/mL	↔
Protein S	Functional: 0.50–1.00 U/mL Antigen: 0.57–1.20 U/mL	↓
AT	0.80–1.25 U/mL	↔
Homocysteine	<10 µmol/L	↓
Ferritin	—	↑
ESR	—	↑

Abbreviations: AT, antithrombin; CBC, complete blood count; ESR, erythrocyte sedimentation rate; Hb, hemoglobin; INR, international normalized ratio; PTT, partial thromboplastin time; VWF, Von Willebrand factor antigen; WBC, leukocytes.

Reprinted from Rodger M. Normal hematologic changes in pregnancy. In: Rosene-Montella K, Keely E, Barbour LA, et al, editors. Medical care of the pregnant patient. 2nd edition. Philadelphia (PA): American College of Physicians; 2008. p. 423. Table 35-1; with permission.

Iron Deficiency Anemia

Iron deficiency anemia accounts for most (>90%) nonphysiologic anemias. During a normal singleton pregnancy, a woman loses 1000 mg of iron to the fetus and placenta, expansion of red blood cells (RBCs), and insensible losses.[8] Studies of the efficacy of iron supplementation on pregnancy outcomes are lacking. Transferrin is usually increased with pregnancy. Serum ferritin is a useful screening test for iron deficiency in pregnancy, with a sensitivity of 90% and specificity of 85%.[9] Iron repletion recommendations are generally the same for pregnant patients as nonpregnant patients. The current recommendation is 15 to 30 mg daily of supplemental elemental iron for all pregnant women. Parental iron can be used for patients who do not absorb or are intolerant of oral iron. Iron sucrose in pregnancy has better safety data and is preferable to iron dextran. Recombinant erythropoietin has been shown to be of some benefit in patients with an inadequate response to iron, but it may cause a hypertensive effect.[10] However, data are limited to only 1 study and this should not be considered standard of care at this point. In patients refractory to standard iron repletion, another cause of anemia should be investigated.

Macrocytic Anemias

Macrocytic anemias are most commonly caused by folate deficiency and, rarely, vitamin B_{12} deficiency. Accurate diagnosis of both folate and B_{12} deficiency in pregnancy usually requires measuring plasma homocysteine and methylmalonic acid levels. Folate deficiency is caused by increased demands from the fetus and erythropoiesis from the expansion of maternal red cell mass. Hormonal changes of pregnancy can decrease folate absorption and increase urine losses.[11] Folate requirements increase from 50 µg/d in the nonpregnant patient to 150 µg/d in pregnant patients. The current recommendation is 1 mg daily of supplemental folate for all pregnant women. This folate supplementation prevents neural tube defects and folic acid deficiency. Higher doses of folate are recommended in patients on antiepileptic drugs, which further deplete maternal folate levels, and in patients with a previously affected child with a neural tube defect. Repletion for both vitamin B_{12} and folate deficiency are the same as for nonpregnant patients. Other less common causes of macrocytic anemia include alcohol use, medications, hypothyroidism, and liver disease.

Hemoglobinopathies

For most women with hemoglobinopathies, pregnancy is possible and successful with increased monitoring to avoid maternal and fetal complications.

Sickle Cell Disease

Sickle cell syndrome is caused by an inherited single nucleotide (GAG/GTG) mutation in the β-globin gene. Heterozygosity for HbS (sickle cell trait) does not cause disease but homozygous inheritance or compound heterozygous inheritance with another mutant β-globin gene does result in sickle cell disease. At least 17 hemoglobinopathies resulting in sickle cell disease variants exist. The more common types are listed in **Table 2**. Some risks to the mother and fetus are caused by pregnancy. Pregnancy-related increases in adhesion and coagulation proteins, such as Von Willebrand factor, fibrinogen, and factor VIII, may exacerbate RBC adhesion leading to RBC and platelet aggregation.[12] This process results in occlusion of the vessels and a vasoocclusive event, which may be more frequent during pregnancy. The frequency of obstetric complication in women with sickle cell disease is shown in **Table 3**. Sickle cell disease carries approximately a 6.5% risk of spontaneous abortion according to the Cooperative Study of Sickle Disease.[13] Rates of intrauterine growth restriction may be increased in women with sickle cell disease, especially those with acute complications of sickle cell disease during pregnancy.[13,14] Preterm labor, placental abruption, and preeclampsia may be more common in patients with sickle cell anemia (HbSS disease) compared with healthy African American women without sickle cell disease.[13,14]

Table 2
Characteristics of common sickle cell diseases compared with sickle cell trait

Disease	Baseline Hb (g/dL)	MCV	Baseline Reticulocyte (%)	Relative Clinical Severity
HbSS	6.0–9.0	Normal	5–30	++++
HbS-β°-thalassemia	6.0–9.0	Low	5–30	++++
HbSC	10.0–13.0	Normal	3–4	+++
HbS-β⁺-thalassemia	10.0–14.0	Low	3–4	++
Hb AS	14.0–16.0	Normal	0–1	0

Abbreviations: Hb AS, sickle cell trait; HbSC, sickle hemoglobin C disease; HbSS, sickle cell anemia; MCV, mean corpuscular volume.

Reprinted from Hassell K. Hemoglobinopathies, thalassemias, and anemia. In: Rosene-Montella K, Keely E, Barbour LA, et al, editors. Medical care of the pregnant patient. 2nd edition. Philadelphia (PA): American College of Physicians; 2008. p. 486. Table 40-1; with permission.

Table 3
Frequency of obstetric complications in women with sickle cell disease

| | Transfusion Study, 1978–1986 | | | Cooperative Study, 1979–1986 |
	Control	SS	SC	Sβthal	
Number of pregnancies	8981	100	66	23	225
Gestational age at delivery (wk)	40	37.5	38.6	37.1	37.7
Preterm labor (%)	17	26	15	22	9
Placenta previa (%)	0.4	1	2	4	—
Abruptio placenta (%)	0.5	3	2	4	—
Toxemia (%)	4	18	9	13	11
Cesarean section (%)	14	29	30	26	—

Abbreviations: Sβthal, sickle β thalassemia; SC, sickle hemoglobin C; SS, sickle cell anemia.
Reprinted from Hassell K. Hemoglobinopathies, thalassemias, and anemia. In: Rosene-Montella K, Keely E, Barbour LA, et al, editors. Medical care of the pregnant patient. 2nd edition. Philadelphia (PA): American College of Physicians; 2008. p. 489. Table 40-2; with permission.

Patients should be followed in a high-risk clinic in conjunction with a health care provider familiar with the care of patients with sickle cell disease. A complete blood count, reticulocyte count, urinalysis, and blood pressure monitoring are recommended with each visit. A prenatal vitamin without iron and with additional folate should be prescribed.[15] During the first trimester, preventing nausea and volume depletion may decrease sickle cell–related complications. Close monitoring for the development of sickle cell pain events such as acute chest syndrome, acute splenic sequestration, splenic infarct, and acute multiorgan failure is recommended during pregnancy, labor, and the postpartum period. Pain crises are treated similarly to nonpregnant patients and are outlined in **Table 4**. Adequate intravenous fluid administration and oxygenation should be maintained during labor. Analgesia doses may exceed those usually required for obstetric pain because of increased tolerance of pain medications used for pain crises.[16] Indications for cesarean section are obstetric and the same as for patients without sickle cell disease.

Table 4
Management of acute sickle cell pain episodes in pregnant women

IV fluids: correct dehydration, then maintain euvolemia
Oxygen therapy: maintain normal oxygen saturation
Investigation and treatment of infection
Pain control: IV on a regular schedule (not as needed)
Monitor for complications of sickle cell disease:
    Daily complete blood count and reticulocyte count
    Baseline chemistry profile; repeat as needed for clinical deterioration
    Frequent pulse oximetry

Narcotics (IV)	Nonnarcotic Adjuncts (First-Second Trimester)
Morphine sulfate	Nonsteroidal antiinflammatory drugs
Hydromorphone	Diphenhydramine
Fentanyl	

Abbreviation: IV, intravenous.
Reprinted from Hassell K. Hemoglobinopathies, thalassemias, and anemia. In: Rosene-Montella K, Keely E, Barbour LA, et al, editors. Medical care of the pregnant patient. 2nd edition. Philadelphia (PA): American College of Physicians; 2008. p. 491. Table 40-3; with permission.

Chronic anemia associated with sickle cell disease is exacerbated by the usual dilution effect of pregnancy. Iron repletion does not correct the anemia and should be avoided because many patients are already iron overloaded from repeat transfusions. The use of prophylactic blood transfusions is not supported.[17,18] Simple or exchange transfusions should be instituted for the same indications as for nonpregnant patients, including stroke, ocular events, severe acute chest syndrome, splenic sequestration, symptomatic aplastic crisis, and cerebrovascular accident (**Box 1**).[19]

Pregnant patients with suspected sickle cell trait should be confirmed by hemoglobin electrophoresis. These women are at increased risk of bacteruria that may lead to urinary tract infections or pyelonephritis; thus, even asymptomatic bacteruria should be treated.[20]

Thalassemia

Thalassemias are a result of quantitative disorders of hemoglobin production resulting from decreased or imbalanced production of generally structurally normal globins. In β-thalassemia, a mutation in β-globin leads to decreased production and an excess of α-globins and the reverse for mutations in α-globins in α-thalassemias. These mutations result in membrane damage and red cell fragility, causing microcytosis with target cell morphology and a chronic hemolytic anemia with compensatory reticulocytosis and splenomegaly. α-Thalassemias occur more commonly in Asian, African, or Mediterranean populations. β-Thalassemias occur more commonly in Mediterranean and African populations.

In general, women with α-thalassemia or β-thalassemia trait tolerate pregnancy well. These patients have a mild baseline microcytic anemia and, despite increased iron absorption characteristic of thalassemia, iron deficiency can develop and iron studies may need to be checked during pregnancy.[21] Patients with severe α-thalassemia and β-thalassemia intermedia have compromised fertility, and few pregnancies have been reported. Approximately 50% of pregnancies result in stillbirth, intrauterine growth restriction, and preterm delivery.[22] In a small number of patients, term pregnancy was attained with the use of transfusion support with target hemoglobin of 10 gm/dl.[23]

THROMBOCYTOPENIA

Thrombocytopenia affects 10% of pregnancies and can be isolated or part of a systemic disorder. The thrombocytopenia cause may be specific to or unrelated

---

Box 1
Recommended indications for transfusion in pregnant women with sickle cell disease

- Toxemia

- Severe anemia (decrease to 30% less than the baseline or Hb ≤6.0 g/dL)

- Acute renal failure

- Septicemia/bacteremia

- Acute chest syndrome with hypoxia or other severe sickle cell complication

- Anticipated surgery

Abbreviation: Hb, hemoglobin.
   Reprinted from Hassell K. Hemoglobinopathies, thalassemias, and anemia. In: Rosene-Montella K, Keely E, Barbour LA, et al, editors. Medical care of the pregnant patient. 2nd edition. Philadelphia (PA): American College of Physicians; 2008. p. 492. Table 40-5, with permission.

to pregnancy. Most cases are asymptomatic and detected incidentally by routine screening of blood counts during pregnancy. Manifestations include easy bruising, petechiae, epistaxis, and gingival bleeding. Significant hemorrhage is rare, even when counts decrease to less than 20,000/μL. The major causes of thrombocytopenia in pregnancy are presented in **Table 5**. A 10% decrease in platelets can commonly be seen in pregnancy. For general management, most women can continue routine obstetric care. The mode of delivery for patients with thrombocytopenia should be determined by obstetric indications. No studies have been conducted to determine the optimal platelet count but observational data indicate that a platelet count of more than 50,000/μL to 75,000/μL is adequate for epidural anesthesia, vaginal delivery, and cesarean section.[24,25] However, the treating team and the anesthesiologist should individualize each patient's care.

- Gestational thrombocytopenia is a benign form of thrombocytopenia that represents the most common cause of thrombocytopenia in pregnant woman. Patients typically have platelet counts greater than 70,000/μL. It is not associated with any adverse outcomes for the mother or the fetus. The cause of the thrombocytopenia is not well understood but could be related to diminished platelet survival combined with the physiologic increase in plasma volume. Gestational thrombocytopenia is considered a diagnosis of exclusion and it is often difficult to differentiate from idiopathic thrombocytopenia (ITP).
- ITP is found in approximately 1 in 10,000 pregnancies and usually presents in the first trimester. There have been isolated cases of ITP that cause thrombocytopenia in the neonate. No correlation has been found between maternal and fetal/neonatal platelet counts. Most cases of severe fetal or neonatal thrombocytopenia are related to alloimmune thrombocytopenia (discussed later). There is no evidence to support the need for intrapartum fetal platelet counts in patients with ITP. ITP in pregnancy is generally treated with either corticosteroids or intravenous immunoglobulin (IVIG) for similar indications as in nonpregnant patients, with an attempt to keep platelet counts at more than 50,000 to 70,000/μL near term. For refractory patients, a combination of corticosteroids and IVIG is recommended. Splenectomy can be considered but should be reserved for the second trimester. Rituximab, a pregnancy class C medication, has been used successfully in a limited number of pregnant women, including 1 case of ITP that was associated with asymptomatic neonatal B-lymphocyte suppression.[26–28] The thrombopoietic agents romiplostim and eltrombopag are pregnancy class C medications, and there are no data to recommend use in pregnancy.
- Preeclampsia affects 6% of first pregnancies, and about 50% of these patients have thrombocytopenia. The pathophysiology of the thrombocytopenia is not well understood but accelerated platelet consumption is thought to contribute.
- HELLP (hemolysis, increased liver function tests, and low platelets) syndrome, which affects between 0.1% and 0.89% of pregnancies, shares many clinical features with preeclampsia and is often considered a variant of severe preeclampsia. HELLP has a higher rate of maternal and fetal mortality than preeclampsia, making correct diagnosis and treatment imperative. Patients with HELLP typically have a microangiopathic hemolytic anemia with schistocytes seen on peripheral blood smear, an increased lactate dehydrogenase (LDH), serum levels of aspartate aminotransferase greater than 70 U/L, and platelet counts less than 100,000/μL. HELLP is often difficult to differentiate from thrombotic thrombocytopenic purpura-hemolytic uremic syndrome (TTP-HUS). Treatment of preeclampsia and HELLP consists of stabilization of the

Table 5
Differential diagnosis of thrombocytopenia in pregnancy

	Incidence (%)	Timing of Onset	Degree of Thrombocytopenia	Microangiopathic Chemolytic Anemia	Hypertension	Coagulopathy	Liver Disease	Renal Disease	CNS Disease
ITP	3–4	Most common in first trimester, anytime	Mild to severe	None	None	None	None	None	None
Gestational/ incidental thrombocytopenia	75–80	Second–third trimester	Mild	None	None	None	None	None	None
Preeclampsia	15–20	Late second to third trimester	Mild to moderate	Mild	Moderate to severe	None to mild	None	Proteinuria	Seizures with preeclampsia
HELPP	—	Late second to third trimester	Moderate to severe	Moderate to severe	None to severe	Absent to mild	Moderate to severe	None to moderate	None to moderate
DIC	Rare	Anytime	Moderate to severe	Mild to moderate	None	Mild to severe	Variable	Variable	None
AFLP	Rare	Third trimester	Mild	Mild	None to mild	Severe	Severe	None to mild	None to mild
TTP	Rare	Second to third trimester	Severe	Moderate to severe	None	None	None	None to moderate	None to severe
HUS	Rare	After birth	Moderate to severe	Moderate to severe	None to mild	None	None	Moderate to severe	None to mild

Abbreviations: AFLP, acute fatty liver pregnancy; DIC, disseminated intravascular coagulation; HELPP, hemolysis, elevated liver function tests, low platelets; HUS, hemolytic uremic syndrome; ITP, immune thrombocytopenia; TTP, thrombotic thrombocytopenic purpura.

mother followed by expeditious delivery, which usually results in resolution of the disorder within 3 to 4 days. However, both syndromes, especially HELLP, occasionally worsen or develop in the postpartum period. There are limited data from several small, randomized studies of the use of corticosteroids in the prenatal or postnatal setting. Corticosteroids for HELLP are thought to hasten the resolution of thrombocytopenia and laboratory abnormalities when used 5 to 7 days after delivery for worsening thrombocytopenia or other signs of clinical decline. However, clear efficacy rather than just correction of laboratory abnormalities has not been shown.[29]

- TTP risk increases during pregnancy. Pregnant women comprise 10% to 20% of patients with TTP. TTP typically develops in the second or third trimester. Treatment is plasma exchange. The risk of HUS also increases with pregnancy and most cases develop 3 to 4 weeks after birth. Atypical HUS with renal failure as the predominant manifestation is the most common. The prognosis of postpartum HUS is poor, with more than 25% of patients with persistent renal failure. Plasma exchange is recommended despite low response rates because of the difficulty differentiating HUS from TTP.

- Disseminated intravascular coagulation (DIC) may accompany preeclampsia and may also result from retained fetal products, sepsis, placental abruption, or amniotic fluid embolization. In general, the thrombocytopenia is milder and the degree of microangiopathic hemolysis is less than with TTP, HUS, or HELLP. DIC in pregnancy can be abrupt, severe, and fatal if not addressed appropriately. Therapy is aimed at treating the underlying condition that precipitated the DIC. The British Committee for Standards in Haematology has published guidelines for the management of DIC.[30] Transfusion support should be based on the presence of bleeding from low platelets or a prolonged prothrombin time. Cryoprecipitate may be used for severe hypofibrinogenemia (fibrinogen <100 g/dL) that persists after plasma therapy. Low doses of heparin may be indicated for patients with significant thrombosis.

- Acute fatty liver of pregnancy, another pregnancy-specific cause of thrombocytopenia, usually occurs during the third trimester in primaparas and twin gestations. Typical symptoms are usually nausea, vomiting, right upper quadrant pain, anorexia, jaundice, and increased liver enzymes consistent with cholestasis. Most patients have concurrent DIC. Diabetes insipidus and hypoglycemia are present in more than half of cases. Bleeding is common, caused by coagulopathy resulting from diminished hepatic synthesis of coagulation factors, as well as DIC and acquired antithrombin deficiency.

- Additional causes of thrombocytopenia include pseudothrombocytopenia (caused by platelet aggregation induced by ethylenediamine tetraacetic acid); hypersplenism; congenital platelet disorders such as Bernard-Soulier syndrome, May-Hegglin anomaly, gray platelet syndrome, and Glanzmann thrombasthenia; bone marrow disease; drug-induced, human immunodeficiency virus, and other autoimmune thrombocytopenias; congenital thrombocytopenias; and type 2B Von Willebrand Disease (VWD; discussed later).

PLATELET FUNCTION DISORDERS

Platelet function disorders are a heterogeneous group of bleeding disorders caused by defects in platelet function resulting in a defect in the primary platelet plug of hemostasis. These rare disorders are mainly congenital and include platelet storage disorders (ie, Bernard-Soulier syndrome and Glanzmann thrombasthenia), platelet secretion disorders, and platelet cytoskeletal disorders. Some platelet cytoskeletal disorders are acquired from medications, uremia, liver disease, acquired antiplatelet antibodies, dysproteinemia, myeloproliferative disease, acute myeloid leukemia, acquired storage pool disorders, and acquired VWD. Most patients with platelet function disorders have similar manifestations that include bruising and bleeding from minor lacerations, spontaneous gingival bleeding, epistaxis, and gastrointestinal bleeding.

Treatment of platelet function disorders is based on the underlying disorder and personal bleeding history. Routine cesarean sections are not recommended. Episiotomy, instrumental vaginal delivery, and epidural anesthesia should be avoided. Platelet transfusions are often indicated to prevent or treat bleeding, with prophylactic platelet transfusions reserved for patients with severe disorders.[31] Desmopressin acetate (DDAVP) during labor has been used successfully in some patients with platelet function disorders.[32] The use of recombinant factor VIIa with Bernard-Soulier syndrome and Glanzmann thrombasthenia is recommended to prevent alloimmunization from platelet transfusion or in patients who already have platelet antibodies.[33] These patients require monthly monitoring for antiplatelet antibodies after 20 weeks. If antiplatelet antibodies are identified, then care should be coordinated with maternal fetal medicine to monitor for neonatal alloimmune thrombocytopenia.

VON WILLEBRAND DISEASE (VWD) AND OTHER BLEEDING DISORDERS

Pregnancy normally leads to a shift in the hemostatic balance toward coagulation. However, 10% of maternal deaths are a result of bleeding disorders (this is the leading cause of maternal mortality in developing nations). Patients with known bleeding disorders are at higher risk and may require additional screening and therapy to prevent or stop bleeding complications. Pregnancy is often the first manifestation of an undiagnosed bleeding disorder. Bleeding disorders can be congenital or acquired (**Box 2**) and caused by either low levels of coagulation factors or platelet abnormalities. VWD and deficiencies of factor VIII, IX, and XI are the most common inherited coagulation factor deficiencies complicating pregnancy. General principles for management of congenital bleeding disorders in pregnancy are shown in **Box 3**.

Von Willebrand Disease (VWD)

VWD is the most common inherited bleeding disorder and is found in approximately 1% of the general population.[34] Von Willebrand factor (VWF) is the primary plasma protein required for platelet adhesion and is important for platelet aggregation. Absence or reduced amounts of VWF or an abnormal VWF protein results in defective platelet adhesion and aggregation that leads to mucocutaneous bleeding. There are several variants. Most (75%) patients have type 1 VWD, which is a result of a partial, quantitative deficiency of VWF. Type 2 VWD is less common. It is caused by a qualitative defect and has several subtypes: type 2A, type 2B, type 2N, and type 2M. Types 1 and 2 are autosomal dominant modes of inheritance. Type 3 VWD is autosomal recessive inheritance with incomplete penetrance. It is characterized by severe deficiency in VWF resulting in a deficiency in factor VIII (FVIII) and is the rarest of the three.[35]

The diagnosis of VWD is based on a clinical history of bruising or bleeding. Characteristics and laboratory findings of VWD are shown in **Table 6**. Levels of VWF are also affected by ABO blood groups and levels do not always correspond with bleeding phenotype.[36] A health care provider experienced in bleeding disorders should follow patients.

There is no evidence that VWD affects fertility or the rate of miscarriage.[37] Increased estrogen levels in pregnancy result in an increase in VWF and FVIII beginning in the

---

Box 2
Bleeding disorders in pregnancy

Congenital disorders

- VWD

- Hemophilia A carrier

- Hemophilia B carrier

- Factor XI deficiencies

- Other rare coagulation factor defects

- Hyperfibrinolytic disorders

- Platelet function disorders (eg, Glanzmann thrombasthenia, Bernard-Soulier syndrome)

Acquired disorders

- ITP

- TTP

- HELLP syndrome

- Drug-related thrombocytopenia

- Acquired factor VIII deficiency

- DIC

- Anticoagulants (oral, intravenous, subcutaneous)

- Vitamin K deficiency

- Antiplatelet agents (eg, acetylsalicylic acid, nonsteroidal antiinflammatories)

- Renal failure

Reprinted from Tinmouth AT, Rodger M. Bleeding disorders. In: Rosene-Montella K, Keely E, Barbour LA, et al, editors. Medical care of the pregnant patient. 2nd edition. Philadelphia (PA): American College of Physicians; 2008. p. 461. Table 38-1; with permission.

---

early second trimester and peaking between 29 and 35 weeks. Most patients with type 1 VWD normalize levels of VWF and FVIII during pregnancy but patients with severe disease may not. The response rate of VWF and FVIII in individual pregnancies is unpredictable, and it is recommended that measurement of VWF levels be done between 32 and 34 weeks of pregnancy for delivery planning and both immediately after birth and at 2 to 3 weeks after delivery when plasma levels may decrease rapidly and bleeding may occur.[38,39] Levels of VWF may increase in patients with type 2 VWD but functional levels may not change because of the production of functionally deficient proteins. In type 3 VWD, levels generally do not increase with pregnancy.

VWF and FVIII levels should be 50 IU/dL or greater for epidural anesthesia and delivery. For levels less than 50 IU/dL, prophylactic treatment with DDAVP for type 1 and some type 2 VWDs at the time of parturition, particularly with cesarean delivery, and for approximately 3 to 5 days after birth.[40,41] Both intravenous and intranasal formulations are safe in the second and third trimesters. However, intranasal DDAVP is generally reserved for less serious bleeding in an outpatient setting. Typical intravenous dosing is 0.3 μg/kg every 8 to 12 hours. Judicious administration of fluids is recommended with the use of DDAVP to avoid severe hyponatremia, hypertension, and fluid retention. Tachyphylaxis can occur with repeated doses of DDAVP. For patients with type 3 VWD, VWF levels remain low or unmeasurable during pregnancy and replacement therapy with VWF concentrates is needed during labor and

> **Box 3**
> **General principles for management of pregnancy in patients with congenital bleeding disorders**
>
> - Close liaison between a hematologist/hemophilia treatment center and the obstetric service
> - Prepregnancy counseling including determination of coagulation factor/VWF levels or carrier status
> - Baseline coagulation factor/VWF levels early in pregnancy and at 28 to 32 weeks of gestation
> - Fetal sex determination for hemophilia carriers
> - Prenatal fetal diagnosis for hemophilia carriers
> - Elective cesarean section not routinely indicated
> - Prophylactic therapy for invasive procedures and delivery if coagulation factor levels are decreased
> - Fetal scalp electrodes and blood sampling should be avoided for any potentially affected fetuses
> - Vacuum extraction and forceps delivery should be avoided for any potentially affected fetuses
> - Cord blood sampling for clotting factor levels for any potentially affected fetuses
> - Vitamin K by mouth for any potentially affected fetuses
> - Circumcision should be delayed until coagulation factor level is known and appropriate management arranged
>
> *Reprinted from* Tinmouth AT, Rodger M. Bleeding disorders. In: Rosene-Montella K, Keely L, Barbour LA, et al, editors. Medical care of the pregnant patient. 2nd edition. Philadelphia (PA): American College of Physicians; 2008. p. 466. Table 38-4; with permission.

postpartum.[37] For patients with type 2B VWD, thrombocytopenia may develop or worsen during pregnancy. However, whether this thrombocytopenia exacerbates bleeding is unclear.[42] Some of these patients may require VWF concentrates.

Other Congenital Disorders of Coagulation

Other congenital disorders of coagulation are less common and include hemophilia A and B and factor XI deficiency. All of these can also be sporadic as well as inherited. Hemophilia A and B are X-linked disorders. Female carriers of hemophilia A and B may have decreased levels of factor VIII and IX respectively, with associated bleeding risks. Normally, factor levels in female carriers are greater than 50% but levels can be variable. In 10% to 20% of carriers, coagulation factors are less than 40%. Diagnosis is made by family history of hemophilia and measuring individual coagulation factor levels with or without genetic analysis. In addition, women may be homozygotes for hemophilia A and B. These woman have lower FVII or FIX levels and often require infusion of purified factor concentrates at the time of delivery. In addition, male neonates have hemophilia requiring comprehensive hematologic care. In all cases, hematologists experienced in treating hemophilia and associated with an institution with a hemophilia comprehensive care clinic should follow these women.[43] Factor VIII levels as discussed earlier in VWD tend to increase in the second and third trimester but can be variable. Factor IX levels tend to remain unchanged during pregnancy. Baseline coagulation factor levels should be established early in pregnancy and rechecked in the third trimester and before invasive procedures. No treatment is

Table 6
VWD characteristics and laboratory findings

Type	Characteristic	Diagnostic Laboratory Findings
1	Partial quantitative deficiency	Factor VIII, VWF:Ag, VWF:RCoF proportionately decreased Normal multimer pattern
2A	Loss of high-molecular-weight multimers	VWF:RCoF disproportionately decreased Loss of high-molecular-weight multimers on electrophoresis gel
2B	Increased affinity of VWF multimers to platelet glycoprotein Ib/IX	VWF:RCoF disproportionately decreased Decrease in high-molecular-weight multimers on electrophoresis gel Increased ristocetin-induced platelet aggregation Decreased platelets
2M	Decreased platelet activity with preservation of high-molecular-weight multimers	VWF:RCoF disproportionately decreased Normal multimer pattern Factor VIII disproportionately decreased
2N	Decreased binding of factor VIII	Absent VWF:Ag, VWF:RCoF
3	Absence or near absence of detectable VWF	No multimers on electrophoresis gel

Abbreviation: RCoF, ristocetin cofactor.
Reprinted from Tinmouth AT, Rodger M. Bleeding disorders. In: Rosene-Montella K, Keely E, Barbour LA, et al, editors. Medical care of the pregnant patient. 2nd edition. Philadelphia (PA): American College of Physicians; 2008. p. 465. Table 38-2; with permission.

required for levels of more than 0.5 U/mL. For levels less than 0.5 U/mL, factor should be given before delivery or invasive procedures. General recommendations are to keep the levels at more than 0.5U/mL for 3 to 4 days after vaginal delivery and 4 to 5 days for a cesarean section.

Factor XI deficiency is rare, affecting 5% of all patients with bleeding disorders. Diagnosis is usually made by family history or investigation of a bleeding disorder. In patients with factor XI levels less than 30%, partial thromboplastin time (PTT) can be increased. A factor XI assay is still recommended to confirm diagnosis. In general, patients who are homozygous or compound heterozygotes have factor levels of less than 20%, and bleeding problems with hemostatic challenge. Heterozygotes have factor XI levels between 20% and 60% with variable bleeding complications.[44] Bleeding is less severe and less predictable than with hemophilia A and B.[45] In patients with factor XI deficiency, levels of factor XI during pregnancy have been reported as both increased and decreased.[46–49] Treatment decisions are based on bleeding history and factor XI levels, with a goal factor XI level of 0.7 U/mL during delivery and cesarean section or other procedures.[42] Treatment options include fresh frozen plasma (FFP), factor XI concentrate, and recombinant factor VIIa. Given the limited availability of factor XI concentrate and the small amount of factor XI in FFP, the use of recombinant factor VIIa is favored.[50]

Acquired Disorders

Acquired factor VIII inhibitor (acquired hemophilia A) is a rare disorder that occurs when autoantibodies develop against factor VIII. It is often associated with pregnancy, malignancy, pemphigoid, rheumatoid arthritis, systemic lupus erythematosus, and other autoimmune diseases. However, in about half the patients, no clinical association is identified.[51] Approximately 10% to 15% of cases are associated with pregnancy.[52] Most cases occur during the postpartum period, usually within 4 months of delivery. Bleeding symptoms can vary, are associated with the level of antibody activity, and can be life threatening. Treatment consists of controlling bleeding and therapy to eradicate the inhibitor. For patients with low antibody titer levels (<10 Bethesda units) factor VIII concentrates can be used. Patients with high titer antibodies are treated with bypassing agents. Treatment to eradicate the inhibitor consists of immunosuppressive therapy; usually steroids alone or with cyclophosphamide. Cyclophosphamide and other alkylating agents should be avoided in women who desire future fertility.[53] Rituximab is recommended for second-line treatment. There are limited data on first-line use of rituximab, but large prospective trials are lacking.[54]

THROMBOPHILIA AND THROMBOEMBOLISM

Pregnancy and the puerperium are hypercoagulable states that prepare for the bleeding challenge of delivery. Pregnancy increases the risk of thromboembolism 4 to 5 times and cesarean section doubles that risk.[55] Venodilatation with venous stasis is a progesterone effect that begins early in pregnancy. Most pregnancy-related thrombotic events are venous thromboembolisms (VTEs). Most VTEs occur during pregnancy, but more than one-third occur after birth.[56] Arterial thromboembolism risk is also increased during pregnancy.

Many coagulation factors (fibrinogen; factors V, VII, VIII, X; and VWF) increase during normal pregnancy by 20% to 100% from the first to the third trimester (**Table 7**). Plasminogen activator inhibitor types 1 and 2 are also increased. Factor XI and protein S decrease, whereas other coagulation factors, such as II and IX, remain the same.[57] Fibrinolysis is decreased. Most (>90%) deep vein thromboses

Table 7 Changes in coagulation factor levels in pregnancy	
Coagulation Factor	**Changes in Pregnancy (%)**
Fibrinogen	↑ (175–46)
Thrombin (factor II)	↔
Factor V	↑ (0–30)
Factor VIII	↑ (55–70)
Factor IX	↔
Factor X	↑ (22–23)
Factor XI	↓ (10–40)
VWF antigen	↑ (87–100)
VWF RCoF	↑ (100)
Protein C	↔
Protein S (total)	↓ (7–16)
Protein S (free)	↓ (30–54)
PAI-1	↑ (58)
PAI-2	↑ (385)

Abbreviations: PAI-1, plasminogen activator inhibitor 1; PAI-2, plasminogen activator inhibitor 2; VWF RCoF, Von Willebrand factor ristocetin cofactor.

Reprinted from Rodger M. Normal hematologic changes in pregnancy. In: Rosene-Montella K, Keely E, Barbour LA, et al, editors. Medical care of the pregnant patient. 2nd edition. Philadelphia (PA): American College of Physicians; 2008. p. 424. Table 35-2; with permission.

(DVTs) occur in the left leg, likely caused by compression of the iliac vein by the iliac artery, and later from the compression of the pelvic vessels by the gravid uterus.[58] Pregnancy-associated VTE is associated not only with the acute morbidity from acute DVT and pulmonary embolism (PE) but also long-term morbidity including an 80% risk of postthrombotic syndrome and a 65% risk of deep venous insufficiency.[59] PE continues to be the leading cause of maternal mortality in developed nations, so appropriate thromboprophylaxis and prompt diagnosis and treatment are needed.

Risk factors for VTE in pregnancy can be inherited or acquired (**Table 8**). The most important individual risk factor for VTE in pregnancy is a personal history of thrombosis, followed by congenital or acquired thrombophilia and family history of thrombosis. Approximately 20% to 50% of pregnancy-associated thromboembolic events are associated with a thrombophilic disorder, and 15% to 25% of all cases are recurrent events.[60,61] Factor V Leiden and prothrombin gene mutation are the most commonly inherited thrombophilias and antiphospholipid syndrome is the most common acquired thrombophilia. Indications for a diagnostic evaluation of thrombophilia in pregnancy include previous VTE and family history of thrombophilia. Screening is no longer recommended by the American College of Obstetricians and Gynecologists in all women with placenta-mediated pregnancy complications (ie, pregnancy loss, intrauterine growth retardation, preeclampsia, and placenta abruptions), with the exception of antiphospholipid antibody screening, for which there are data on the efficacy of treatment (**Table 9**). A recommended screening panel is shown in **Box 4**. In women with a prior VTE and thrombophilia, the risk of a recurrent VTE in pregnancy is approximately 20%.[62] The type of thrombophilia aids in selection of treatment plans.

Diagnosis of VTE in pregnancy is made more difficult by a scarcity of published data on diagnostic guidelines including a lack of validation of diagnostic imaging procedures. Guidelines are largely extrapolated from data in nonpregnant patients and there are concerns about radiation exposure to the fetus and mother. However, diagnostic evaluation for PE by V/Q or computed tomography (CT) PE scan exposes the fetus to significantly less than the maximum total pregnancy exposure of 5 rad as allowed by the National Commission on Radiation Protection. Fetal radiation exposure for common diagnostic tests for VTE are shown in **Table 10**. Efforts to limit exposure should be attempted but must be weighed against the risk of an undiagnosed VTE.

Table 8 Classification of hypercoagulable states	
Acquired	**Congenital**
Antiphospholipid antibody syndrome	Protein C deficiency
AT deficiency	Protein S deficiency
Nephrotic syndrome	AT deficiency
Preeclampsia	Activated protein C resistance
Medical illness	Factor V Leiden mutation
Cancer	Fibrinolytic defects
Systemic lupus erythematosus	Prothrombin gene mutation
Drugs (estrogen-containing compounds)	Hyperhomocysteinemia
Hyperhomocysteinemia	

Abbreviation: AT, antithrombin.

Reprinted from Rodger M, Langlois N, Rosene-Montella K. Congenital and acquired thrombophilias. In: Rosene-Montella K, Keely E, Barbour LA, et al, editors. Medical care of the pregnant patient. 2nd edition. Philadelphia (PA): American College of Physicians; 2008. p. 445. Table 37-1; with permission.

Table 9	
Indications for diagnostic evaluation for thrombophilia	
Nonobstetric Indications	**Obstetric Indications**
Family history of thrombophilia or thromboembolism	Early-onset severe preeclampsia
Family history of placenta-mediated pregnancy complications	Fetal demise
History of venous thromboembolism	Intrauterine growth restriction
	Placental thrombosis
	Previous child with cerebral palsy
	Neural tube defect (marker for hyperhomocysteinemia)
	Placental abruption (or severe abruption)
	Recurrent miscarriage

Reprinted from Rodger M, Langlois N, Rosene-Montella K. Congenital and acquired thrombophilias. In: Rosene-Montella K, Keely E, Barbour LA, et al, editors. Medical care of the pregnant patient. 2nd edition. Philadelphia (PA): American College of Physicians; 2008. p. 451. Table 37-4; with permission.

The diagnostic test of choice for DVT during pregnancy is compression ultrasonography. If the ultrasound is negative and clinically suspicion remains high, a repeat study should be performed in 1 week, or earlier for progressive symptoms. Because ileofemoral and pelvic clot can develop de novo in pregnancy, magnetic resonance venogram (MRV) should be considered if repeat ultrasound fails to diagnose pelvic clot and symptoms persist. A proposed algorithm is shown in **Figs. 1** and **2**. The diagnosis of PE in pregnancy, as in nonpregnant patients, can be a diagnostic challenge. Most pregnant patients with documented PE have a normal A-a gradient so other diagnostic testing is required for all patients suspected of having a PE. For suspected PE, initial work-up with a ventilation/perfusion (V/Q) scan is recommended or CT angiography with bismuth breast shields to reduce maternal breast irradiation. Nondiagnostic V/Q scans require further evaluation with CT angiography. D-dimer levels are unreliable in pregnancy because they increase throughout normal pregnancy and remain increased in the postpartum period, but they have some clinical usefulness in guiding diagnostic tests in patients with a high clinical suspicion of VTE.[63]

Box 4
Recommended thrombophilia screening tests
Factor V Leiden
Protein C deficiency
Protein S deficiency
AT deficiency
Prothrombin gene mutation G20210A
Anticardiolipin antibodies
Lupus anticoagulant
Hyperhomocysteinemia

Reprinted from Rodger M, Langlois N, Rosene-Montella K. Congenital and acquired thrombophilias. In: Rosene-Montella K, Keely E, Barbour LA, et al, editors. Medical care of the pregnant patient. 2nd edition. Philadelphia (PA): American College of Physicians; 2008. p. 452. Table 37-5; with permission.

Table 10
Fetal radiation exposures associated with diagnostic imaging for venous thromboembolism

Diagnostic Test	Exposure (rad)[a]
Leg compression ultrasonography	0
Magnetic resonance venography	0
Bilateral venography	0.628
Limited venography with abdominal shielding	<0.05
Pulmonary angiography via femoral route	0.37
Pulmonary angiography via brachial route	<0.05
V/Q scanning	≤0.58
CT PE angiogram	0.01 (2–4 to maternal breast)
Low-dose perfusion scanning alone	<0.012

[a] The National Commission on Radiation Protection recommends 5 rad as the maximum allowable exposure for the pregnancy.
Adapted from Rodger M, Rosene-Montella K, Barbour LA. Acute thromboembolic disease. In: Rosene-Montella K, Keely E, Barbour LA, et al, editors. Medical care of the pregnant patient. 2nd edition. Philadelphia (PA): American College of Physicians; 2008. p. 431. Table 36-3; with permission.

VTE in pregnancy warrants immediate anticoagulation. Warfarin is teratogenic and should be avoided throughout pregnancy. Therapeutic intravenous or subcutaneous unfractionated heparin (UFH) may be used as initial therapy. UFH carries a substantial risk of osteoporosis and a 2% to 3% incidence of vertebral fractures when used throughout pregnancy.[64] Low-molecular-weight heparin (LMWH) is the preferred long-term anticoagulant in pregnancy. It has a better pharmacokinetic profile and a substantially lower risk of heparin-induced thrombocytopenia. Dose adjustments are required as pregnancy progresses and glomerular filtration rate and weight increase. LMWH is contraindicated in renal failure and has limited use in patients with high bleeding risk or who need imminent surgery. When LMWH is used, anti-Xa levels should be closely monitored. Recommended anti-Xa levels for prophylaxis are 0.2 to 0.6 units/mL and, for therapeutic doses of LMWH, are 0.5 to 1.2 units/mL.[65]

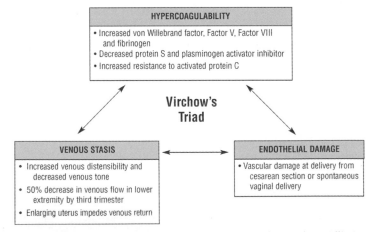

Fig. 1. Thrombotic changes associated with pregnancy. (*From* McLeod AG, Ellis C. Prevention and treatment of venous thromboembolism in high risk situations in pregnancy. Fetal Maternal Med Rev 2005;16:51–70; with permission.)

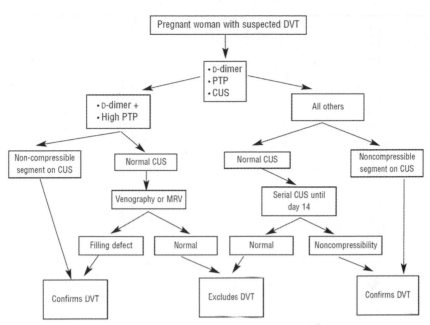

Fig. 2. Management of suspected DVT in pregnancy. CUS, venous compression ultrasound imaging; DVT, deep vein thrombosis; PTP, pretest probability. (*From* Rodger MA, Walker M, Wells PS. Diagnosis and treatment of venous thromboembolism in pregnancy. Best Pract Res Clin Haematol 2003;16:279–96; with permission.)

Patients who are on LMWH may be converted to unfractionated heparin at 34 to 36 weeks, because of its shorter half-life and reversibility to increase the likelihood that a patient can receive epidural anesthesia and also to decrease bleeding risk at delivery. Resumption of anticoagulation 4 to 6 hours after a vaginal delivery, and 6 to 12 hours after cesarean section, is recommended. In patients who have acute (within 1 month of delivery) or high-risk thrombosis close to term, a temporary inferior vena cava filter may be used when anticoagulation is interrupted.

There is a paucity of clinical trials regarding preventative management of primary and recurrent thrombosis in pregnancy. Most guidelines recommend thromboprophylaxis in pregnant patients with prior thrombosis without a transient risk factor, or in whom the transient risk factor was estrogen-containing oral contraceptives or pregnancy. The American College of Obstetricians and Gynecologists recently released guidelines recommending the prophylactic use of pneumatic compression devices before cesarean section for all women not already receiving anticoagulation because of the substantial risk of VTE in these patients.[55] **Table 11** reviews recommended thromboprophylaxis for pregnant patients with thrombophilias.

Other Thromboses

Pregnancy is also associated with unusual anatomic sites of thromboses. Ovarian vein thrombosis may occur in postpartum patients, usually in the setting of infection, and may present as fever and flank pain. It predominantly occurs on the right side. Because of reported cases of propagation into the inferior vena cava and embolization, treatment should be the same as for a lower extremity DVT.[66] Pregnancy and the postpartum period are associated with an increased risk of cerebral venous thrombosis, which

Table 11
Recommended thromboprophylaxis for pregnancies complicated by inherited thrombophilias

Clinical Scenario	Antepartum Management	Postpartum Management
Low-risk thrombophilia without previous VTE	Surveillance without anticoagulation therapy or prophylactic LMWH or UFH	Surveillance without anticoagulation therapy or postpartum anticoagulation therapy if the patient has additional risks factors
Low-risk thrombophilia with a single previous episode of VTE; not receiving long-term anticoagulation therapy	Prophylactic or intermediate-dose LMWH/UFH or surveillance without anticoagulation therapy	Postpartum anticoagulation therapy or intermediate-dose LMWH/UFH
High-risk thrombophilia without previous VTE	Prophylactic LMWH or UFH	Postpartum anticoagulation therapy
High-risk thrombophilia with a single previous episode of VTE; not receiving long-term anticoagulation therapy	Prophylactic, intermediate-dose, or adjusted-dose LMWH/UFH regimen	Postpartum anticoagulation therapy or intermediate or adjusted-dose LMWH/UFH for 6 wk (therapy level should be at least as high as antepartum treatment)
No thrombophilia with previous single episode of VTE associated with transient risk factor that is no longer present; excludes pregnancy-related or estrogen-related risk factor	Surveillance without anticoagulation therapy	Postpartum anticoagulation therapy
No thrombophilia with previous single episode of VTE associated with transient pregnancy-related or estrogen-related risk factor	Prophylactic-dose LMWH or UFH	Postpartum anticoagulation therapy
No thrombophilia with previous single episode of VTE without an associated risk factor (idiopathic); not receiving long-term anticoagulation therapy	Prophylactic-dose LMWH or UFH	Postpartum anticoagulation therapy
Thrombophilia or no thrombophilia with 2 or more episodes of VTE not receiving long-term anticoagulation therapy	Prophylactic or therapeutic-dose LMWH or prophylactic or therapeutic-dose UFH	Postpartum anticoagulation therapy or therapeutic-dose LMWH/UFH for 6 wk

From Practice bulletin: thromboembolism in pregnancy. The American College of Obstetricians and Gynecologists; Women's Health Care Physicians. Obstet Gynecol 2001:118(3):721. Table 2; with permission.

frequently presents as a severe headache that may or may not have neurologic symptoms. Pregnant woman with the prothrombin gene mutation or factor V Leiden have a greater risk. Magnetic resonance imaging (MRI/MRV) is recommended for diagnosis.

HEMATOLOGIC MALIGNANCIES

Hematologic malignancies are a rare complication in pregnancy. However, in the United States, malignancy is the second leading cause of maternal death. Hematologic malignancies represent 25% of malignancies diagnosed in pregnancy.[67] Hodgkin lymphoma is the most common, affecting 1 in 1000 to 6000 pregnancies,[68] followed by non-Hodgkin lymphoma and acute and chronic leukemias. Management of hematologic malignancies requires balancing the need for immediate therapy and its maternal and fetal effects with the effect of the natural progression of the disease on the fetus and the pregnancy. Treatment decisions must take into consideration gestational age, clinical stage of disease, and patient preferences. Within these limitations, diagnostic and therapeutic decisions should try to mimic those of nonpregnant patients, so that the necessary diagnostic and therapeutic management is optimized during pregnancy. A multispecialty team including hematologists/oncologists, high-risk obstetricians, social workers, geneticists, and clergy is recommended.

Diagnosis and staging can be challenging in pregnancy. An excisional biopsy of a lymph node is preferred for lymphomas. Bone marrow aspiration and biopsy may safely be performed. Radiographs and noncontrast MRIs, both with abdominal shielding and ultrasound, are preferred to CT scans. Positron emission tomography scans and bone scans should be used when their usefulness in guiding treatment outweighs the risk of exposure.

Whenever possible, treatment should be deferred until the second trimester after fetal organogenesis is completed. Chemotherapy in the first trimester has been associated with spontaneous abortion and carries a significant risk of congenital abnormalities. The risk of congenital malformations in the first trimester is estimated at 10% for single-agent chemotherapy and 15% to 35% with combination therapy.[69,70] Vincristine has the lowest risk and alkylating agents and antimetabolites the highest risk.[70] Therapeutic abortion is recommended if chemotherapy cannot be delayed. The risk of congenital malformations approaches that of the nonpregnant population for most chemotherapeutic agents after the first trimester. To date, studies of offspring have not shown significant short-term or long-term effects on the exposed fetus when chemotherapy is given after the first trimester.[71–73]

Treatment regimens should be individually tailored and based on the latest available data. Standard doses of drugs should be used adjusted to continuing weight gain. Melphalan and procarbazine, both alklylating agents, should not be used in pregnancy because of data showing a significant risk of early and late spontaneous abortion and congenital malformations.[74] Thalidomide and lenalidomide are contraindicated in pregnancy because they are highly teratogenic. Most experts recommend avoidance of the antimetabolite methotrexate (which has both a dose-dependent and trimester-dependent effect) during pregnancy, unless no alternative exists.[75] The use of newer agents, including monoclonal antibodies and tyrosine kinase inhibitors, lacks data for teratogenesis. Interferon therapy seems to be safe in pregnancy, with 40 published cases of successful use. There has been 1 case of fetal malformation with concurrent use of interferon and hydroxyurea.[74] However, interferon therapy may adversely affect future fertility. The choice of chemotherapeutic agents must be weighed against the benefit and availability of alternative therapies. Radiation therapy is generally avoided but can be used in certain limited situations with extreme precautions.[76]

Delivery indications are usually the same as for normal pregnancy. However, delivery should be planned at least 2 weeks after chemotherapy to allow for recovery of maternal and fetal blood counts. The placenta should be sent for pathologic examination at delivery. Most pregnant women presenting with a hematologic malignancy have prognoses similar to nonpregnant patients and normal pregnancy outcomes.[74]

Aplastic Anemia

Aplastic anemia, defined as pancytopenia with a hypocellular bone marrow, has an annual incidence in the general population estimated at 2 per million in North America, with higher rates in east Asia. Diagnosis is suspected with persistent pancytopenia and confirmed with bone marrow biopsy. During pregnancy, aplastic anemia may be caused by chance but other causes should be ruled out. The disease often progresses during pregnancy. For patients previously treated with immunsuppressives, the relapse risk is significant but patients with prior allogeneic bone marrow transplant do not seem to have a significant risk of relapse during pregnancy. Patients require frequent blood counts and a multidisciplinary team. However, counseling of the potentially serious risks to both the mother and baby should be discussed and therapeutic abortion may be considered. Successful pregnancy is possible with supportive care, namely transfusion therapy.

Alloimmunization to platelet and blood transfusions is increased during pregnancy. Antithymocyte globulin is contraindicated but cyclosporine seems to be safe according to data derived from patients who have had renal transplants. For transfusion-dependent patients or patients with blood counts that are declining toward transfusion-dependent levels, cyclosporine at a dose of 5 mg/kg/d can be used to maintain levels between 150 and 250/μL. However, responses can take 6 to 12 weeks.[76]

SUMMARY

Evaluation and treatment of hematologic disorders in pregnancy requires an understanding of normal physiologic changes during pregnancy. Hematologic disorders may be caused by preexisting conditions, normal physiologic changes, or can be acquired. A multidisciplinary approach is often necessary for monitoring and treatment of both the mother and the fetus. In general, outcomes are good for both the mother and the fetus.

REFERENCES

1. Taylor DJ, Lind T. Red cell mass during and after normal pregnancy. Br J Obstet Gynaecol 1979;86:364–70.
2. Whittaker PG, McPhail S, Lind T. Serial hematologic changes and pregnancy outcome. Obstet Gynecol 1996;88:33–9.
3. Centers for Disease Control and Prevention (CDC). CDC criteria for anemia in children and childbearing-aged women. MMWR Morb Mortal Wkly Rep 1989; 38:400–4.
4. Messer RH. Pregnancy anemias. Clin Obstet Gynecol 1974;17:163–84.
5. Carles G, Tobal N, Raynal P, et al. Doppler assessment of the fetal cerebral hemodynamic response to moderate or severe maternal anemia. Am J Obstet Gynecol 2003;188:794–9.
6. Sifakis S, Pharmakides G. Anemia in pregnancy. Ann N Y Acad Sci 2000;900: 125–36.
7. Brabin BJ, Hakimi M, Pelletier D. An analysis of anemia and pregnancy-related maternal mortality. J Nutr 2001;131:604S.

8. Mani S, Duff TP. Anemia in pregnancy. Clin Perinatol 1995;22:593–606.
9. Bridges KR, Seligman PA. Disorders of iron metabolism. In: Handin RI, Lux SE, Stossel TP, editors. Blood: principles & practice of hematology. London: JB Lippincott; 1995. [Chapter: 49].
10. Breymann C, Visca E, Huch R, et al. Efficacy and safety of intravenously administered iron sucrose with and without adjuvant recombinant human erythropoietin for the treatment of resistant iron-deficiency anemia during pregnancy. Am J Obstet Gynecol 2001;184:662–7.
11. Shojania AM. Folic acid and vitamin B12 deficiency in pregnancy and in the neonatal period. Clin Perinatol 1984;11:433–59.
12. Cines DB, Pollak ES, Buck CA, et al. Endothelial cells in physiology and in the pathophysiology of vascular disorders. Blood 1998;91:3527–61.
13. Smith JA, Espeland M, Bellevue R, et al. Pregnancy in sickle cell disease: experience of the Cooperative Study of Sickle Cell Disease. Obstet Gynecol 1996;87:199–204.
14. Hassell K. Pregnancy and sickle cell disease. Hematol Oncol Clin North Am 2005;19:903–16.
15. Rappaport VJ, Velazquez M, Williams K. Hemoglobinopathies in pregnancy. Obstet Gynecol Clin North Am 2004;31:287–317.
16. Rathmell JP, Viscomi CM, Ashburn MA. Management of nonobstetric pain during pregnancy and lactation. Anesth Analg 1997;85:1074–87.
17. Koshy M, Burd L, Wallace D, et al. Prophylactic red-cell transfusion in pregnant patients with sickle cell disease. A randomized cooperative study. N Engl J Med 1988;319:1447–52.
18. Mahomed K. Prophylactic versus selective blood transfusion for sickle cell anaemia during pregnancy (Review). Cochrane Database Syst Rev 2005;1:CD000040.
19. Wanko SO, Telen MJ. Transfusion management in sickle cell disease. Hematol Oncol Clin North Am 2005;19:803–26.
20. Tuck SM, Studd JW, White JM. Pregnancy in women with sickle cell trait. BJOG 1983;90:108–11.
21. Hassell K. Hemoglobinopathies, thalassemias, and anemia: I. Hemoglobinopathies and anemia. In: Rosene-Montella K, Keely E, Barbour AL, et al, editors. Medical care of the pregnant patient. 2nd edition. Philadelphia: American College of Physicians; 2008. p. 486–506.
22. Kilpatrick SJ, Laros RK. Thalassemia in pregnancy. Clin Obstet Gynecol 1995;38: 485–96.
23. Mordel N, Birkenfeld A, Golfarb AN, et al. Successful full-term pregnancy in homozygous beta-thalassemia major: case report and review of the literature. Obstet Gynecol 1989;73:837–40.
24. Neunert C, Lim W, Crowther M, et al. The American Society of Hematology 2011 evidence-based practice guideline for immune thrombocytopenia. Blood 2011; 17:4190–207.
25. Karovitch A, Rodger M. Thrombocytopenia. In: Rosene-Montella K, Keely E, Barbour AL, et al, editors. Medical care of the pregnant patient. 2nd edition. Philadelphia (PA): American College of Physicians; 2008. p. 476–85.
26. Herold M, Schnohr S, Bittrich H. Efficacy and safety of a combined rituximab chemotherapy during pregnancy [letter]. J Clin Oncol 2001;19:3439.
27. Kimby E, Sverrisdottir A, Elinder G. Safety of rituximab therapy during the first trimester of pregnancy: a case history. Eur J Haematol 2004;72:292–5.
28. Klink DT, van Elburg RM, Schreurs MW, et al. Rituximab administration in third trimester of pregnancy suppresses neonatal B-cell development. Clin Dev Immunol 2008;2008:271–363.

29. Woudstra DM, Chandra S, Hofmeyr GJ, et al. Corticosteroids for HELLP (hemolysis, elevated liver enzymes, low platelets) syndrome in pregnancy. Cochrane Database Syst Rev 2010;9:CD008148.

30. Levi M, Toh C, Thachill J, et al. Guidelines for the diagnosis and management of disseminated intravascular coagulation. Br J Haematol 2009;145:24–33.

31. Bolton-Maggs PH, Chalmers EA, Collins PW, et al. A review of inherited platelet disorders with guidelines for their management on behalf of the UKHCDO. Br J Haematol 2006;135:603–33.

32. Schulman S, Johnson H, Egberg N, et al. DDAVP-induced correction of prolonged bleeding time in patients with congenital platelet function defects. Thromb Res 1987;45:165–74.

33. International Data Collection on Recombinant Factor VIIa and Congenital Platelet Disorders Study Group. Prophylactic and therapeutic recombinant factor VIIa administration to patient with Glanzmann's thrombasthenia: results of an international survey. J Thromb Haemost 2004;2:1096–103.

34. Rodeghiero F, Castaman G, Dini E. Epidemiological investigation of the prevalence of von Willebrand's disease. Blood 1987;69:454–9.

35. Sadler JE. A revised classification of von Willebrand disease. For the Subcommittee on von Willebrand Factor of the Scientific and Standardization Committee of the International Society on Thrombosis and Haemostasis. Thromb Haemost 1994;71:520–5.

36. Gill JC, Endres-Brooks J, Bauer PJ, et al. The effect of ABO blood group on the diagnosis of von Willebrand disease. Blood 1987;69:1691–5.

37. Lak M, Peyvandi F, Mannucci PM. Clinical manifestations and complications of childbirth and replacement therapy in 385 Iranian patients with type 3 von Willebrand disease. Br J Haematol 2000;111:1236–9.

38. Conti M, Mari D, Conti E, et al. Pregnancy in women with different types of von Willebrand disease. Obstet Gynecol 1986;68:282–5.

39. Roqué H, Funai E, Lockwood CJ. von Willebrand disease and pregnancy. J Matern Fetal Med 2000;9:257–66.

40. Mannucci PM. How I treat patients with von Willebrand disease. Blood 2009;97:1915–9.

41. Pacheco LD, Costantine MM, Saade GR, et al. von Willebrand disease and pregnancy: a practical approach for the diagnosis and treatment. Am J Obstet Gynecol 2010;302:194–200.

42. Pareti FI, Federici AB, Cattaneo M, et al. Spontaneous platelet aggregation during pregnancy in a patient with vWD type II B can be blocked by monoclonal antibodies to both platelet glycoproteins Ib and IIb/IIIa. Br J Haematol 1990;75:86–91.

43. Tinmouth AT, Rodger M. Bleeding disorders. In: Rosene-Montella K, Keely E, Barbour AL, et al, editors. Medical care of the pregnant patient. 2nd edition. Philadelphia: American College of Physicians; 2008. p. 476–85.

44. Bolton-Maggs PH. Factor XI deficiency and its management. Haemophilia 2000;6(Suppl 1):100–9.

45. Bolton-Maggs PH. Bleeding problems in factor XI deficient women. Haemophilia 1999;5:155–9.

46. Condie RG, Ogston D. Sequential studies on components of the haemostatic mechanism in pregnancy with particular reference to the development of preeclampsia. Br J Obstet Gynaecol 1976;83:938–42.

47. Bremme KA. Haemostatic changes in pregnancy. Best Pract Res Clin Haematol 2003;16:153–68.

48. Clark P, Brennand J, Conkie JA, et al. Activated protein C sensitivity, protein C, protein S and coagulation in normal pregnancy. Thromb Haemost 1998;79: 1166–70.

49. Nossel HL, Lanzkowsky P, Levy S, et al. A study of coagulation factor levels in women during labour and in their newborn infants. Thromb Diath Haemorrh 1966;16:185–97.

50. Myers B, Pavord S, Kean L, et al. Short communication: pregnancy outcome in Factor XI deficiency: incidence of miscarriage, antenatal and postnatal haemorrhage in 33 women with Factor XI deficiency. Br J Obstet Gynaecol 2007;114: 643–6.

51. Green D, Lechner K. A survey of 214 non-hemophilic patients with inhibitors to factor VIII. Thromb Haemost 1981;45:200–3.

52. Delgado J, Jimenez-Yuste V, Hernandez-Navarro F. Acquired hemophilia: review and meta-analysis focused on therapy and prognostic factors. Br J Haematol 2003;121:21–35.

53. Hay CRM, Brown S, Collins PW, et al. The diagnosis and management of factor VIII and IX inhibitors: a guideline from the United Kingdom Haemophilia Centre Doctors Organisation. Br J Haematol 2006;133:591–605.

54. Franchini M, Lippi G. How I treat acquired factor VIII inhibitors. Blood 2008;112: 250–5.

55. Wright JD, Pawar N, Gonzalez JS, et al. Scientific evidence underlying the American College of Obstetricians and Gynecologists' practice bulletins. Obstet Gynecol 2011;118:505–12.

56. Gherman RB, Goodwin TM, Leung B, et al. Incidence, clinical characteristics, and timing of objectively diagnosed venous thromboembolism during pregnancy. Obstet Gynecol 1999;94:730–4.

57. Williams MD, Wheby MS. Anemia in pregnancy. Med Clin North Am 1992;76: 631–47.

58. Ray JG, Chan WS. Deep vein thrombosis during pregnancy and the puerperium: a meta-analysis of the period of risk and the leg of presentation. Obstet Gynecol Surv 1999;54:265–71.

59. Bergqvist A, Bergqvist D, Lindhagen A, et al. Late symptoms after pregnancy-related deep vein thrombosis. Br J Obstet Gynaecol 1990;97:338–41.

60. Robertson L, Wu O, Langhorne P, et al. Thrombosis: Risk and Economic Assessment of Thrombophilia Screening (TREATS) Study. Thrombophilia in pregnancy: a systematic review. Br J Haematol 2005;132:171–96.

61. Gerhardt A, Scharf RE, Beckmann MW, et al. Prothrombin and factor V mutations in women with a history of thrombosis during pregnancy and the puerperium. N Engl J Med 2000;342:374–80.

62. Brill-Edwards P, Ginsberg JS, Gent M, et al. Safety of withholding heparin in pregnant women with a history of venous thromboembolism. Recurrence of Clot in This Pregnancy Study Group. N Engl J Med 2000;343:1439–44.

63. Kjellberg U, Andersson NE, Rosen S, et al. APC resistance and other haemostatic variables during pregnancy and puerperium. Thromb Haemost 1999;81:527–31.

64. Ginsburg JS, Hirsh J. Use of antithrombotic agents during pregnancy. Chest 1998;114:524S–30S.

65. Bates SM, Greer IA, Hirsh J, et al. Use of antithrombotic agents during pregnancy: the seventh ACCP conference on antithrombotic and thrombolytic therapy. Chest 2004;126(Suppl):627S–44S.

66. DHSS. Report on confidential inquiries: maternal deaths in England and Wales 1986-1988. London: Her Majesty's Station Office; 1991.

67. Hurley TJ, McKinnell JV, Irani MS. Hematologic malignancies in pregnancy. Obstet Gynecol Clin North Am 2005;32:595–614.
68. Stewart HL Jr, Monto RW. Hodgkin's disease and pregnancy. Am J Obstet Gynecol 1952;63:570–8.
69. Doll DC, Ringenberg QS, Yarbro JW. Management of cancer during pregnancy. Arch Intern Med 1988;148:2058–64.
70. Doll DC, Ringenberg QS, Yarbro JW. Antineoplastic agents and pregnancy. Semin Oncol 1989;16:337–46.
71. Kalter H, Warkany J. Medical progress. Congenital malformations: etiologic factors and their role in prevention (first of two parts). N Engl J Med 1983;308: 424–31.
72. Shapira T, Pereg D, Lishner M. How I treat acute and chronic leukemia in pregnancy. Blood Rev 2008;22:247–59.
73. Aviles A, Neri N. Hematological malignancies and pregnancy: a final report of 84 children who received chemotherapy in utero. Clin Lymphoma 2001;2:173–7.
74. Perez-Encinas M, Bello JL, Perez-Crespo S, et al. Familial myeloproliferative syndrome. Am J Hematol 1994;46:225–9.
75. Feldkamp M, Carey JC. Clinical teratology counseling and consultation case report: low dose methotrexate exposure in the early weeks of pregnancy. Teratology 1993;47:533–9.
76. Marsh JC, Ball SE, Darbyshire P, et al. Guidelines for the diagnosis and management of acquired aplastic anaemia. Br J Haematol 2003;123:782–801.

Index

Note: Page numbers of article titles are in **boldface** type.

A

Acquired bleeding disorders, clinical manifestations of, 325, 328
    diagnostic algorithm for, 336–337
Acquired coagulation inhibitors, diagnostic algorithm for, 337
Acquired Von Willebrand syndrome, diagnostic algorithm for, 337–338
Acute lymphoblastic leukemia, leukocytosis in, 313
Acute myelogenous leukemia, leukocytosis in, 312–313
Age, and risk of anemia, 206–207
Alcohol abuse, bone marrow suppression and anemia due to, 224
    thrombocytopenia due to, 237
Alloimmune hemolysis, due to transfused RBC, 218
Altitude, polycythemias associated with high, 270–271
Ancillary tests. *See* Laboratory tests.
Anemia, consultation for, **205–230**
        consequences of, 209
        determinants of hemoglobin concentration, 206–209
            age, 206–207
            diseases and medications, 209
            gender, 208–209
            genetics, 206
            geography, 209
            race, 207–208
        diagnostic workup, 209–226
            anemia of inflammation, 225–226
            decreased RBC production, 220–225
            initial, 209–212
            RBC loss or dilution anemia, 212–220
        in pregnant patients, 409–413
            hemoglobinopathies, 411
            iron deficiency, 410
            macrocytic, 410–411
            sickle cell disease, 411–413
            thalassemia, 413
Anticoagulation therapy, for venous thrombosis, 348–355, 359–361
        bridging for invasive procedures, 359–361
        duration of, 349–354
        initial treatment, 348–349
        new oral anticoagulants, 354–355
Antiphospholipid-antibody syndrome, catastrophic, life- or limb-threatening
    thrombocytopenia in, 377
    secondary immune thrombocytopenia in, 242
Aplastic anemia, in pregnant patients, 428

Hematol Oncol Clin N Am 26 (2012) 433–445
doi:10.1016/S0889-8588(12)00034-2
0889-8588/12/$ – see front matter © 2012 Elsevier Inc. All rights reserved.

hemonc.theclinics.com

Autoimmune disorders, neutropenia, 257–260
     primary, 257–258
     pure white cell aplasia, 258
     secondary, 259–260
          chronic idiopathic, 259–260
          hyperthyroidism (Graves' disease), 259
          rheumatoid arthritis and Felty syndrome, 259
          systemic lupus erythematosus, 259
Autoimmune hemolytic anemias, 215, 216–218

B

Bacterial infections, neutropenia related to, 263
Bernard-Soulier syndrome, thrombocytopenia in, 239
Bleeding, consultation for patient with bruising or, **321–344**
     clinical manifestations, 325–328
          abnormalities of connective tissue/collagen, 325, 328
          acquired disorders, 328
          defects of primary hemostasis, 325
          defects of secondary hemostasis, 325
     diagnostic algorithm and differential diagnosis, 332–338
          acquired bleeding disorders, 336–337
          acquired coagulation inhibitors, 337
          acquired Von Willebrand syndrome, 337–338
          Ehlers-Danlos syndrome, 333
          inherited coagulation disorders, 333–335
          platelet function disorders, 333
          thrombocytopenia, 333
          Von Willebrand disease, 332–333
     laboratory testing, 328–332
          screening tests, 329–331
          second line of testing, 331–332
          third line of testing, 332
     patient history, bleeding assessment tests, 323–325
          bleeding history, 322–323
     physical examination, 325
     treatment, 338–340
          direct/replacement therapies, 339
          for bleeding of unknown cause, 340
          indirect therapies, 338–339
Bleeding disorders, anemia in pregnant patients with, 417–421
Bone marrow disorders, inability to produce RBCs due to, 223–225
     bone marrow suppression, 224–225
     primary disorders, 223–224
     secondary dysfunction, 224
Bruising. *See* Bleeding.

C

Cardiac care unit, thrombocytopenia in, 244–245
Cardiopulmonary bypass, thrombocytopenia and, 245
Catastrophic antiphospholipid-antibody syndrome, life- or limb-threatening
   thrombocytopenia in, 377

Chronic myeloid leukemia, thrombocytosis in, 295
Coagulation disorders, congenital, in pregnant patients, 419–420
   inherited, diagnostic algorithm and differential diagnosis, 333–335
      hemophilia, 333–335
      recessive, 335
Coagulation factors, clinical manifestations of defects or deficiencies of, 325
Coagulation inhibitors, acquired, diagnostic algorithm for, 337
Cobalamin deficiency, anemia due to, 221–222
Collagen, clinical manifestations of abnormalities of, 325, 328
Congenital disorders, coagulation disorders in pregnant patients, 419–420
   neutropenia, 255–257
      cyclic, 255–257
      severe (Kostmann's syndrome), 257
   polycythemias, 269–270, 272–273
   thrombocytopenia in, 238–239
Connective tissue, clinical manifestations of abnormalities of, 325, 328
Consultative hematology, 205–432
   anemia, consequences of, 209
      definition, 206
      determinants of hemoglobin concentration, 206–209
      diagnostic workup, 209–226
         anemia of inflammation, 225–226
         decreased RBC production, 220–225
         initial, 209–212
         RBC loss or dilution anemia, 212–220
      in pregnant patients, 409–413
   bleeding and bruising, **321–344**
      clinical manifestations, 325–328
      diagnostic algorithm and differential diagnosis, 332–338
      laboratory testing, 328–332
      patient history, 322–325
      physical examination, 325
      treatment, 338–340
   erythrocytosis, **267–283**
      absolute polycythemias, 269–278
      regulation of erythropoiesis, 268–269
      relative polycythemias, 269
   in pregnant patients, **409–432**
      anemia, 409–413
      hematologic malignancies, 427–428
      platelet function disorders, 416–417
      thrombocytopenia, 413–416
      thrombophilia and thromboembolism, 421–427
      Von Willebrand disease and other bleeding disorders, 417–419
   leukocytosis, **303–319**
      causes of secondary, 306–312
         drug effect, 308–309
         infections, 306–308
         lymphocytosis, 309–311
         noninfectious causes of, 308
         nonmalignant hematologic disorders associated with, 311–312

Consultative (*continued*)

    classification of, 305–306

    development, maturation, and survival of granulocytes, 304

    diagnostic workup of, 315–317

    distinguishing a primary from a reactive (secondary), 306

    drug effect, 308–309

    evaluation of, 305

    hematologic malignancies and, 312–315

        acute lymphoblastic leukemia, 313

        acute myelogenous leukemia, 312–313

        chronic leukemia, 313–315

    lymphocyte development, 305

    monocyte development, 304

    white blood cell development, 303–304

life- or limb-threatening thrombocytopenia, **369–382**

    in heparin-induced thrombocytopenia, 369–371

    in post-transfusion purpura, 378–380

    in thrombotic microangiopathies, 371–377

lymphadenopathy, **895–408**

    evaluation of, 400–402

    location of, 396–400

    mechanisms of, 395–396

monoclonal spikes and multiple myeloma, **383–393**

    clinical presentation, 387

    diagnostics, 389–390

    epidemiology and diagnostic criteria for multiple myeloma variants, 386–387

    importance of early diagnosis of multiple myeloma, 390

    monoclonal gammopathy of undetermined significance, 383–386

    suspecting multiple myeloma in patient with M spike, 387–389

neutropenia, **253–266**

    causes, 255, 256, 257, 258

    congenital, 255–257

    diagnostic workup, 254–255

    drug-induced, 260–262

    ethnic variation, 255

    immune-related, 257–260

    infections causing, 262–263

    malignancy causing, 263–264

    overview, 253

splenomegaly, **895–408**

    causes of, 402–403

    evaluation of, 403–405

    indications for removal of enlarged spleen, 405

    mechanisms of, 396

thrombocytopenia, **231–252**

    ancillary tests, 232–233

    associated with infections, 243, 244

    drug-induced, 239–240

    in patients with a solid tumor, 246

    in patients with hematologic malignancy, 246

    in pregnant patients, 413–416

in the cardiac care unit, 244–245
in the intensive care unit, 243
in the internal medicine patient, 237–239
in the stem cell and solid organ transplant patient, 247
mechanisms of, 234–237
pertinent history in patient with, 231
physical examination, 231–232
post-transfusion purpura, 242–243
primary immune, 240–241
secondary immune, 241–242
thrombocytosis, **285–301**
  chronic myeloid leukemia, 295
  essential, 288–294
  polycythemia vera, 295
  primary myelofibrosis, 296
  reactive, 285–288
venous thromboembolism, **345–367**
  anticoagulant bridging for invasive procedures, 359–361
  diagnosis, 347–348
  duration of anticoagulant treatment, 349–354
  hypercoagulable workup, 358–359
  initial treatment, 348–349
  new oral anticoagulants, 354–355
  presentation, 347
  superficial venous thrombosis, 355–357
  travel-related venous thrombosis, 357–358
Cyanotic heart disease, polycythemias associated with, 270
Cyclic neutropenia, 255–257

D

Deep vein thrombosis, in pregnant patients, 421–427
  overview of venous thromboembolism, **345–367**
Dilution anemia, diagnostic workup of, 212–220
    due to RBC destruction, 214–220
Disseminated intravascular coagulation (DIC), limb- or life-threatening thrombocytopenia
  in, 371–373
Drug-induced disorders, leukocytosis, 308–309
  neutropenia, 260–262
  polycythemia, 271–272
Drug-mediated hemolysis, 218

E

Ehlers-Danlos syndrome, clinical manifestations of, 325, 328
  diagnostic algorithm and differential diagnosis, 333
Endocrine disorders, polycythemias associated with, 271–272
Environmental toxins, anemia due to, 225
Enzyme deficiencies, hemolysis due to, 218–220
Erythrocytosis, consultation for, **267–283**
    absolute polycythemias, 269–278

Erythrocytosis (*continued*)
    regulation of erythropoiesis, 268–269
    relative polycythemias, 269
Erythropoiesis, regulation of, 268–269
Essential thrombocytosis. *See* Thrombocytosis, essential.

F

Felty syndrome, secondary autoimmune neutropenia in, 259
Folic acid deficiency, anemia due to, 222

G

Gender, and risk of anemia, 208–209
Genetics, of hemoglobin concentration, 206
Geography, and risk of anemia, 209
Granulocytes, development, maturation, and survival of, 304
Graves disease, secondary autoimmune neutropenia in, 259

H

Heavy metal toxicity, anemia due to, 225
Helicobacter pylori, secondary immune thrombocytopenia in, 242
HELPP syndrome, in pregnancy, life-or limb-threatening thrombocytopenia in, 376
Hematologic disorders, consultation for. *See* Consultation.
    malignant, associated with leukocytosis, 312–315
    nonmalignant, associated with leukocytosis, 311–312
Hematologic malignancies, in pregnant patients, 427–428
    lymphadenopathy and splenomegaly, **395–408**
    thrombocytopenia in patients with, 246
Hematology, consultative. *See* Consultation, hematologic.
Hemoglobin concentration, determinants of, 206–209
        age, 206–207
        diseases and medications, 209
        gender, 208–209
        genetics, 206
        geography, 209
        race, 207–208
Hemoglobinopathies, in pregnant patients, 411
Hemolytic uremic syndrome, limb- or life-threatening thrombocytopenia in, 374–375
Heparin-induced thrombocytopenia, in the intensive care unit, 243
    life- or limb-threatening, 369–371
Hepatitis C, secondary immune thrombocytopenia in, 242
Hereditary disorders, increased RBC destruction due to, 218–220
History, clinical, in initial workup of anemic patient, 210
    in patient with thrombocytopenia, 231
    in patients with bleeding or bruising, 322–325
    in workup of anemia of inflammation, 226
    in workup of leukocytosis, 315–314
HIV infection, neutropenia related to, 262–263
    secondary immune thrombocytopenia in, 242

Hypercoagulable workup, for venous thrombosis, 358–359
Hypertension, malignant, limb- or life-threatening thrombocytopenia in, 376–377
Hyperthyroidism, secondary autoimmune neutropenia in, 259

I

Immune disorders, neutropenia, 257–260
    primary autoimmune, 257–258
    pure white cell aplasia, 258
    secondary autoimmune, 259–260
        chronic idiopathic, 259–260
        hyperthyroidism (Graves' disease), 259
        rheumatoid arthritis and Felty syndrome, 259
        systemic lupus erythematosus, 259
    thrombocytopenia (ITP), primary, 240–241
        secondary, 241–242
Immune-mediated hemolysis, anemia due to, 215, 216–218
Infections, bone marrow suppression and anemia due to, 224
    neutropenia due to, 262–263
        bacterial, 263
        HIV, 262–263
        other viruses, 263
        parasites, 263
    secondary leukocytosis due to, 306–308
    thrombocytopenia associated with, 243
Inflammation, anemia of, 225–226
Intensive care unit, thrombocytopenia in, 243
Internal medicine patients, causes of thrombocytopenia seen in, 237–239
    alcohol abuse and, 237
    congenital, 238–239
    iron deficiencies, 237
    liver disease and, 239
    nutritional deficiencies, 237
Iron deficiency, anemia due to, 220–221
    in pregnant patients, 410
    thrombocytopenia due to, 237

J

JAK2 mutations, in polycythemia vera, 274

K

Kostmann's syndrome, 257

L

Laboratory studies, in initial workup of anemic patient, 210–212
    in neutropenia workup, 254–255
    in patients with bleeding or bruising, 328–332
    in workup of anemia of inflammation, 226

Laboratory (*continued*)
   in workup of dilution anemia, 214
   in workup of leukocytosis, 316–317
   in workup of patient with thrombocytopenia, 232–233
Large granulocytic lymphocytic leukemia, neutropenia in, 263
Leukemia, chronic myeloid, thrombocytosis in, 295
   large granulocytic lymphocytic, neutropenia in, 263
   leukocytosis in, acute lymphoblastic, 313
      acute myelogenous, 312–313
      chronic, 313–315
Leukocytosis, consultation on, **303–319**
      causes of secondary, 306–312
         drug effect, 308–309
         infections, 306–308
         lymphocytosis, 309–311
         noninfectious causes of, 308
         nonmalignant hematologic disorders associated with, 311–312
      classification of, 305–306
      development, maturation, and survival of granulocytes, 304
      diagnostic workup of, 315–317
      distinguishing a primary from a reactive (secondary), 306
      drug effect, 308–309
      evaluation of, 305
      hematologic malignancies and, 312–315
         acute lymphoblastic leukemia, 313
         acute myelogenous leukemia, 312–313
         chronic leukemia, 313–315
      lymphocyte development, 305
      monocyte development, 304
      white blood cell development, 303–304
Liver disease, thrombocytopenia due to, 238
Lymphadenopathy, consultation for, **895–408**
      evaluation of, 400–402
      location of, 396–400
      mechanisms of, 395–396
Lymphocytes, development of, 305
Lymphocytosis, leukocytosis related to, 309–311

M

Macrocytic anemias, in pregnant patients, 410–411
Malignant hypertension, limb- or life-threatening thrombocytopenia in, 376–377
Mechanical hemolysis, anemia due to, 214–215, 216
Medications, affecting hemoglobin concentration, 209
   bone marrow suppression and anemia due to, 224
   drug-induced leukocytosis, 308–309
   drug-induced neutropenia, 260–262
   drug-induced thrombocytopenia, 239–240
Microangiopathies, thrombotic, life- or limb-threatening thrombocytopenia in, 371–377
      catastrophic antiphospholipid-antibody syndrome, 377
      disseminated intravascular coagulation, 371–373

    hemolytic uremic syndrome, 374–375
    malignant hypertension, 375–377
    preeclampsia/HELPP, 375
    thrombotic thrombocytopenic purpura, 373–374
Monoclonal gammopathy of undetermined significance (MGUS), 383–386
    diagnosis and follow-up of patients with, 385
    epidemiology, 383–385
    risk factors and models for progression of, 385–386
Monoclonal spikes, consultation for possible multiple myeloma in patients with, **383–393**
    clinical presentation, 387
    diagnostics, 389–390
    epidemiology and diagnostic criteria for multiple myeloma variants, 386–387
    importance of early diagnosis of multiple myeloma, 390
    monoclonal gammopathy of undetermined significance, 383–386
    suspecting multiple myeloma in patient with M spike, 387–389
Monocytes, development of, 304
Multiple myeloma, consultation for possible, in patients with monoclonal spikes, **383–393**
    clinical presentation, 387
    diagnostics, 389–390
    epidemiology and diagnostic criteria for multiple myeloma variants, 386–387
    importance of early diagnosis of multiple myeloma, 390
    monoclonal gammopathy of undetermined significance, 383–386
    suspecting multiple myeloma in patient with M spike, 387–389
Myelodysplastic syndromes, neutropenia in, 263–264
Myelofibrosis, primary, thrombocytosis in, 296
MYH9-related diseases, thrombocytopenia in, 239

N

Neutropenia, consultation for, **253–266**
    causes, 255, 256, 257, 258
    congenital, 255–257
        cyclic, 255–257
        severe (Kostmann syndrome), 257
    diagnostic workup, 254–255
    drug-induced, 260–262
        rituximab, 262
    ethnic variation, 255
    immune-related, 257–260
        primary, 257–258
        pure white cell aplasia, 258
        secondary, 258–259
    infections causing, 262–263
        bacterial, 263
        HIV, 262–263
        other viruses, 263
        parasites, 263
    malignancy causing, 263–264
        large granulocytic lymphocytic leukemia, 263
        myelodysplastic syndromes, 263–264
    overview, 253

Nutritional deficiencies, RBC production and, 220–222
    cobalamin, 221–222
    folic acid, 222
    iron, 220–221
    other, 222
  thrombocytopenia and, 237

O

Obstructive sleep apnea, polycythemias associated with, 270
Organ dysfunction, RBC production and, 222–223
Organ transplant patients, thrombocytopenia in, 247

P

Parasites, neutropenia related to, 263
Pickwickian syndrome, polycythemias associated with, 270
Plasma cell dyscrasia variant, of multiple myeloma, epidemiology and diagnostic
    criteria, 386–387
Platelet function disorders, clinical manifestations of, 325
  diagnostic algorithm and differential diagnosis, 333
  in pregnant patients, 416–417
Platelets, decreased production of, thrombocytopenia due to, 236
  destruction of, thrombocytopenia due to, 235–236
    immune, 235–236
    increased, 235
    nonimmune, 236
  sequestration of, thrombocytopenia due to, 236–237
Polycythemia vera, 273–278, 295
  clinical manifestations, 274–276
  epidemiology, 273
  JAK2 mutations in, 274
  pathobiology, 273–274
  therapy, 277–278
  thrombocytosis in, 295
Polycythemias, absolute, 269–278
    polycythemia vera, 273–278
    primary familial and congenital, 269–270
    secondary, 270–273
  relative, 269
Post-transfusion purpura, 242–243
  life- or limb-threatening thrombocytopenia in, 378–380
Preeclampsia, limb- or life-threatening thrombocytopenia in, 376
Pregnancy, consultation for special hematologic issues in, **409–432**
    anemia, 409–413
    hematologic malignancies, 427–428
    life- or limb-threatening thrombocytopenia in preeclampsia/ HELPP, 376
    platelet function disorders, 416–417
    thrombocytopenia, 413–416
    thrombophilia and thromboembolism, 421–427
    Von Willebrand disease and other bleeding disorders, 417–419

Pseudoleukocytosis, true leukocytosis *versus,* 306
Pseudothrombocytopenia, 235
Pulmonary embolism, overview of venous thromboembolism, **345–367**

R

Race, and risk of anemia, 207–208
Reactive thrombocytosis. *See* Thrombocytosis, reactive.
Red blood cells (RBCs), destruction of, as cause of anemia, 214–220
    enzyme deficiencies, abnormal hemoglobins, and membrane abnormalities,
      218–220
    immune-mediated, 215, 216–218
    mechanical, 214–215, 216
  failure of production of, as cause of anemia, 220–225
    bone marrow dysfunction leading to, 223–225
    nutrient deficiencies leading to, 220–222
    organ dysfunction leading to, 222–223
  loss of, initial workup for, 212–214
Renal transplantation, polycythemias associated with high, 271
Rheumatoid arthritis, secondary autoimmune neutropenia in, 259
Rituximab, drug-induced neutropenia with, 260–262

S

Severe cyclic neutropenia, 257
Sickle cell disease, in pregnant patients, 411–413
Smoking, polycythemias associated with high, 271
Smoldering multiple myeloma, epidemiology and diagnostic criteria, 386–387
Solid tumors, thrombocytopenia in patients with, 246
Splenomegaly, consultation for, **895–408**
    causes of, 402–403
    evaluation of, 403–405
    indications for removal of enlarged spleen, 405
    mechanisms of, 396
Stem cell transplant patients, thrombocytopenia in, 247
Superficial venous thrombosis, 355–357
Systemic lupus erythematosus, secondary autoimmune neutropenia in, 259

T

Thalassemia, in pregnant patients, 413
Thrombocytopenia, consultation for, **231–252**
    ancillary tests, 232–233
    associated with infections, 243, 244
    drug-induced, 239–240
    in patients with a solid tumor, 246
    in patients with hematologic malignancy, 246
    in pregnant patients, 413–416
    in the cardiac care unit, 244–245
      cardiopulmonary bypass and, 245
    in the intensive care unit, 243

Thrombocytopenia (*continued*)
    heparin-induced, 243
   in the internal medicine patient, 237–239
     alcohol abuse and, 237
     congenital, 238–239
     iron deficiencies, 237
     liver disease and, 239
     nutritional deficiencies, 237
   in the stem cell and solid organ transplant patient, 247
   life- or limb-threatening, **369–382**
     in heparin-induced thrombocytopenia, 369–371
     in post-transfusion purpura, 378–380
     in thrombotic microangiopathies, 371–377
   mechanisms of, 234–237
     decreased production of platelets, 236
     dilutional, 237
     immune destruction of platelets, 235–236
     increased platelet destruction, 235
     nonimmune destruction of platelets, 236
     pseudothrombocytopenia, 235
     sequestration of platelets, 236–237
   pertinent history in patient with, 231
   physical examination, 231–232
   post-transfusion purpura, 242–243
   primary immune, 240–241
   secondary immune, 241–242
     antiphospholipid antibody syndrome, 242
     Helicobacter pylori and, 242
     hepatitis C and, 242
     HIV infection and, 242
     systemic lupus erythematosus and, 241–242
  diagnostic algorithm and differential diagnosis, 333
Thrombocytosis, consultation on, **285–301**
   chronic myeloid leukemia, 295
   essential, 288–294
     and myeloproliferative states, 288
     clinical features, 290–293
     diagnosis, 293
     distinction from other causes, 288–289
     epidemiology, 288
     pathophysiology, 289–290
     prognosis, 293
     treatment, 294
   polycythemia vera, 295
   primary myelofibrosis, 296
   reactive, 285–288
     pathogenesis, 286–287
     prevalence and relevance, 285–286
     versus essential thrombocytosis, 287–288
Thromboembolism, in pregnant patients, 421–427
  overview of venous, **345–367**

Thrombophilia, in pregnant patients, 421–427
Thrombotic thrombocytopenic purpura, limb- or life-threatening, 373–374
Travel, venous thrombosis related to, 357–358
Tumors, solid, thrombocytopenia in patients with, 246

V

Venous thromboembolism, in pregnant patients, 421–427
    overview of, **345–367**
        anticoagulant bridging for invasive procedures, 359–361
        diagnosis, 347–348
        duration of anticoagulant treatment, 349–354
        hypercoagulable workup, 358–359
        initial treatment, 348–349
        new oral anticoagulants, 354–355
        presentation, 347
        superficial venous thrombosis, 355–357
        travel-related venous thrombosis, 357–358
Viruses, neutropenia related to, 262–263
Von Willebrand disease, anemia in pregnant patients with, 417–419
    clinical manifestations of, 325
    diagnostic algorithm and differential diagnosis, 332–333
Von Willebrand syndrome, acquired, diagnostic algorithm and differential diagnosis, 337–338

W

White blood cells (WBCs), development of, 303–304